Y0-EII-109

Advancing Responsible Adolescent Development

Series Editor
Roger J.R. Levesque
Indiana University, Bloomington, IN, USA

More information about this series at http://www.springer.com/series/7284

Kristin C. Thompson • Richard J. Morris

Juvenile Delinquency and Disability

Springer

Kristin C. Thompson
University of Arizona
Tuscon, AZ, USA

Richard J. Morris
University of Arizona
Tuscon, AZ, USA

ISSN 2195-089X   ISSN 2195-0903   (electronic)
Advancing Responsible Adolescent Development
ISBN 978-3-319-29341-7   ISBN 978-3-319-29343-1   (eBook)
DOI 10.1007/978-3-319-29343-1

Library of Congress Control Number: 2016931437

© Springer International Publishing Switzerland 2016
This work is subject to copyright. All rights are reserved by the Publisher, whether the whole or part of the material is concerned, specifically the rights of translation, reprinting, reuse of illustrations, recitation, broadcasting, reproduction on microfilms or in any other physical way, and transmission or information storage and retrieval, electronic adaptation, computer software, or by similar or dissimilar methodology now known or hereafter developed.
The use of general descriptive names, registered names, trademarks, service marks, etc. in this publication does not imply, even in the absence of a specific statement, that such names are exempt from the relevant protective laws and regulations and therefore free for general use.
The publisher, the authors and the editors are safe to assume that the advice and information in this book are believed to be true and accurate at the date of publication. Neither the publisher nor the authors or the editors give a warranty, express or implied, with respect to the material contained herein or for any errors or omissions that may have been made.

Printed on acid-free paper

This Springer imprint is published by Springer Nature
The registered company is Springer International Publishing AG Switzerland

*In memory of Jacqueline Anne Morris
and her interests in juvenile delinquency
and related public policy issues*

Preface

Over the last century, society has made considerable progress in how it responds to juvenile offenders. Prior to the twentieth century, children and adolescents who committed illegal acts were punished in a manner similar to that of adults, with little regard given to how their age or developmental immaturity may be impacting their misbehaviors. However, as child advocates and various professionals became increasingly vocal in the mid- to late 1800s regarding the need to separate juvenile offenders from adult criminals, policy-makers began to understand that children and adolescents were emotionally, developmentally, and cognitively different from that of adults. The most obvious result of this understanding was the establishment in 1899 of the first juvenile court in Cook County, Illinois, with this juvenile justice system being a distinctly different judicial entity from the adult criminal justice system. This new judicial system was so different that it did not even use the word "criminal" when describing children and adolescents who committed illegal acts, preferring instead to use the term "juvenile delinquent" or "juvenile offender." This new judicial system also differed from the adult criminal justice system in that it emphasized a "rehabilitation" approach versus the "punishment" approach that was used in the adult correctional system.

Although the juvenile justice system began as an entity focused on rehabilitating youth offenders, the degree or emphasis on rehabilitative practices has fluctuated over the last century, with juvenile courts instituting at times a more punitive approach based largely on society's frustration with the significant increases in juvenile offending and increases in the rates of re-offending. As a result of this societal frustration, as well as the increased interest on the part of social and behavioral scientists, research has steadily increased over the years as researchers and practitioners have tried to better understand the factors associated with juvenile offending and re-offending. The result has been the publication of thousands of studies, scholarly writings, books, and position papers that have focused on incidence and prevalence, assessment and diagnosis, education, vocational training, and risk assessment in the area of juvenile delinquency. In addition to research, a substantial number of theories have been published regarding the etiology of juvenile delinquency, and several laws have been enacted and lawsuits filed that have focused on protecting the rights of juvenile delinquents.

Many professionals and researchers who work directly with or have studied adjudicated delinquents have also begun focusing their efforts on developing effective treatment and prevention programs for reducing recidivism in these youth. In this regard, research findings have identified several commonalities among these youth. For example, one area of commonality that has emerged over the past 25–30 years of empirical research and is the focus of this book is the unmistakable positive relationship between youth who engage in illegal acts and the presence of cognitive, developmental, educational, and mental health disabilities. In fact, emerging research has suggested that if particular youth manifest certain types of disability plus present with certain demographic characteristics, then they are at a higher risk for becoming juvenile offenders and/or re-offending once they have been released from custody. In this regard, we will describe in this book the particular disabilities that have been found to be associated with juvenile delinquency, as well as present some case studies that are illustrative of the types of disabilities and difficulties that youth experience both before and after they become involved in the juvenile justice system. We report not only the findings and theoretical perspectives regarding the relationship between various types of disability and juvenile delinquency but also provide some recommendations and guidelines for mental health professionals, educators, and juvenile justice personnel to consider in their respective work with juvenile offenders.

The book provides an overview of the relationship between disability and delinquency, but more importantly it discusses the various impacts that a disability can have on offending and the processing of a youth through the juvenile justice system. It is intended for individuals who have entered or plan to enter the field of juvenile justice or who will be working with juvenile delinquents in some capacity. It will be especially useful to those who are or will be providing mental health services, special education, or vocational and rehabilitation training to these youth.

Preparation for this book began 15 years ago with a foundation grant from Drs. Lee Meyerson and Nancy Kerr to the second author (RJM) and the University of Arizona's School Psychology Program. The grant supported disability-focused research and public policy and advocacy work, and funds enabled the second author to begin collaboration with local juvenile court personnel and others to plan an organized and systematic program of research and work that centered on understanding the high prevalence of intellectual, cognitive, developmental, learning, emotional, and language disabilities among juvenile delinquents. The funds also permitted the sponsoring of dissertation research and the hiring of graduate students over the years to assist in these research, public policy, and advocacy endeavors. In this regard, we would like to acknowledge the work of the following current and former school psychology doctoral students on the various projects: Priscilla Bade-White, Ph.D.; Julie Duvall, J.D., Ph.D.; Roxanne Edwinson, Ph.D.; Sara Glennon, Ph.D.; Toby Laird, Ph.D.; Emery Mahoney, Ph.D.; Erin Aldrich, Ed.S.; Kimberly Morris, Ph.D.; Katie

Stoll, M.A.; Gretchen Schoenfield, Ph.D.; and Christina Vasquez, Ph.D. In addition, the first author (KCT) was a doctoral student during the early to later phases of the project, and her participation led to ongoing research, policy work, and psychological practice in the area of juvenile delinquency and disability.

We would also like to acknowledge and thank Garth Haller at Springer, for showing interest in our work and for his support in the preparation of this book, and Roger Levesque, J.D., Ph.D., series editor of *Advancing Responsible Adolescent Development*, for his very helpful feedback on an earlier draft of this book. We also wish to acknowledge the indexing work of Ms. Megan Beardmore, who is a doctoral student in the School Psychology Program at the University of Arizona.

Finally, the first author (KCT) wants to thank the second author (RJM) for his guidance and mentoring both during graduate school and as she has begun to establish herself in her career. She would also like to thank her parents for their support and encouragement throughout the years. And to her dear friend Nelson, thank you for the fire. The second author (RJM) wants to acknowledge the support of his wife, Yvonne, who has always been a great friend, confidant, and professional colleague, and thank his children and their respective spouses, Stephanie (Michael) and Michael (Lindsay), for their support over the years.

Tucson, AZ, USA
Kristin C. Thompson
Richard J. Morris

About the Authors

Kristin C. Thompson, Ph.D. is an assistant professor of practice in the School Psychology Program at the University of Arizona. She received her Ph.D. in school psychology from the University of Arizona after completing an APA-accredited psychology internship within the Wisconsin Department of Corrections (Ethan Allen School for delinquent youth). Dr. Thompson has worked with the juvenile court system in Arizona, and she also maintains a private practice that focuses on assessment, diagnosis, and treatment of child and adolescents with learning, emotional, and behavioral problems. She is a member of the American Psychological Association and the National Association of School Psychologists and is a licensed psychologist and a nationally certified school psychologist. Dr. Thompson has published several research articles and book chapters, as well as presented many professional papers and workshops, in the areas of juvenile delinquency and child and adolescent mental health. Her current research interests include the relationship between juvenile delinquency and disability, juvenile justice policy, and interventions for students with emotional and behavioral disorders.

Richard J. Morris, Ph.D. is the Meyerson Foundation distinguished professor emeritus of disability and rehabilitation and professor emeritus of school psychology in the Department of Disability and Psychoeducational Studies, College of Education, the University of Arizona. He has been elected a fellow of the American Psychological Association (APA), charter fellow of the Association for Psychological Science, and a fellow of the American Association on Intellectual and Developmental Disabilities. He has authored or edited 14 books, written more than 120 journal articles and book chapters, and made more than 150 professional presentations in the areas of child and adolescent psychotherapy, child and adult psychopathology, juvenile delinquency, school-based mental health services, professional and ethical issues in the delivery of psychological services to children and adults, and disability policy issues. His books include *The Practice of Child Therapy*, 4th edition (with Thomas R. Kratochwill), *Evidenced-Based Interventions for Students with Learning and Emotional Difficulties* (with Nancy Mather), *Disability Research and Policy: Current Perspectives*, *Handbook of Psychotherapy with Children and Adolescents* (with Thomas R. Kratochwill), and *Treating Children's Fears and Phobias: A Behavioral Approach* (with Thomas R. Kratochwill). His current research interests include the relationship between disability and juvenile delinquency, managing childhood aggressive and disruptive behaviors in the classroom, and legal and ethical issues associated with the delivery of children's mental health services. Dr. Morris is a former chair and board member of the State of Arizona, Board of Psychologist Examiners; past member of the APA Ethics Committee; past chair of the APA Membership Committee; and past board trustee of the American Insurance Trust (formerly, the "American Psychological Association Insurance Trust"). At present, Dr. Morris serves as a member of the board of directors of the Potomac National Security Reinsurance Company, Ltd., focusing on professional liability insurance.

Contents

Part I Introduction to Juvenile Delinquency

1 Introduction and Overview of Book 3
    Impact of Disabilities in the Juvenile Justice System 5
    Purpose and Overview of Book 6
    References 8

2 Characteristics of Juvenile Delinquents 9
    Characteristics and Risk Factors of Juvenile Delinquency 11
        Sex 12
        Ethnicity 13
        Socioeconomic Status 14
        Family Background and Childhood Abuse and Neglect 15
        School Achievement 16
        Cognitive Functioning 17
    Risk Factors of Recidivism 21
        Offense History 22
        Academic Achievement 23
        Sex 23
    Conclusion 24
    References 24

3 Juvenile Delinquency and Disability 31
    What Is a Disability? 32
    Prevalence and Incidence of Juveniles with Disabilities 33
    Conclusion 37
    References 37

4 Theories of Juvenile Delinquency 41
    Theories of Juvenile Delinquency 42
        Classical Theories 42
        Psychological Theories 43
        Sociological Theories 45

	Control Theories	47
	Biological Theory	48
	Conclusion	49
	References	50
5	**History of the Juvenile Justice System**	**55**
	Development of the Juvenile Justice System	56
	Relevant Case Law and Statutes	58
	Processing of Youth and Adults Within the Justice System	63
	Processing of a Youth Within the Juvenile Justice System	63
	Processing of an Adult Within the Criminal Justice System	66
	Impact of Having a Disability in the Processing of Youth Within the Juvenile Justice System	67
	Risk Assessment	68
	Competency	69
	Conclusion	70
	References	71
6	**Disability Law**	**73**
	Disability Law	74
	Individuals with Disabilities Education Improvement Act	76
	Section 504 of the Rehabilitation Act	81
	Americans with Disabilities Act	82
	Section 504 and ADA in Juvenile Correctional Settings	82
	Conclusion	83
	References	84

Part II Developmental and Educational Disabilities

7	**Developmental Disabilities**	**87**
	Intellectual Disability	88
	Impact on Functioning	89
	Etiology and Treatment	90
	Juvenile Delinquents with Intellectual Disabilities	91
	Autism Spectrum Disorder	94
	The Case of Andrew	94
	Diagnostic Symptoms and Characteristics of Autism Spectrum Disorder	96
	Etiology	99
	Impact on Cognitive Functioning	100
	Diagnosis and Treatment of ASD	102
	Juvenile Delinquents with ASD	102
	Communication Disorders	107
	Types of Communication Disorders	108
	Etiology and Treatment	109
	Implications on Functioning	110
	Communication Disorders and Juvenile Delinquency	112
	References	115

8 Learning and Emotional Disabilities ... 121
Specific Learning Disability ... 122
Reading Disabilities ... 123
Math Disabilities ... 126
Writing Disabilities ... 128
Impact of Specific Learning Disability on Functioning ... 132
Emotional Disabilities ... 133
Impact on Functioning ... 135
School-Based Interventions for Emotional Disabilities ... 138
Learning and Emotional Disabilities and Juvenile Delinquency ... 140
Impact on Risk and Risk Assessment ... 142
Competency ... 144
References ... 144

Part III Mental Health Disabilities

9 Mental Health Disorders ... 153
What Is a Mental Health Disorder? ... 154
Commonly Used Terms ... 154
Mental Health Disorders in the Juvenile Justice System ... 156
References ... 160

10 Mood Disorders ... 163
Depressive Disorders ... 163
Etiology and Treatment ... 165
Implications on Functioning ... 167
Mood Dysregulation Disorder ... 168
Diagnosis and Treatment ... 170
Implications on Functioning ... 170
Bipolar Disorder ... 171
Diagnosis and Treatment ... 173
Implications on Functioning ... 174
Mood Disorders in the Juvenile Justice System ... 176
Impact on Offending and Risk Assessment ... 178
Competency ... 180
References ... 181

11 Anxiety and Trauma-Related Disorders ... 187
Generalized Anxiety Disorder ... 187
Generalized Anxiety Disorder and Juvenile Delinquency ... 189
Trauma and Stressor-Related Mental Health Disorders ... 191
The Case of Brianna ... 191
Post-Traumatic Stress Disorder ... 192
Adjustment Disorder ... 196
Reactive Attachment Disorder ... 197

	Trauma and Stressor-Related Disorders in the Juvenile Justice System	200
	Impact on Risk and Risk Assessment	202
	Competency	203
	References	203
12	**Externalizing Disorders**	209
	Attention Deficit Hyperactivity Disorder	209
	Etiology	211
	Implications on Functioning	212
	Treatment of ADHD	214
	Disruptive Behavior Disorders	216
	Oppositional Defiant Disorder	216
	Conduct Disorder	217
	Etiology of Disruptive Behavior Disorders	218
	Implications on Functioning	220
	Treatment of Disruptive Behavior Disorders	221
	Intermittent Explosive Disorder	223
	Etiology and Treatment	223
	Implications on Functioning	224
	Externalizing Disorders and Juvenile Delinquency	225
	Impact on Risk and Risk Assessment	226
	Competency	227
	References	228

Part IV Conclusion

13	**Conclusion**	239
	Impact of Disability in the Juvenile Justice System	240
	Initial Contact with Law Enforcement	240
	Diversion	241
	Hearing and Trial Reviews	242
	Adjudication and Placement	244
	Coordinating Services for Youth Offenders Having a Disability	245
	References	247
Index		249

List of Figures

Fig. 5.1	Processing of a youth through the juvenile justice system	64
Fig. 5.2	Processing of an adult in the criminal justice system	65
Fig. 8.1	Writing sample of a 14-year-old boy with dysgraphia. "I do not like to write"	129
Fig. 8.2	Writing sample of a 10-year-old girl with attention deficit hyperactivity disorder and a SLD in written expression. "The boy is skating"	129
Fig. 8.3	Writing sample from a 13-year-old boy who was diagnosed with attention deficit hyperactivity disorder and a reading disability. "A flashlight provides a single beam of light in the dark"	129
Fig. 9.1	Causal model for mental health in delinquents (Defoe et al., 2013)	159

List of Tables

Table 1.1 Prevalence (in percentages) of common disabilities in the juvenile justice system.. 4

Part I
Introduction to Juvenile Delinquency

Chapter 1
Introduction and Overview of Book

Since the inception of the juvenile justice system in 1899, the process of adjudicating youth offenders has evolved into a series of procedures that endeavor to provide juveniles with many of the same basic rights under the US Constitution that are provided to adult offenders. These procedures are carried out formally while also trying to respect and understand the developmental immaturity of children and adolescents. The juvenile justice system has worked for more than a century to provide a rehabilitative approach to adjudicating juvenile offender cases rather than emphasizing only an approach that is punitive in nature (Zimring, 2005). Protecting the rights of juvenile offenders has emerged as a result of changes in federal laws (e.g., *Juvenile Justice and Delinquency Prevention Act*, 1974) and various court decisions (e.g., *Kent v. United States*, 1966; *Miller v. Alabama*, 2012), particularly court decisions that take into consideration the immature brain development of children and adolescents and how this immaturity may affect youth behaviors (e.g., *Roper v. Simmons*, 2005).

This development in how the juvenile justice system responds to juveniles has also occurred as researchers and professionals working with these youth have begun to better understand the common characteristics and risk factors associated with juvenile delinquency. For example, research has demonstrated that these youth are largely characterized as being from low-income families, are more likely to be from a minority group, and are more likely to have a history of abuse or neglect, poor academic achievement, and low verbal skills (e.g., Hong, Huang, Golden, Patton, & Washington, 2014; Sickmund & Puzzanchera, 2014; Thompson & Morris, 2013). Subsequently, the justice system has began to integrate this knowledge into prevention and intervention programs that aim to address at-risk youth, such as federal acts focused on reducing police officer's disproportionate minority contact (i.e., *Juvenile Justice and Delinquency Prevention Act*, 2002).

In addition to the characteristics listed above, recent research has also indicated that there is a high prevalence of cognitive, developmental, educational, and/or mental health disabilities in youth being processed through the juvenile justice system. Specifically, as can be seen in Table 1.1, the research literature has shown that

Table 1.1 Prevalence (in percentages) of common disabilities in the juvenile justice system

Type of disability	General population[a]	Juvenile offenders
Intellectual disability	1	8–10[b]
Autism spectrum disorder	1–2	Unknown
Communication disorder	3–6	14–50[c]
Educational disability (e.g., learning disability and emotional disability)	10	26–75[d]
Major depressive disorder	5	10–30[e]
Bipolar disorder	1	3–7[f]
Post-traumatic stress disorder	4–9	32–52[g]
Attention deficit/hyperactivity disorder	5–10	40–50[h]
Oppositional defiant disorder	1–11	50–75[h]
Conduct disorder	2–10	50–75[h]

[a]American Psychiatric Association [APA] (2013)
[b]Stahlberg, Anckarsater, and Nilsson (2010)
[c]Bryan, Freer, and Furlong (2007)
[d]Morris and Morris (2006)
[e]Fazel, Doll, and Langstrom (2008)
[f]Mallett, Stoddard-Dare, and Seck (2009)
[g]Wilson, Berent, Donenberg, Emerson, Rodriguez, and Sandesara (2013)
[h]Teplin, Abram, McClelland, Dulcan, and Mericle (2002)

there is an overrepresentation of disabilities among delinquents as compared to the general population of youth.

Although the research literature has demonstrated that there is an overrepresentation of juveniles with disabilities, related prevention and intervention programs are scarce. While the exact reasons for this are unclear, many factors may contribute to the court's limited responsiveness. First, while evidence suggests disabilities are overrepresented, it is unknown whether the relationship is causal versus correlational, as the majority of youth with disabilities do *not* become involved with the juvenile justice system. For example, while statistics suggest that upward of 50 % of juvenile delinquents meet the criteria for an attention deficit/hyperactivity disorder (e.g., Teplin et al., 2002), only a small percentage of those with an attention deficit disorder actually become involved with the legal system (APA, 2013). Second, resources that help the juvenile justice system understand the impact a disability may have on a youth's processing through the juvenile justice system are scarce, and therefore, many professionals do not fully understand the mitigating factors a disability can have on one's behavior. Finally, there is limited evidence regarding what empirically based interventions may help decrease the probability that a juvenile offender with a disability will reoffend, likely making it difficult for court systems to justify spending on such programs. Therefore, while it is understood that disabilities are common among the juvenile offender population, the exact implications of this need further exploration and critical discussion, as thus far court responsiveness to the issues appears minimal.

Impact of Disabilities in the Juvenile Justice System

While empirical evidence is limited regarding the specific implications that disabilities may have on the juvenile justice system, our knowledge of the difficulties related to various disabilities is not. Therefore, having an understanding of the cognitive, social, and behavioral characteristics of various disabilities can help professionals begin to understand the profound impact that the overrepresentation of disabilities may have on the juvenile justice system. For example, this high prevalence has an impact on the laws that focus on the juvenile justice system and on the manner in which juveniles having a disability are processed by police and within the court system. Specifically, a youth's disability may impact common practices within the court system such as risk assessment, competency to stand trial, and court-required sanctions such as placing a youth on probation.

The presence of a disability in a youth may also impact the manner in which police investigate and arrest the youth. Moreover, given the high prevalence of disabilities in youth within the juvenile justice system, this may create greater stress on court personnel since, in addition to their typical workload, they need to receive further training and understanding regarding the nature of specific disabilities in youth. Finally, the high prevalence of disabilities among juvenile offenders has considerable implications on intervention and treatment programs commonly utilized by mental health professionals, educators, and rehabilitation counselors, since many of the "typical procedures" used for nondisabled youth may not be appropriate for individuals having particular types of disability.

Given the above implications, we believe that the juvenile justice system's responsiveness to and understanding of issues related to the presence of a disability in many youth offenders are critical to the manner in which these youth are processed through the system and to the subsequent educational, mental health, rehabilitative, and social services provided to these youth. An example of the possible problems and difficulties that may occur when a youth having a disability may encounter in the juvenile justice system involves the case of Alex[1]. He was arrested over 20 times since his first arrest at 9 years of age. In addition to several domestic violence charges, Alex had two arrests for sex-related offenses. At 15 years of age, he was placed in a long-term correctional facility, since he was found guilty of molestation of a minor and had a history of failing to respond to court-ordered interventions such as individual therapy, family therapy, and sex offender group therapy. In addition, Alex failed to complete most court-required programs for reasons such as "refusing to talk," "being noncompliant with activities," or "pretending not to understand."

During Alex's adjudication hearing, his attorney requested a psychological evaluation because of her concerns regarding Alex's cognitive capacity to participate

---

[1] The case descriptions presented throughout this book are based on real cases and events; however, the names and details of the cases have been changed substantially to protect the confidentiality of the youth and families involved.

and understand matters relating to his trial and the adjudication process. As a result of the psychological evaluation, Alex was identified as having a mild intellectual disability (previously referred to in the psychological literature as "mild mental retardation"), with the psychologist concluding that Alex did not have the intellectual capacity to learn or understand to the same degree as his same-age peers. The court was informed that Alex had an intellectual disability and that his repeated failure in therapeutic and restoration programs was likely not due mainly to poor motivation, but to his severe learning and communication impairments. The court was also informed that if the goal was to help Alex have a chance at long-term success, a long-term correctional facility would be an inappropriate placement as Alex's intellectual disability meant that he would have a difficult time adapting to, functioning in, and learning from an environment having few personnel trained in providing services to individuals with disabilities. Instead, it was recommended that Alex would best be served by placing him in a secure facility that would protect the public from him while also providing him with appropriate mental health and educational and vocational counseling that is appropriate for his level of cognitive functioning.

Unfortunately for Alex, there were no local placements available that could offer the services recommended by the psychologist, and financial limitations within the juvenile court system also prevented him from being placed in an appropriate out-of-state setting. Therefore, he was placed in a local long-term correctional setting that did not include the level of services that were recommended, since it was deemed by court staff that what was most important in terms of public safety was that Alex needed intensive supervision until he turned 18 years old. By making this decision, it was understood that Alex would likely not receive the level of mental health and vocational services that were recommended, although he would certainly receive some of those services plus educational services. Protecting the public was of utmost importance given Alex's offense history.

Purpose and Overview of Book

Complex cases like that of Alex are not unusual given the high prevalence of disability in youth in the juvenile justice system. In addition, the negative outcome experienced by Alex is not unusual given the fact that, in our opinion, the juvenile court system across the United States does not yet understand and/or have not responded to the findings from the social and behavioral sciences and cognitive neuroscience regarding the various cognitive, social, and behavioral implications of disabilities. In this regard, this book explores the research surrounding the most common types of disabilities presented by youth within the juvenile justice system. In addition, the book explores the concomitant issues related to juvenile delinquency and disability, including how the current system responds to (or fails to respond to) these individuals and how various disabilities may impact a juvenile's ability to participate in his or her court trial or respond to standard treatments and interventions.

In the case of Alex, for example, the system provided a number of services for him, including case management for both him and his family, psychiatric and counseling services, family therapy, therapeutic day programming, in-home services, respite care, and placement in group homes. However, little improvement was observed as a result of these services, since most of the services were not tailored to Alex's unique cognitive, learning, and communication deficits. Had his severe deficits been given more serious consideration when determining intervention programs or if his intellectual disability had been identified earlier than during his adjudication hearing, sex offender therapy or other programs could have been tailored more appropriately to his level of functioning. In addition, the professional staff interacting with him would have known that his "noncompliance" and "low motivation" were probably not due to behavioral problems or to "antisocial thinking," but more likely related to his significant cognitive impairments.

Part I of this book provides a basis for our current understanding of the relationship between disability and delinquency. Characteristics of juvenile delinquents are provided, as well as characteristics of delinquents with disabilities and theories related to the etiology of delinquency. This section also provides an overview of the history of the juvenile justice system, including a general discussion of how a disability may impact a youth's processing within the juvenile justice system, as well as a chapter related to disability law and its relevance to juvenile delinquents.

Parts II and III of this book provide information on the most common disabilities reported within the juvenile justice system, including diagnostic characteristics of each disability and how they may affect an individual's cognitive, developmental, social, academic, emotional, and/or behavioral functioning. In discussing the various disabilities, this book provides a discussion of the thinking and behavioral impairments related to these disabilities, as well as a critical analysis of how these impairments may impact a juvenile's real or perceived level of risk to himself or herself or the community, their competency and ability to participate in a trial, and their ability to comply with or benefit from typical educational, mental health, and rehabilitative intervention programs.

Part IV provides the reader with concluding comments and our perspectives on the relationship between juvenile delinquency and disability. It is important to note here that although structural or functional neurological impairments have been found to be related to many disabilities in youth, and many disabilities have been found to cause impairments in the behavioral and cognitive functioning of youth, it cannot be concluded that all youth having a disability will commit illegal acts. In fact, most youth having a disability *do not* engage in illegal behavior.

In this regard, there is no implied argument being advanced in this book that disability is a *cause* of juvenile delinquency, particularly since determining factors associated with juvenile delinquency is a complex, difficult process. Rather, it is hoped that by helping professionals who work with youth offenders understand the relationship between disability and delinquency, these professionals will be able to provide youth having a disability with effective and individualized intervention programs that will decrease the probability they will reoffend and, therefore, give them a better chance of becoming productive citizens and living a successful life with less likelihood of future involvement in the juvenile justice or adult criminal court systems.

References

American Psychiatric Association. (2013). *Diagnostic and statistical manual for mental disorders (DSM-5)*. Washington, DC: Author.

Bryan, K., Freer, J., & Furlong, C. (2007). Language and communication difficulties in juvenile offenders. *International Journal of Language and Communication Disorders, 42*(5), 505–520. doi:10.1080/13682820601053977.

Hong, J. S., Huang, H., Golden, M., Patton, D. U., & Washington, T. (2014). Are community violence-exposed youth at risk of engaging in delinquent behavior? A review and implications for residential treatment research and practice. *Residential Treatment for Children and Youth, 31*, 266–283. doi:10.1080/0886571X.2014.958343.

Juvenile Justice and Delinquency Prevention Act. (1974). Pub. L. No. 93-415. Washington, DC: Coalition for Juvenile Justice.

Kent v. United States, 383 U.S. 541 (1966).

Mallett, C. A., Stoddard-Dare, P. A., & Seck, M. M. (2009). Predicting juvenile delinquency: The nexus of childhood maltreatment, depression, and bipolar disorder. *Criminal Behavior and Mental Health, 19*(4), 235–246. doi:10.1002/cbm.737.

Miller v. Alabama, 567 U.S. (2012)

Morris, K., & Morris, R. J. (2006). Disability and juvenile delinquency: Issues and trends. *Disability and Society, 21*(6), 613–627. doi:10.1080/09687590600918339.

Roper v. Simmons, 543 U.S. 551 (2005).

Sickmund, M., & Puzzanchera, C. (2014). *Juvenile offenders and victims: 2014 national report*. Pittsburgh, PA: National Center for Juvenile Justice.

Stahlberg, O., Anckarsater, H., & Nilsson, T. (2010). Mental health problems in youth committed to juvenile institutions: Prevalence and treatment needs. *European Child & Adolescent Psychiatry, 19*(12), 893–903. doi:10.1007/s00787-010-0137-1.

Teplin, L. A., Abram, K. M., McClelland, G. M., Dulcan, M. K., & Mericle, A. A. (2002). Psychiatric disorders in youth in juvenile detention. *Archives of General Psychiatry, 59*(12), 1133–1143. doi:10.1001/archpsyc.59.12.1133.

Thompson, K. C., & Morris, R. J. (2013). Predicting recidivism in juvenile offenders: Comparison of risk factors predictive of recidivism in adolescent male versus female juvenile offenders. *Journal of Juvenile Justice, 3*, 36–47.

Wilson, H. W., Berent, E., Donenberg, G. R., Emerson, E. M., Rodriguez, E. M., & Sandesara, A. (2013). Trauma history and PTSD symptoms in juvenile offenders on probation. *Victims & Offenders, 8*(4), 465–477. doi:10.1080/15564886.2013.835296.

Zimring, R. E. (2005). *American juvenile justice*. New York, NY: Oxford University Press.

Chapter 2
Characteristics of Juvenile Delinquents

In 2010, there were nearly 1.6 million arrests of juveniles (Snyder & Mulako-Wangota, 2013). While this appears to be a staggering number of juvenile arrests, it actually represents a considerable decline from previous years. For example, in the late 1980s and early 1990s, the number of juvenile arrests in the United States peaked at over two million arrests, particularly for violent crimes (Snyder & Sickmund, 2006). Since 2001, however, the rates have dropped nearly 21 %, with the number of arrests for violent crimes having the greatest decline (Puzzanchera, 2013). In 2010, juveniles were involved in about one in ten arrests for murder; one in four arrests for robbery, burglary, and disorderly conduct; and nearly one in five arrests for larceny-theft and motor vehicle theft. When examining arrest data and comparing the rates of juvenile arrests to adults, however, it is important to take into consideration that arrest data represent the *total number of arrests* of youth offenders, not the number of youth arrested; therefore, it is possible that the same youth may have had multiple arrests in the same year. Consequently, the total number of arrests does not necessarily translate into the total number of juveniles involved in crimes in a given year. Also, since many crimes go unreported or no arrest is made, the reported numbers may be an underestimate of the actual number of illegal acts committed by youth offenders. Finally, in comparing arrest rates for youth to those of adults, it is likely that youth are overrepresented, since they are more easily apprehended than adults (Puzzanchera, 2013).

Of the total number of juvenile offender arrests, violent offenses accounted for approximately 4.6 % of all juvenile arrests in 2010, with the number of violent crimes being the lowest it has been since at least 1980 (Snyder & Mulako-Wangota, 2013). Violent crimes include murder and nonnegligent manslaughter, forcible rape, robbery, and aggravated assault. Aside from a peak in violent crimes between 2004 and 2006, violent crimes have steadily declined since the early 1990s. In the case of forcible rape, for example, the number of juvenile arrests in

2010 was the lowest since 1980, at nearly one-third of what its high was in 1991. Juveniles were involved in approximately 14 % of all forcible rape arrests in 2010, with the majority of those youth being between 15 and 17 years of age (Puzzanchera, 2013). The number of aggravated assault arrests was also lower than it has been in over 20 years, with more than a 50 % decrease since its peak in 1997. Interestingly, however, the number of juvenile arrests for robbery increased nearly 43 % from 2002 through 2009 and then declined by 21 % in 2010 (Puzzanchera, 2013).

Property offenses, which include burglary, larceny-theft, motor vehicle theft, and arson, accounted for nearly 22 % of the total juvenile arrests. There was a decrease in juvenile property offenses in 2010, while an increase in adult property offenses was observed (Snyder & Mulako-Wangota, 2013). In regard to arson, nearly 40 % of all individuals arrested for arson are youth, with over half of these individuals being younger than 15 years old. In regard to offenses against person, simple assault is the most common for which individuals are arrested. Between 1980 and 1997, the arrest rate of juveniles for simple assault increased dramatically, nearly 200 %. The arrest rate for simple assault has declined some in the past few years; however, rates remain high as compared to arrests for other offenses.

The majority of juvenile arrests are of youth over the age of 15, with youth younger than this accounting for approximately 27 % of total arrests. Specifically, youth under the age of 10 accounted for less than 1 % of total juvenile arrests; approximately 5 % of arrests were youth between the ages of 10 and 12 years of age, with youth between the ages of 13 and 14 accounting for approximately 21 % of all juvenile arrests (Snyder & Mulako-Wangota, 2013).

With respect to sex, adolescent males comprise a significant proportion of juvenile arrests, accounting for nearly 71 % of all juvenile arrests. Despite the disparity between sexes in regard to total juvenile arrests, females have not necessarily experienced the same decline in offending as has been observed in males (Puzzanchera, 2013). In addition, although overall rates of juvenile crimes have decreased over the past decade, rates of offenses committed by females have risen or the declines have been considerably less than that found in males. For example, while the incidence of violent crimes has decreased considerably for males, it has remained consistent for females, and the incidence of aggravated assault arrests by females has increased. The rate of arrests for simple assaults has also remained relatively high for females. There were also increases observed in property crimes by females, particularly in larceny-theft, and while the male arrest rate for burglary has declined by nearly 75 % since 1980, the arrest rate for female juveniles has decreased around 50 %.

In regard to ethnicity, minority youth are overrepresented in the juvenile justice system, as is discussed in more detail in the following section. Minority youth are disproportionately arrested for crimes, with this disparity in minority representation in offending being most notable for robbery, in which Black youth were arrested at a rate of ten times that of White youth (Puzzanchera, 2013).

Characteristics and Risk Factors of Juvenile Delinquency

There is a substantial amount of research literature that has investigated a variety of risk factors and characteristics that are common among most delinquent youth. While juvenile delinquents are largely a complex group of children and adolescents with no verifiable cause(s) of delinquency identified, research has recognized several common characteristics found among the juvenile delinquency population. In addition, research has identified characteristics that appear to place certain children and adolescents at a greater risk of committing illegal acts and reoffending once they have been adjudicated and released or placed on probation.

Characteristics and/or risk factors are generally considered those factors that are associated with an increased probability that a juvenile will engage in illegal acts (Hoge, 2001). A variable may be identified as a "risk factor" if it is associated with the youth before he or she is adjudicated as a juvenile delinquent and if it still exists after other possible confounding variables have been controlled. A variety of risk factors appear to place certain youth at risk for engaging in illegal acts, although the mere presence of such risk factors does not imply causation or indicate that a particular individual will, in fact, engage in such acts. Such risk factors only suggest that there will be an increase in the probability that a youth will engage in delinquent behavior—they do not make it a certainty. It is notable, however, that research has found a cumulative effect of risk factors, in that having multiple risk factors places a youth at a greater risk of engaging in illegal acts and problematic behaviors. For example, a study by Herrenkohl et al. (2000) found that a 10-year-old with six or more risk factors was ten times more likely to engage in violent behavior before age 18 than a 10-year-old with only one risk factor. Therefore, risk assessment instruments, which are frequently used by professionals during the evaluation of juveniles and adults who have been arrested in an attempt to classify the person's likelihood of reoffending, are typically based on the number of risk factors that the individual possesses at the time of the evaluation. Numerical scores are assigned to sets of risk factors, and those scores are used to rank an individual's likelihood of re-offending, ranging from low to high risk (Hoge, 2002; Schwalbe, 2007). These instruments rely on research examining factors related to delinquency and are used both for prevention and intervention programs for youth offenders and at-risk youth.

Numerous investigations have been conducted to identify variables associated with juvenile delinquency, with one of the first major studies being conducted by Glueck and Glueck (1950). These researchers examined 500 delinquents and 500 nondelinquents between 11 and 17 years of age. Their research identified several factors associated with increased juvenile delinquency, including poor parenting skills in the household, family criminal history, and defiant attitudes of the youth. Glueck and Glueck also reported that there was an additive nature to the factors, with the more factors being present the higher the likelihood of a youth offending. A variety of other studies have also appeared in the literature, and common risk factors or characteristics that are prevalent among these youth appear to include the following: ethnicity, with a disproportionate number of youth across the United

States who are arrested being identified as belonging to a minority group; lower socioeconomic status; below average intelligence; having an educational disability; low academic achievement levels in reading and math; and, the presence of a mental health diagnosis (Beebe & Mueller, 1993; Morris & Morris, 2006; Skowyra & Cocozza, 2007).

Despite the availability of literature examining risk factors associated with delinquency, inconsistent findings are still present in the research. These inconsistencies are due, in part, to the various methodologies and samples used in studies, as the majority of studies utilize only all-male samples, are limited to groups of juveniles who have committed either relatively minor or severe offenses, include only incarcerated youth or only detained youth, or rely on self-reported delinquency while other studies rely on court records of arrest histories. In addition, many studies utilize samples of primarily male delinquents or combine male and female delinquents into one sample, despite ample available evidence that suggests male and female delinquents differ in their risk factors (e.g., Thompson & Morris, 2013; Tille & Rose, 2007; Vitopoulos, Peterson-Badali, & Skilling, 2012).

The following sections provide an overview of the risk factors research has found to be associated with juvenile delinquency. In addition to the factors listed below, the juvenile delinquency research literature clearly suggests that there is an overrepresentation of youth having a disability within the juvenile justice system, with studies finding prevalence values ranging from 20 to 750 % (e.g., Bullis & Yovanoff, 2005; Bullock & McArthur, 1994; Morgan, 1979; Morris & Morris, 2006). This relationship is discussed in brief below, with a more thorough discussion of the relationship between juvenile delinquency and disability (i.e., cognitive, developmental, educational, and mental health disabilities) appearing in Parts II and III of this book.

Sex

As previously noted, males are more represented in the juvenile justice system than females. This is likely due to a variety of factors. First, males are more likely to be arrested for committing such illegal acts as theft or assault, while females are more likely to be detained for status offenses—that is, those offenses which would *not* be illegal if the individual was an adult, such as running away from home or truancy (Puzzanchera, 2013). Some suggest that this may be related to the fact that females are often treated differently than males at the initial point of contact with the law (e.g., when stopped by a police officer, females may be less likely to be formally arrested). However, the literature does show that the overall number of delinquency cases for females has risen dramatically over the past few decades, with the number of cases involving females increasing by 92 % between 1985 and 2002 (e.g., Snyder & Sickmund, 2006). In addition, the percentage of female delinquents being arrested for violent crimes has risen dramatically in the past decade. For example, in the 1980s, males were four times as likely as females to be arrested for a violent crime, whereas they are now only twice as likely (Snyder & Sickmund, 2006). Some have argued that this is due to declining rates of violent offenses on the part of males, while others argue that this is because females are, in fact, involved in more violent crimes. Others maintain that this closing of the gender gap between males and females only means that the "arrest culture" on the part of police has changed, with law enforcement being less reluctant than in earlier years to arrest females who have engaged in delinquent acts (Zahn et al., 2010).

Risk factors of delinquency have been found to be significantly different for male and female offenders, which may also contribute to the disproportionate representation of males and females in the juvenile justice system. For example, studies have found that female delinquents are significantly more likely to have been exposed to trauma than male delinquents, with more than 60 % of females reporting that they have been raped or are fearful of being raped. In addition, females may be more negatively impacted by a disruptive home environment than males (Zahn et al., 2010).

Interestingly, as will be mentioned in subsequent chapters of this book, many of the disabilities common among the juvenile delinquent population are also more prevalent among males versus females. This is particularly true for impulse control and disruptive behavior disorders, as ADHD, oppositional defiant disorder, and conduct disorder are all more common among males than females (American Psychiatric Association [APA], 2013), and these are also the most common disabilities found among juvenile delinquents (Teplin, Abram, McClelland, Dulcan, & Mericle, 2002).

Ethnicity

Minority youth have been overrepresented in the juvenile justice system for a number of years. In 2004, for example, the Office of Juvenile Justice and Delinquency Prevention reported that of all juvenile arrests for violent crimes, 52 % were White, 46 % were Black, 1 % were Asian-American, and 1 % were Native American (Snyder & Sickmund, 2006), whereas the general composition of child and adolescent population was 78 % White, 17 % Black, 4 % Asian, and 1 % Native American. Unfortunately, many government agencies have historically combined into one category "White" and "Hispanic" youth, so data specifically related to Hispanic youth are not available nationwide. Some states, however, do differentiate between Hispanic and White youth and have reported disproportional representation of Hispanic youth among those juveniles who have been arrested. For example, in 2007, the Arizona Department of Juvenile Corrections (2008) reported that there was an overrepresentation of minority youth, particularly Hispanic youth, who were adjudicated within their system. Specifically, 51.1 % of adjudicated youth were classified as Hispanic, 30.1 % were Caucasian, 12.8 % were African-American, 4.8 % were Native American, and 0.7 % were Asian. This is compared to the general youth population of 75.5 % Caucasian, 25.3 % Hispanic, 3.1 % African-American, 5 % Native American, and 1.8 % Asian.

In regard to types of offenses, available literature suggests significantly more minorities are adjudicated for violent versus nonviolent offenses (van Wijk et al., 2005), and some studies have found that Caucasians are more prevalent in the specific category of sex offenses (e.g., van Wijk, Van Horn, Bullens, Bijleveld, & Doreleijers, 2005; Veneziano, Veneziano, LeGrand, & Richards, 2004).

In 1988, amendments were made to the *Juvenile Justice and Delinquency Prevention Act of 1974* that required those states participating in federal programs to determine if minority youth were overrepresented and, if so, to make an effort at reducing the disproportionate representation. Studies have found mixed results regarding whether this program has been effective (e.g., Barrett, Katsiyannis, & Zhang, 2006; Jones, Harris, Fader, & Grubstein, 2001; Rodriguez, 2007; Wu, Cernkovich, & Dunn, 1997). A review of studies between 1989 and 2001 that looked at minority contact within the juvenile justice system concluded that despite some alleviation in the disproportionate representation of minorities in the juvenile justice system, ethnicity and race still affected the processing of youth through the juvenile justice system (Pope, Lovell, & Hsia, 2002).

Socioeconomic Status

A significant correlation has been found between juvenile delinquency and low socioeconomic status (SES; Loeber & Farrington, 2012; Hay, Fortson, Hollist, Altheimer, & Schaible, 2007). A theoretical explanation for why low socioeconomic status may have an impact on delinquency is evident in different sociological theories, such as *strain theory* and *social control theory*, and some researchers have indicated that economic background may be the best predictor for which juveniles will become incarcerated (Johnson et al., 1999). In this regard, Snyder and Sickmund (2006) found that in 2002, one out of every six juveniles lived in poverty. Directly related to ethnicity, African-American and Hispanic youth—two ethnic groups already overrepresented in the juvenile justice system—were also three times more likely to live in poverty compared to Caucasian juveniles. Some researchers have posited that the direct relationship between poverty and low academic achievement, which itself has been linked to delinquency, may also increase the risk of youth from low socioeconomic classes being likely to be arrested (Cohen, 1955; Lawrence, 1998; Pagani, Boulerice, Vitaro, & Tremblay, 1999). In this regard, Pagani et al. (1999) examined the impact that poverty may have on academic achievement and delinquency for adolescent males living in low-income neighborhoods, with results suggesting that poverty level significantly predicted delinquency. Jarvelin, Laara, Rantakallio, and Moilanen (1994) also concluded in their investigation of adolescent males that the incidence of delinquency is higher for those who are from lower socioeconomic classes, and highest for those from a low socioeconomic background with a history of poor academic performance.

Despite evidence supporting low socioeconomic status as being a strong primary risk factor for juvenile delinquency, some later research suggested that it may actually be a moderator variable, having a more indirect effect. For example, a study by Defoe, Farrington, and Loeber (2013) used advanced statistical modeling to explore causal factors of delinquency and found that low socioeconomic status was not a direct cause of delinquency, but rather an indirect influence and was a contributing factor only in relation to other variables. A study by Low, Sinclair, and Shortt (2012) also suggested that socioeconomic status might be more of a moderator variable rather than a direct contributing factor to delinquency. In this study, the researchers found that low socioeconomic status placed more strain on family relationships, which therefore contributed to delinquency.

Family Background and Childhood Abuse and Neglect

Some studies have also reported that nearly one-quarter of juvenile delinquents live in single-parent households (e.g., Sickmund & Puzzanchera, 2014). Consistent with this, studies looking at the relationship between single-parent households and delinquency have found that those delinquents whose fathers were not involved in their life were more likely to reoffend (Barrett, Katsiyannis, & Zhang, 2010). Other family characteristics that research has associated with juvenile delinquency include a family history of involvement with the juvenile or adult criminal justice system (Farrington, 1989), as well as limited parental involvement in the youth's upbringing (Farrington, Loeber, Yin, & Anderson, 2002).

While the relationship between a history of childhood abuse or neglect and juvenile delinquency is far from understood, research has consistently found that there is a higher prevalence of youth with a history of abuse or neglect than found in the general population (e.g., Ford, Chapman, Mack, & Pearson, 2006; Hong, Huang, Golden, Patton, & Washington, 2014). Studies have found that more than 60 % of first-time offenders have a history of family involvement in the child welfare system (Sickmund & Puzzanchera, 2014). Involvement with the child welfare system has also been associated with repeat offending and an earlier age of first offense for youth (Barrett, Katsiyannis, Zhang, & Zhang, 2014). There has also been some evidence to suggest that a history of physical abuse may be related to violent offending in youth (Hawkins et al., 2000; Maas, Herrenkohl, & Sousa, 2008).

Related to the high prevalence of childhood abuse and neglect reported among juvenile offenders, research has found significantly more youth offenders qualifying for a diagnosis of a trauma-related disorder, such as posttraumatic stress disorder (PTSD) and reactive attachment disorder, than in the equivalent general population of youth. For example, while it is estimated that approximately 4–9 % of children and adolescents in the general population meet the criteria for PTSD (Kilpatrick et al., 2003), studies have found that from 32 to 52 % of incarcerated juvenile delinquents may meet the criteria for PTSD (e.g., Kerig, Moeddel, & Becker, 2010; Wilson et al., 2013). The high incidence of trauma-related disorders in the youth offender population is largely attributed to the fact that many of these youth have been exposed to violence, abuse, or trauma during childhood (Chen, Voisin, & Jacobson, 2013).

For example, Stimmel, Cruise, Ford, and Weiss (2014) found that 86 % of their sample of youth offenders had been exposed to at least one traumatic event, with those meeting criteria for PTSD having a greater number of emotional and behavioral problems. A more detailed discussion of the implications of PTSD and other trauma-related disorders in the juvenile delinquency population is presented in Chap. 11.

School Achievement

For nearly a century, research has investigated the association between delinquency and academic achievement, consistently finding that juvenile delinquents tend to perform lower in academic achievement than their same-age peers. In 1950, Glueck and Glueck found that nearly 85 % of juvenile delinquents were behind their peers academically, with more recent studies reporting similar estimates (Beebe & Mueller, 1993; Zamora, 2005). A later study by Thompson and Morris (2013) examined a large sample of over 1000 delinquent youth and found that less than half of male delinquents were passing state standardized achievement tests in reading, writing, and math.

Research has also suggested that a failure to properly develop basic reading and writing skills may be a strong predictor of later incarceration (e.g., Drakeford, 2002; Rogers-Adkinson, Melloy, Stuart, Fletcher, & Rinaldi, 2008). Reading and mathematics are the most commonly researched areas, with findings suggesting that in some cases, as many as 70 % of incarcerated delinquents read at or below the fourth grade level (U.S. Bureau of Justice Statistics, 1997). A meta-analysis conducted by Foley (2001) for articles published between 1975 and 1999 found that the average reading level of delinquents was between the fourth and seventh grades, significantly below the expected reading level for the age of these youth. A study by Baltodano, Mathur, and Rutherford (2005) concurred with the lower-than-average reading level for juvenile delinquents, finding that delinquents have significantly lower standardized test scores in reading. Some research has even investigated a link between severity of offense and academic achievement levels, suggesting that youth who engage in violent offenses display the greatest academic deficits when compared to those engaging in nonviolent offenses (Beebe & Mueller, 1993; van Wijk, Loeber et al., 2005). On the other hand, findings have been different for juvenile sex offenders, with it being suggested that these youth display fewer academic weaknesses than other types of juvenile offenders (Jacobs, Kennedy, & Meyer, 1997; Milloy, 1994). van Wijk, Van Horn et al. (2005) also reported that a smaller percentage of sex offenders displayed low academic achievement than violent offenders.

Related to these latter findings, research has shown that there is a significant overrepresentation of youth with educational disabilities (i.e., learning and emotional disabilities) in the juvenile justice system. For example, within the public school system across the United States, it is estimated that between 10 and 13 % of students receive special education services for educational disabilities (U.S. Department of Education, 2014), while studies have shown that between 30 and 75 % of youth in the juvenile justice system qualify for an educational disability and are eligible to receive special education services (e.g., Morris & Morris, 2006; Quinn, Rutherford, Leone, Osher, & Poirier, 2005). As is discussed in more detail in Chapter 8, research has also found a relationship between the type of educational disability and offense patterns in juveniles (e.g., Cruise, Evans, & Pickens, 2011).

Additional support for a relationship between low academic achievement and juvenile delinquency has been provided by studies demonstrating that academic interventions lead to decreased rates of recidivism (Archwamety & Katsiyannis, 2000; Katsiyannis & Archwamety, 1997; Malmgren & Leone, 2000). For example, a study by Blomberg, Bales, and Piquero (2012) examined academic achievement in a sample of 4146 delinquents and found that those with average academic achievement were significantly more likely to return to school after being released and were less likely to be rearrested in a one-year post-release period. As previously mentioned, a study by Defoe et al. (2013) used structural equation modeling to identify causal factors of delinquency, including low socioeconomic status, academic achievement, hyperactivity, and mental health issues in their model. Their results found low academic achievement to be the only direct causal variable of delinquency, with other variables such as SES and hyperactivity having indirect effects, but moderated by academic achievement. These authors proposed that academic achievement should be a primary focus on interventions for juvenile delinquents given the strong causal relationship between low achievement and delinquency.

Youth who drop out of school are significantly more likely to be involved with the juvenile justice system than those who remain in school, with high school dropouts being 3.5 times more likely to be arrested than those who do not dropout (U.S. Department of Education, 1994). In this regard, throughout the entire US correctional system, it has been reported that approximately 82 % of adult prison inmates are high school dropouts (Ysseldyke, Algozzine, & Thurlow, 1992). Moreover, approximately 10.9 % of young adults are not enrolled in school and have not completed high school (Snyder & Sickmund, 2006). These numbers vary slightly between male and female adolescents (12.0 and 9.9 % dropout rates, respectively), but substantial variations are seen when focusing on ethnicity. For example, the dropout rate for Hispanic youth was reported by Snyder and Sickmund (2006) to be 27.8 %, 13.1 % for African-American youth, 6.9 % for Caucasian youth, and 3.8 % for Asian youth. As previously mentioned, Hispanic and African-American youth are also significantly overrepresented in the juvenile delinquency population.

Cognitive Functioning

The cognitive functioning of juvenile offenders has become an area of increasing focus in recent research literature, though explorations of the relationship between general intelligence (IQ) and delinquency have been present for decades. Several researchers have identified a link between low IQ and delinquency (Fergusson & Horwood, 2002; Hirschi & Hindelang, 1977; Koolhof, Loeber, Wei, Pardini, & D'escury, 2007; Lynam, Moffitt, & Stouthamer-Loeber, 1993; Moffitt & Silva, 1988). Early studies suggested that delinquents performed as much as 15–20 points below the general population in intellectual functioning (Caplan, 1965), while later studies have found more varied results, with some suggesting that it is a deficit in Verbal IQ that characterizes delinquents rather than a general Full Scale IQ deficit (Culberton, Feral, & Gabby, 1989; Raine et al., 2005). Little research exists, however, that has examined the actual causal link between IQ and juvenile delinquency. Lynam et al. (1993) explored the relationship between IQ and delinquency by controlling for several other risk factors, with their research suggesting that low IQ may have a more indirect link to delinquency, in that low IQ contributes to low academic achievement which, in turn, is related to delinquency. Other explanations vary regarding why lower IQ is correlated with juvenile delinquency, but include the negative relationship between low IQ and academic achievement, as well as the notion that juveniles with low IQs may not as easily evade detection from law enforcement and, therefore, are arrested and/or incarcerated at a higher rate (Vold & Bernard, 1986).

In regard to types of offenders, the literature is mixed as to whether IQ level can differentiate violent offenders from nonviolent offenders. In an analysis of intellectual, behavioral, and personality correlates of violent versus nonviolent juvenile offenders, Kennedy, Burnett, and Edmonds (2011) found that verbal intelligence differentiated between types of offenders, but other studies have not found such a relationship (e.g., van Wijk, Vermeiren, Loeber, Doreleijers, & Bullens, 2006).

With respect to intellectual disability, research has reported that there is a higher prevalence of intellectual disability among juvenile delinquents than there is in the general public school population. Specifically, while intellectual disabilities exist in approximately 1 % of the general school population (U.S. Department of Education, 2014), studies have found that approximately 10 % of juvenile offenders have an intellectual disability (Quinn et al., 2005; Stahlberg, Anckarsater, & Nilsson, 2010).

In addition to general intelligence, studies have revealed that juvenile delinquents display other cognitive deficits, such as memory, abstract reasoning, receptive and expressive language, and executive functioning deficits. One theory of delinquency is biological theory, which posits that that criminal behavior may be due, in part, to neuropsychological deficits (Shoemaker, 2005). While there are a variety of neuropsychological variables that can be measured, such as auditory and visual memory, visual-spatial skills, and motor skills, two major areas that the research literature suggests may be related to juvenile delinquency are executive functioning skills and verbal processing skills. Specifically, within the construct of executive functioning, deficits in juvenile offenders have been suggested in such area as attention, response inhibition, and planning. Within the construct of verbal skills, specific deficits have been suggested in the areas of receptive language and language comprehension (Bryan, Freer, & Furlong, 2007).

Executive Functioning. The frontal lobe of the human brain controls systems that implement a variety of different behavioral strategies in response to the environment

(Kolb & Whishaw, 2008). Behavioral functions controlled by the frontal lobe include aspects such as (but not limited to) planning, self-awareness, regulation of behavior, attention, concentration, working memory, reasoning, cognitive flexibility, inhibitory control, and problem solving, collectively known as executive functioning (e.g., Kolb & Whishaw, 2008; Zillmer & Spiers, 2001). Deficits in executive functioning may lead to problems with environmental control of behavior, including poor response inhibition, risk taking, rule breaking and failure to comply with instructions, gambling, self-regulatory problems, and poor problem solving skills (e.g., Kolb & Whishaw, 2008; Milner, 1964). Some studies suggest that frontal lobe functions may also control emotional responses such as regulation of emotion, aggression, and antisocial personality traits (Bauer, O'Connor, & Hesselbrock, 1994; Yeudall & Fromm-Auch, 1979).

Given that executive functioning is responsible for regulation of an individual's behavior, many studies have examined executive functioning skills in juvenile offenders. There is some empirical support that these youth do, in fact, display a relative weakness in executive functioning, with some researchers maintaining that executive functioning deficits can distinguish between juvenile delinquents and nondelinquents and, more specifically, violent from nonviolent youth (e.g., Raine et al., 2005). However, not all researchers have agreed, and it is argued by some that the deficits may be the result of other confounding variables such as the presence of attention deficit hyperactivity disorder in these youth (e.g., Cauffman, Steinberg, & Piquero, 2005; Sequin, Pihl, Hardin, Tremblay, & Boulerice, 1995). Available research does vary to some extent in regard to what specific executive functioning deficits exist and to what magnitude, but, in general, common executive functioning deficits include poor attention and concentration, impulsivity, response perseveration, poor flexibility, poor response inhibition, poor planning of actions, and poor organization.

Lueger and Gill (1990) conducted a study on executive functioning in juvenile delinquents, finding that delinquents experienced deficits in problem solving, cognitive flexibility (e.g., ability to quickly adapt to changing demands in the environment), sustained attention, working memory (e.g., ability to retain information while completing a task, such as following multistep instructions), and related motor tasks. Participants included 21 adolescents between 13 and 17 years of age, who were residents in a facility for the treatment of court-referred behaviorally disordered and emotionally disturbed youth and 20 normal controls. Participants were administered a variety of neuropsychological measures associated with frontal lobe functioning, including the *Wisconsin Card Sorting Test* (WCST), a task to measure problem solving and cognitive flexibility; the *Sequential Matching Memory Test*, which measures the ability to sustain attention; the *Kaufman Assessment Battery for Children Hand Movements Test*, a measure of sequential motor memory; the *Trail Making Test*, a widely used measurement of sequential processing, planning, and visual-motor performance; and the *Auditory Verbal Learning Test*, a memory test. Results indicated that youth diagnosed with conduct disorder did, in fact, perform more poorly on measures of frontal lobe functioning than did controls. Specifically, youth having a conduct disorder performed more poorly on tasks of cognitive flexibility, sustained attention, sequencing of memory, and motor tasks. A later study by Raine et al. (2005) also examined problem solving and attention in a sample of 500 teenage boys and found that those with a history of violent and aggressive behavior displayed deficits in attention. A number of other studies have also been conducted to measure executive functioning skills, such as response inhibition (e.g., impulse control), finding that delinquents perform significantly lower in this skill area than their nondelinquent peers (e.g., Dery, Toupin, Pauze, Mercier, & Fortin, 1999; Moffitt, Lynam, & Silva, 1994; Wolff, Waber, Bauermeister, Cohen, & Ferber, 1982; Yeudall, Fromm-Auch, & Davies, 1982).

Verbal Skills. David Wechsler, a prominent psychologist during the mid-twentieth century, was among the first to suggest that "adolescent psychopaths" displayed deficits in verbal abilities (Wechsler, 1944). Although his initial observation was subjective and based only on clinical experience and case studies, his observations were subsequently empirically confirmed (e.g., Graham & Kamano, 1958; Raine et al., 2005; Vermeiren, Schwab-Stone, Ruchkin, De Clippele, & Deboutte, 2002; Yeudall et al., 1982). These deficits in verbal skills have been found across many domains, including a Performance IQ versus Verbal IQ discrepancy on various Wechsler scales of intelligence (e.g., the *Wechsler Intelligence Scale for Children* and the *Wechsler Adult Intelligence Scale*) and specific deficits in receptive verbal skills, verbal memory, and language comprehension (e.g., Braggio, Plshkln, Gameros, & Brooks, 1993; Dery et al., 1999; Linz, Hooper, Hynd, Isaac, & Gibson, 1990; Lynam et al., 1993; Moffitt & Silva, 1988; Olvera, Semrud-Clikeman, Pliszka, & O'Donnell, 2005). For example, in a long-term study conducted on a birth cohort of several hundred New Zealand adolescents, researchers found specific verbal and nonverbal memory abilities to be the factors most strongly related to predicting delinquency by 18 years of age (Moffitt et al., 1994). In this study of over 1000 children, males and females were administered a psychological evaluation every 2 years between 3 and 18 years of age, with a neuropsychological evaluation administered at age 18. Verbal measures included verbal subsets from a Wechsler intelligence test as well as a verbal memory test. A self-reported delinquency scale was administered to participants at age 13, as well as at 18 years of age, to determine whether there was evidence of delinquency. Results found that those participants with a history of delinquent behavior displayed significant deficits in verbal skills and verbal memory abilities when tested at age 13.

It is unknown exactly why there may be a relationship between verbal deficits and juvenile delinquency. One explanation is that individuals with expressive language deficits struggle to express their needs, wants, and frustrations, which can lead to engaging in disruptive behavior (e.g., Conti-Ramsden & Botting, 2008). Other explanations have suggested the link between poor verbal ability and academic achievement, given that these abilities and skills are highly correlated, and research has consistently reported a link between low academic achievement and delinquency. Another hypothesis is that an information-processing deficit exists, directly affecting antisocial behavior (e.g., Nas, Orobio De Castro, & Koops, 2005). The possible link between these cognitive deficits and disability cannot be ignored since, as we discuss in various chapters in this book, cognitive deficits are commonly observed with many of the disabilities that are prevalent in the juvenile offender population. In this regard, the field of cognitive neuroscience has been increasingly demonstrating that impairments in, for example, executive functioning skills are a common weakness in individuals with attention deficit hyperactivity disorder (Coghill, Hayward, Rhodes, Grimmer, & Matthews, 2014). Deficits in executive functions have also been found in youth with bipolar disorder and other mood disorders such as depression (Lundy, Silva, Kaemingk, Goodwin, & Quan, 2010; Nieto & Castellanos, 2011). Similarly, language impairments are typically observed in individuals with developmental disabilities such as autism spectrum disorder and intellectual disability (APA, 2013).

Risk Factors of Recidivism

Juvenile delinquents as a population consist mainly of minority youth from low-income families who have a variety of educational and/or mental health disabilities (e.g., Pagani et al., 1999; Teplin et al., 2002). These youth also show a high frequency of reoffending (e.g., Cottle, Lee, & Heilbrun, 2001). In this regard, a major area of concern surrounding the problem of juvenile delinquency is that of recidivism or, generally speaking, the repetition of criminal behavior or repeated arrests by an individual. Although the overall arrest rates of youth have declined to some extent over the past decade, recidivism percentages among youth offenders remain high and stable, and it is estimated that 70 to 90 % of these youth will reoffend (e.g., McMackin, Tansi, & LaFratta, 2004; Trulson, Marquart, Mullings, & Caeti, 2005; Van Der Geest & Bijleveld, 2008). There is a lack of consensus, however, in the literature regarding a standard definition of recidivism. For example, it is not clear from the available literature whether a probation violation counts as a separate arrest, given that some states include probation violations as an additional offense while others do not during their respective collection of data on these youth. As a result of this type of variation in data collection, no nationally based recidivism data are tracked for juveniles and, therefore, comparison between states on rates of recidivism is difficult to perform. In addition, the only recidivism data available for various juvenile courts are the official court records for the particular jurisdiction, which represents recidivism that came to the attention of that particular court and only for those offenses that took place again in that same jurisdiction (Snyder & Sickmund, 2006). The lack of a standard definition of recidivism is also a methodological consideration when examining empirical studies of recidivism, as rates tend to change depending on the definition of recidivism used. Despite these limitations, some national data that do exist suggest that nearly six out of every ten juveniles return to juvenile court before they turn 18 years of age. In fact, Snyder and Sickmund (2006) reported that at age 17, nearly 84 % of juveniles referred to the court have had at least one prior referral, and 53 % of those referred at age 17 have had seven or more referrals. These numbers highlight the societal concerns related to juvenile offender recidivism and are suggestive of the need for more effective psychosocial intervention and prevention programs for youth offenders.

Another factor to take into consideration when analyzing recidivism percentages is the period of time analyzed to determine whether recidivism actually took place with certain youth. Since longitudinal studies are rare and difficult to carry out, recidivism must often be determined over a relatively short period of time and may not include a youth's entire offense history. Also, because of privacy laws it is difficult to track the offenses of youth into adulthood, so most available data are only related to the recidivism of youth during the time that they are considered legally as a "juvenile," that is, until the youth become 18 years of age.

There are a variety of explanations and studies available which discuss factors related to youth who recidivate. Risk factors that have been consistently found to be associated with higher recidivism rates include the following: age of first offense, type(s) of offense committed, and academic achievement levels (e.g., Archwamety & Katsiyannis, 2000; Cottle et al., 2001; Dembo et al., 1995; Jones et al., 2001; Katsiyannis, Ryan, Zhang, & Spann, 2008). A variety of other factors have also been found to be predictive of recidivism, but these factors have been inconsistently supported in the literature. These lesser supported factors include the presence of a history of substance abuse, single-parent family background, being an ethnic minority, lower socioeconomic status, level of intelligence, and a history of conduct behavior problems (e.g., Dembo et al., 1995, 1998; Duncan, Kennedy, & Patrick, 1995; Katsiyannis & Archwamety 1997; Myner, Santman, Cappelletty, & Perlmutter, 1998; Repo & Virkkunen, 1997; Wierson & Forehand, 1995).

Offense History

One factor found to be a stable predictor of recidivism is the child's or adolescent's age at the time of first offense. Specifically, research consistently suggests that the earlier a youth begins committing illegal acts, the greater the likelihood that the person will continue to reoffend (e.g., Cottle et al., 2001; Jones et al., 2001; Trulson et al., 2005). As mentioned earlier, due to privacy laws, these findings are typically limited to youth under 18 years of age; therefore, more recidivism data are available for those who begin offending early since there is a greater time period before they reach 18 years of age. Nevertheless, the age of first offense has been described as "…the single most important predictor in recidivism" (Hoge, 2001, p. 28).

In addition to age of first offense, research suggests that youth who commit more severe crimes are likely to reoffend (e.g., Archwamety & Katsiyannis, 1998; Cottle et al., 2001; Dembo et al., 1995, 1998; Myner et al., 1998). In this regard, Cottle et al. (2001) conducted a meta-analysis of studies examining risk factors that best predicted juvenile recidivism. The results showed that offense history was found to be the strongest predictor of recidivism, with those committing more serious crimes having a higher risk of recidivism.

Academic Achievement

Researchers have also repeatedly linked academic achievement with recidivism, with the juvenile delinquency population being overwhelmingly represented by those in need of academic remediation. For example, Archwamety and Katsiyannis (2000) examined juvenile delinquents in remedial math and reading groups and found that these youth were twice as likely to recidivate as those in the control group. In addition, a literature review by Vacca (2008) that focused on reading achievement and delinquency concluded that if more time was spent on teaching delinquents to read, then recidivism rates would decrease. A review of relevant studies by Katsiyannis et al. (2008) also reported that a significant relationship existed between low academic achievement levels and higher rates of recidivism. Related to this, educational disabilities have also been found to be related to recidivism (Zhang, Barrett, Katsiyannis, & Yoon, 2011).

Sex

Studies that have differentiated between males and females in data analyses have suggested that sex may be a major contributing factor in recidivism, with male juvenile delinquents being more likely to be rearrested than females (e.g., Baffour, 2006; Steketee, Junger, & Junger-Tas, 2013; Thompson & Morris, 2013; Trulson et al., 2005). For example, Archwamety and Katsiyannis (1998) conducted a study that focused solely on female delinquents and recidivism. They found that age of first offense and the age that a female delinquent was first committed to either a detention or correctional facility significantly predicted female recidivists from non-recidivists. The study also indicated that gang affiliation, history of child abuse, and length of stay in a correctional facility were predictive of recidivism. Archwamety and Katsiyannis (1998) also found that like the results reported for males in the literature, females had poor math skills that were significantly related to recidivism; however, unlike the results reported for males, no significant relationship was found in females between reading skills level and recidivism.

A study by Tille and Rose (2007) also identified factors unique to female delinquents between 13 and 18 years of age, finding that female recidivists were more likely to have emotional and behavioral problems and come from an unstable family situation in comparison to the same-age first-time female offenders that they studied. Another study by Thompson and Morris (2013) examined risk factors of recidivism for male versus female delinquents, finding that time spent in detention, dual involvement within the juvenile court system, emotional disability, adjudication status, and socioeconomic status were all significant risk factors regarding recidivism for females, while these factors, as well as low writing and math achievement, were risk factors for male delinquents. In this study, poor academic achievement was not predictive of recidivism for females, and learning disabilities were not predictive of recidivism for males or females; however, the presence of an emotional disability was a significant predictor of recidivism for both sexes.

Conclusion

There are a variety of risk factors and characteristics associated with juvenile delinquency and recidivism. While these factors do not explain fully the cause of juvenile delinquency, they do provide those working with youth offenders additional knowledge and directions for the initiation of prevention and intervention programs. As mentioned in the introduction to this chapter, there are a variety of other risk factors or characteristics of youth offenders that relate to the high prevalence of disabilities among these individuals. The relationship between juvenile delinquency and disability is further discussed in Chap. 3, and the impact that various disabilities have on delinquency will be the focus of the remainder of this book.

References

American Psychiatric Association. (2013). *Diagnostic and statistical manual for mental disorders, (DSM-5)*. Washington, DC: Author.

Archwamety, T., & Katsiyannis, A. (1998). Factors related to recidivism among delinquent females at a state correctional facility. *Journal of Child and Family Studies, 7*(1), 59–67. doi:10.1023/a:1022960013342.

Archwamety, T., & Katsiyannis, A. (2000). Academic remediation, parole violations, and recidivism rates among delinquent youth. *Remedial and Special Education, 21*(3), 161–170. doi:10.1177/074193250002100306.

Arizona Department of Juvenile Corrections. (2008). *Annual report 2008*. Phoenix, AZ: Arizona Department of Juvenile Corrections.

Baffour, T. D. (2006). Ethnic and gender differences in offending patterns: Examining family group conferencing interventions among at-risk adolescents. *Child and Adolescent Social Work Journal, 23*, 557–578. doi:10.1007/s10560-006-0075-4.

Baltodano, H. M., Mathur, S. R., & Rutherford, R. B. (2005). Transition of incarcerated youth with disabilities across systems and into adulthood. *Exceptionality, 13*(2), 103–124. doi:10.1207/s15327035ex1302_4.

Barrett, D. E., Katsiyannis, A., & Zhang, D. (2006). Predictors of offense severity, prosecution, incarceration, and repeat violations for adolescent male and female offenders. *Journal of Child and Family Studies, 15*(6), 709–719. doi:10.1007/s10826-006-9044-y.

Barrett, D. E., Katsiyannis, A., & Zhang, D. (2010). Predictors of offense severity, adjudication, incarceration and repeat referrals for juvenile offenders: A multi-cohort replication study. *Remedial and Special Education, 31*, 261–275. doi:10.1177/0741932509355990.

Barrett, D. E., Katsiyannis, A., Zhang, D., & Zhang, D. (2014). Delinquency and recidivism: A multicohort, matched-control study of the role of early adverse experiences, mental health problems, and disabilities. *Journal of Emotional and Behavioral Disorders, 22*, 3–15. doi:10.1177/1063426612470514.

References

Bauer, L. O., O'Connor, S., & Hesselbrock, V. M. (1994). Frontal P300 decrements in anti-social personality disorder. *Alcoholism, Clinical and Experimental Research, 18*(6), 1300–1305. doi:10.1111/j.1530-0277.1994.tb01427.x.

Beebe, M. C., & Mueller, F. (1993). Categorical offenses of juvenile delinquents and the relation to achievement. *Journal of Correctional Education, 44*, 193–198.

Blomberg, T. G., Bales, W. D., & Piquero, A. R. (2012). Is educational achievement a turning point for incarcerated delinquents across race and sex? *Journal of Youth and Adolescence, 41*, 202–216. doi:10.1007/s10964-011-9680-4.

Braggio, J. T., Plshkln, V., Gameros, T. A., & Brooks, D. L. (1993). Academic achievement in substance-abusing and conduct-disordered adolescents. *Journal of Clinical Psychology, 49*(2), 282–291. doi:10.1002/1097-4679(199303)49:2<282::aid-jclp2270490223>3.0.co;2-n.

Bryan, K., Freer, J., & Furlong, C. (2007). Language and communication difficulties in juvenile offenders. *International Journal of Language and Communication Disorders, 42*(5), 505–520. doi:10.1080/13682820601053977.

Bullis, M., & Yovanoff, P. (2005). More alike than different? Comparison of formerly incarcerated youth with and without disabilities. *Journal of Child and Family Studies, 14*, 127–139.

Bullock, L. M., & McArthur, P. (1994). Correctional special education: Disability prevalence estimates and teachers' preparation programs. *Education and Treatment of Children, 17*, 347–355.

Caplan, N. S. (1965). Intellectual functioning. In H. C. Quay (Ed.), *Juvenile delinquency: Research and theory* (pp. 100–138). Princeton, NJ: D. Van Nostrand.

Cauffman, E., Steinberg, L., & Piquero, A. R. (2005). Psychological, neuropsychological and physiological correlates of serious antisocial behavior in adolescence: The role of self-control. *Criminology, 43*(1), 133–176. doi:10.1111/j.0011-1348.2005.00005.x.

Chen, P., Voisin, D. R., & Jacobson, K. C. (2013). Community violence exposure and adolescent delinquency: Examining a spectrum of promotive factors. *Youth & Society*. doi:10.1177/0044118X13475827.

Coghill, D. R., Hayward, D., Rhodes, S. M., Grimmer, C., & Matthews, K. (2014). A longitudinal examination of neuropsychological and clinical functioning in boys with attention deficit hyperactivity disorder (ADHD): Improvements in executive functioning do not explain clinical improvement. *Psychological Medicine, 44*(5), 1087–1099. doi:10.1017/s0033291713001761.

Cohen, A. (1955). *Delinquent boys: The culture of the gang*. Glencoe, IL: The Free Press of Glencoe.

Conti-Ramsden, G. M., & Botting, N. (2008). Emotional health in adolescents with and without a history of specific language impairment. *Journal of Child Psychology and Psychiatry, 49*, 516–525.

Cottle, C. C., Lee, R. J., & Heilbrun, K. (2001). The prediction of criminal recidivism in juveniles: A meta-analysis. *Criminal Justice and Behavior, 28*(3), 367–394. doi:10.1177/0093854801028003005.

Cruise, K. R., Evans, L. J., & Pickens, I. B. (2011). Integrating mental health and special education needs into comprehensive service planning for juvenile offenders in long-term custody settings. *Learning and Individual Differences, 21*(1), 30–40. doi:10.1016/j.lindif.2010.11.004.

Culberton, F. M., Feral, C. H., & Gabby, S. (1989). Pattern analysis of Wechsler Intelligence Scale for Children—Revised profiles of delinquent boys. *Journal of Clinical Psychology, 45*(4), 651–660. doi:10.1002/1097-4679(198907)45:4<651::aid-jclp2270450423>3.0.co;2-m.

Defoe, I. N., Farrington, D. P., & Loeber, R. (2013). Disentangling the relationship between delinquency and hyperactivity, low achievement, depression, and low socioeconomic status: Analysis of repeated longitudinal data. *Journal of Criminal Justice, 41*(2), 100–107. doi:10.1016/j.jcrimjus.2012.12.002.

Dembo, R., Schmeidler, J., Nini-Gough, B., Sue, C. C., Borden, P., & Manning, D. (1998). Predictors of recidivism to a juvenile assessment center: A three year study. *Journal of Child and Adolescent Substance Abuse, 7*(3), 57–77. doi:10.1300/j029v07n03_03.

Dembo, R., Turner, G., Sue, C. C., Schmeidler, J., Bordon, P., & Manning, D. (1995). Predictors of recidivism to a juvenile assessment center. *Substance Use and Misuse, 30*, 1425–1452. doi:10.3109/10826089509055841.

Dery, M., Toupin, J., Pauze, R., Mercier, H., & Fortin, L. (1999). Neuropsychological characteristics of adolescents with conduct disorder: Association with attention-deficit-hyperactivity and aggression. *Journal of Abnormal Child Psychology, 27*(3), 225–236. doi:10.1023/a:1021904523912.

Duncan, R. D., Kennedy, W. A., & Patrick, C. J. (1995). Four-factor model of recidivism in male juvenile offenders. *Journal of Clinical Child Psychology, 24*(3), 250–257. doi:10.1207/s15374424jccp2403_1.

Drakeford, W. (2002). The impact of an intensive program to increase the literacy skills of youth confined to juvenile corrections. *Journal of Correctional Education, 53*, 139–144.

Farrington, D. P. (1989). Early predictors of adolescent aggression and adult violence. *Violence and Victims, 4*(2), 79–100.

Farrington, D. P., Loeber, R., Yin, Y., & Anderson, S. J. (2002). Are within-individual causes of delinquency the same as between-individual causes? *Criminal Behaviour and Mental Health, 12*(1), 53–68. doi:10.1002/cbm.486.

Fergusson, D. M., & Horwood, L. (2002). Male and female offending trajectories. *Development and Psychopathology, 14*(1), 159–177. doi:10.1017/s0954579402001098.

Foley, R. M. (2001). Academic characteristics of incarcerated youth and correctional educational programs: A literature review. *Journal of Emotional and Behavioral Disorders, 9*(4), 248–259. doi:10.1177/106342660100900405.

Ford, J. D., Chapman, J., Mack, M., & Pearson, G. (2006). Pathway from traumatic child victimization to delinquency: Implications for juvenile and permanency court proceedings and decisions. *Juvenile and Family Court Journal, 57*, 13–26.

Glueck, S., & Glueck, E. T. (1950). *Unraveling juvenile delinquency*. Cambridge, MA: Harvard University Press.

Graham, E. E., & Kamano, D. (1958). Reading failure as a factor in the WAIS subtest patterns of youthful offenders. *Journal of Clinical Psychology, 14*(3), 302–305. doi:10.1002/1097-4679(195807)14:3<302::aid-jclp2270140324>3.0.co;2-l.

Hawkins, J. D., Herrenkohl, T. I., Farrington, D. P., Brewer, D., Catalano, R. F., Harachi, T. W., & Cothern, L. (2000). *Predictors of youth violence*. Washington, DC: Office of Juvenile Justice and Delinquency Prevention, U.S. Department of Justice.

Hay, C., Fortson, E. N., Hollist, D. R., Altheimer, I. J., & Schaible, L. M. (2007). Compounded risk: The implications for delinquency of coming from a poor family that lives in a poor community. *Journal of Youth and Adolescence, 36*(5), 593–605. doi:10.1007/s10964-007-9175-5.

Herrenkohl, T. I., Maguin, E., Hill, K. G., Hawkins, J. D., Abbott, R. D., & Catalano, R. F. (2000). Developmental risk factors for youth violence. *Journal of Adolescent Health, 26*(3), 176–186. doi:10.1016/s1054-139x(99)00065-8.

Hirschi, T., & Hindelang, M. J. (1977). Intelligence and delinquency: A revisionist review. *American Sociological Review, 42*(4), 571–587. doi:10.2307/2094556.

Hoge, R. D. (2001). *The juvenile offender* (Vol. 5). New York, NY: Springer Science & Business Media.

Hoge, R. D. (2002). Standardized instruments for assessing risk and need in youthful offenders. *Criminal Justice and Behavior, 29*(4), 380–396. doi:10.1177/009385480202900403.

Hong, J. S., Huang, H., Golden, M., Patton, D. U., & Washington, T. (2014). Are community violence-exposed youth at risk of engaging in delinquent behavior: A review and implications for residential treatment research and practice. *Residential Treatment for Children and Youth, 31*, 266–283. doi:10.1080/0886571X.2014.958343.

Jacobs, W. L., Kennedy, W. A., & Meyer, J. B. (1997). Juvenile delinquents: A between-group comparison study of sexual and nonsexual offenders. *Sexual Abuse: A Journal of Research and Treatment, 9*(3), 201–217. doi:10.1007/bf02675065.

Jarvelin, M. R., Laara, E., Rantakallio, P., & Moilanen, I. (1994). Juvenile delinquency, education, and mental disability. *Exceptional Children, 61*, 230–241.

Johnson, C. J., Beitchman, J. H., Young, A., Escobar, M., Atkinson, L., Wilson, B., ... & Wang, M. (1999). Fourteen-year follow-up of children with and without speech/language impairments: Speech/language stability and outcomes. *Journal of Speech, Language and Hearing, 42*(3), 744-760. doi:10.1044/jslhr.4203.744.

Jones, P. R., Harris, P. W., Fader, J., & Grubstein, L. (2001). Identifying chronic juvenile offenders. *Justice Quarterly, 18*(3), 479–507. doi:10.1080/07418820100094991.

Kerig, P. K., Moeddel, M. A., & Becker, S. P. (2010). Assessing the sensitivity and specificity of the MAYSI-2 for detecting trauma among youth in juvenile detention. *Child and Youth Care Forum, 40*(5), 345–362. doi:10.1007=s10566-010-9124-4.

Kilpatrick, D. G., Ruggiero, K. J., Acierno, R., Saunders, B. E., Resnick, H. S., & Best, C. L. (2003). Violence and risk of PTSD, major depression, substance abuse/dependence, and comorbidity: Results from the National Survey of Adolescents. *Journal of Consulting and Clinical Psychiatry, 71*(4), 692–700. doi:10.1037/0022-006x.71.4.692.

Katsiyannis, A., & Archwamety, T. (1997). Factors related to recidivism among delinquent youth in a state correctional facility. *Journal of Child and Family Studies, 6*(1), 43–55. doi:10.1023/a:1025068623167.

Katsiyannis, A., Ryan, J., Zhang, D., & Spann, A. (2008). Juvenile delinquency and recidivism: The impact of academic achievement. *Reading & Writing Quarterly: Overcoming Learning Difficulties, 24*, 177–196. doi:10.1080/10573560701808460.

Kennedy, T. D., Burnett, K. F., & Edmonds, W. A. (2011). Intellectual, behavioral, and personality correlates of violent versus non-violent juvenile offenders. *Aggressive Behavior, 37*(4), 315–325. doi:10.1002/ab.20393.

Kolb, B., & Whishaw, I. Q. (2008). *Fundamentals of human neuropsychology*. New York, NY: Worth.

Koolhof, R., Loeber, R., Wei, E. H., Pardini, D., & D'escury, A. C. (2007). Inhibition deficits of serious delinquent boys of low intelligence. *Criminal Behaviour and Mental Health, 17*(5), 274–292. doi:10.1002/cbm.661.

Lawrence, R. (1998). *School crime and juvenile justice*. New York, NY: Oxford University Press.

Linz, T. D., Hooper, S. R., Hynd, G. W., Isaac, W., & Gibson, L. J. (1990). Frontal lobe functioning in conduct disordered juveniles: Preliminary findings. *Archives of Clinical Neuropsychology, 5*(4), 411–416. doi:10.1093/arclin/5.4.411.

Loeber, R., & Farrington, D. P. (2012). *From juvenile delinquency to adult crime: Criminal careers, justice policy and prevention*. New York, NY: Oxford University Press.

Low, S., Sinclair, R., & Shortt, J. W. (2012). The role of economic strain on adolescent delinquency: A microsocial process model. *Journal of Family Psychology, 26*(4), 576–584. doi:10.1037/a0028785.

Lueger, R. J., & Gill, K. J. (1990). Frontal-lobe cognitive dysfunction in conduct disorder adolescents. *Journal of Clinical Psychology, 46*, 696–706.

Lundy, S. M., Silva, G. E., Kaemingk, K. L., Goodwin, J. L., & Quan, S. F. (2010). Cognitive functioning and academic performance in elementary school children with anxious/depressed and withdrawn symptoms. *The Open Pediatric Medical Journal, 14*, 1–9. doi:10.2174/1874309901004010001.

Lynam, D., Moffitt, T., & Stouthamer-Loeber, M. (1993). Explaining the relation between IQ and delinquency: Class, race, test motivation, school failure, or self-control? *Journal of Abnormal Psychology, 102*(2), 187–196. doi:10.1037//0021-843x.102.2.187.

Maas, C., Herrenkohl, T. I., & Sousa, C. (2008). Review of research on child maltreatment and violence in youth. *Trauma, Violence & Abuse, 9*(1), 56–67. doi:10.1177/1524838007311105.

McMackin, R. A., Tansi, R., & LaFratta, J. (2004). Special section: Studies in the rehabilitation of juvenile offenders: Recidivism among juvenile offenders over periods ranging from one to twenty years following residential treatment. *Journal of Offender Rehabilitation, 28*, 1–15. doi:10.1300/j076v38n03_01.

Malmgren, K., & Leone, P. (2000). Effects of a short-term auxiliary reading program on the reading skills of delinquent youth. *Education and Treatment of Children, 28*, 239–247.

Milloy, C. D. (1994). *A comparative study of juvenile sex offenders and non-sex offenders*. Olympia, WA: Washington State Institute for Public Policy.

Milner, B. (1964). Some effects of frontal lobectomy in man. In J. M. Akert & K. Warren (Eds.), *The frontal granular cortex and behavior* (pp. 313–334). New York, NY: McGraw-Hill.

Moffitt, T. E., Lynam, D. R., & Silva, P. A. (1994). Neuropsychological tests predicting persistent male delinquency. *Criminology, 32*(2), 277–300. doi:10.1111/j.1745-9125.1994.tb01155.x.

Moffitt, T. E., & Silva, P. A. (1988). Self-reported delinquency, neuropsychological deficit, and history of attention deficit disorder. *Journal of Abnormal Child Psychology, 16*(5), 553–569. doi:10.1007/bf00914266.

Morgan, D. I. (1979). Prevalence and types of handicapping conditions found in juvenile correctional institutions: A national survey. *Journal of Special Education, 13,* 283–295.

Morris, K. A., & Morris, R. J. (2006). Disability and juvenile delinquency: Issues and trends. *Disability and Society, 21*(6), 613–627. doi:10.1080/09687590600918339.

Myner, J., Santman, J., Cappelletty, G. G., & Perlmutter, B. F. (1998). Variables related to recidivism among juvenile offenders. *International Journal of Offender Therapy and Comparative Criminology, 42*(1), 65–80. doi:10.1177/0306624x98421006.

Nas, C. N., Orobio De Castro, B., & Koops, W. (2005). Social information processing in delinquent adolescents. *Psychology, Crime & Law, 11*(4), 363–375. doi:10.1080/10683160500255307.

Nieto, R. G., & Castellanos, F. X. (2011). A meta-analysis of neuropsychological functioning in patients with early onset schizophrenia and pediatric bipolar disorder. *Journal of Clinical Child and Adolescent Psychology, 40,* 266–280. doi:10.1080/15374416.2011.546049.

Olvera, R. L., Semrud-Clikeman, M., Pliszka, S. T., & O'Donnell, L. (2005). Neuropsychological deficits in adolescents with conduct disorder and comorbid bipolar disorder: A pilot study. *Bipolar Disorders, 7*(1), 57–67. doi:10.1111/j.1399-5618.2004.00167.x.

Pagani, L., Boulerice, B., Vitaro, F., & Tremblay, R. E. (1999). Effects of poverty on academic failure and delinquency in boys: A change and process model approach. *Journal of Child Psychology and Psychiatry, 40*(8), 1209–1219. doi:10.1111/1469-7610.00537.

Pope, C. E., Lovell, R., & Hsia, H. M. (2002). *Disproportionate minority confinement: A review of the research literature from 1989 through 2001.* Washington, DC: Office of Juvenile Justice and Delinquency Prevention.

Puzzanchera, C. (2013). *Juvenile Arrests 2010. Juvenile offenders and victims: National reports series.* Washington, DC: Office of Juvenile Justice and Delinquency Prevention.

Quinn, M. M., Rutherford, R. B., Leone, P. E., Osher, D. M., & Poirier, J. M. (2005). Youth with disabilities in juvenile corrections: A national survey. *Exceptional Children, 71*(3), 339–345. doi:10.1177/001440290507100308.

Raine, A., Moffitt, T. E., Caspi, A., Loeber, R., Stouthamer-Loeber, M., & Lynam, D. (2005). Neurocognitive impairments in boys on the life-course persistent antisocial path. *Journal of Abnormal Psychology, 114*(1), 38. doi:10.1037/0021-843x.114.1.38.

Repo, E., & Virkkunen, M. (1997). Young arsonists: History of conduct disorder, psychiatric diagnoses and criminal recidivism. *Journal of Forensic Psychiatry, 8*(2), 311–320. doi:10.1080/09585189708412013.

Rodriguez, N. (2007). Restorative justice at work: Examining the impact of restorative justice resolutions on juvenile recidivism. *Crime & Delinquency, 53*(3), 355–379. doi:10.1177/0011128705285983.

Rogers-Adkinson, D., Melloy, K., Stuart, S., Fletcher, L., & Rinaldi, C. (2008). Reading and written language competency of incarcerated youth. *Reading & Writing Quarterly, 24*(2), 197–218. doi:10.1080/10573560701808502.

Schwalbe, C. S. (2007). Risk assessment for juvenile justice: a meta-analysis: Predictive validity by gender. *Law and Human Behavior, 31*(5), 1367–1381. doi:10.1007/s10979-006-9071-7.

Sequin, J. R., Pihl, R. O., Hardin, P. W., Tremblay, R. E., & Boulerice, B. (1995). Cognitive and neuropsychological characteristics of physically aggressive boys. *Journal of Abnormal Psychology, 104,* 614–624.

Shoemaker, D. (2005). *Theories of delinquency: An examination of explanations of delinquent behavior* (5th ed.). New York, NY: Oxford University Press.

Sickmund, M., & Puzzanchera, C. (2014). *Juvenile offenders and victims: 2014 national report.* Pittsburgh, PA: National Center for Juvenile Justice.

Skowyra, K. R., & Cocozza, J. J. (2007). *Blueprint for change: A comprehensive model for the identification and treatment of youth with mental health needs in contact with the juvenile justice system.* Washington, DC: National Center for Mental Health and Juvenile Justice.

Snyder, H. N., & Mulako-Wangota, J. (2013). *Arrest data analysis tool*. Washington, DC: Bureau of Justice Statistics.

Snyder, H. N., & Sickmund, M. (2006). *Juvenile offenders and victims: 2006 national report*. Pittsburgh, PA: National Center for Juvenile Justice.

Stahlberg, O., Anckarsater, H., & Nilsson, T. (2010). Mental health problems in youth committed to juvenile institutions: Prevalence and treatment needs. *European Child & Adolescent Psychiatry, 19*(12), 893–903. doi:10.1007/s00787-010-0137-1.

Steketee, M., Junger, M., & Junger-Tas, J. (2013). Sex differences in the predictors of juvenile delinquency. *Journal of Contemporary Criminal Justice, 29*(1), 88–105. doi:10.1177/1043986212470888.

Stimmel, M. A., Cruise, K. R., Ford, J. D., & Weiss, R. A. (2014). Trauma exposure, posttraumatic stress disorder symptomatology, and aggression in male juvenile offenders. *Psychological Trauma: Theory, Research, Practice, and Policy, 6*(2), 184–191. doi:10.1037/a0032509.

Teplin, L. A., Abram, K. M., McClelland, G. M., Dulcan, M. K., & Mericle, A. A. (2002). Psychiatric disorders in youth in juvenile detention. *Archives of General Psychiatry, 59*(12), 1133–1143. doi:10.1001/archpsyc.59.12.1133.

Thompson, K. C., & Morris, R. J. (2013). *Predicting recidivism among juvenile delinquents: Comparison of risk factors for male and female offenders*. Washington, DC: Office of Juvenile Justice and Delinquency Prevention.

Tille, J. E., & Rose, J. C. (2007). Emotional and behavioral problems of 13-to-18-year-old incarcerated female first-time offenders and recidivists. *Youth Violence and Juvenile Justice, 5*(4), 426–435. doi:10.1177/1541204007300355.

Trulson, C. R., Marquart, J. W., Mullings, J. L., & Caeti, T. J. (2005). In between adolescence and adulthood: Recidivism outcomes of a cohort of state delinquents. *Youth Violence and Juvenile Justice, 3*(4), 355–387. doi:10.1177/1541204005278802.

United States Bureau of Justice Statistics. (1997). *Research brief: Education as crime prevention*. Washington, DC: The Center on Crime, Community, and Culture.

U.S. Department of Education. (1994). *Mini-digest of education statistics, 1994*. Washington, DC: National Center for Education Statistics.

U.S. Department of Education. (2014). *Thirty-sixth annual report to Congress on the implementation of the Individuals with Disabilities Education Act*. Washington, DC: Author.

Vacca, J. S. (2008). Crime can be prevented if schools teach juvenile offenders to read. *Children and Youth Services Review, 30*(9), 1055–1062. doi:10.1016/j.childyouth.2008.01.013.

Van Der Geest, V., & Bijleveld, C. (2008). Personal, background and treatment characteristics associated with offending after residential treatment: A 13-year follow up in adolescent males. *Psychology, Crime & Law, 14*(2), 159–176. doi:10.1080/10683160701483609.

van Wijk, A., Loeber, R., Vermeiren, R., Pardini, D., Bullens, R., & Doreleijers, T. (2005). Violent juvenile sex offenders compared with violent juvenile nonsex offenders: Explorative findings from the Pittsburgh youth study. *Sexual Abuse: A Journal of Research and Treatment, 17*(3), 333–352. doi:10.1177/107906320501700306.

van Wijk, A., Van Horn, J., Bullens, R., Bijleveld, C., & Doreleijers, T. (2005). Juvenile sex offenders: A group on its own? *International Journal of Offender Therapy and Comparative Criminology, 49*(1), 25–36.

van Wijk, A., Vermeiren, R., Loeber, R., Doreleijers, T., & Bullens, R. (2006). Juvenile sex offenders compared to non-sex offenders a review of the literature 1995-2005. *Trauma, Violence & Abuse, 7*(4), 227–243. doi:10.1177/1524838006292519.

Veneziano, C., Veneziano, L., LeGrand, S., & Richards, L. (2004). Neuropsychological executive functions of adolescent sex offenders and nonsex offenders. *Perceptual and Motor Skills, 98*(2), 661–674. doi:10.2466/pms.98.2.661-674.

Vermeiren, R., Schwab-Stone, M., Ruchkin, V., De Clippele, A., & Deboutte, D. (2002). Predicting recidivism in juvenile adolescents from psychological and psychiatric assessment. *Comprehensive Psychiatry, 43*(2), 142–149. doi:10.1053/comp.2002.30809.

Vitopoulos, N. A., Peterson-Badali, M., & Skilling, T. A. (2012). The relationship between matching service to criminogenic need and recidivism in male and female youth examining the RNR principles in practice. *Criminal Justice and Behavior, 39*(8), 1025–1041. doi:10.1177/0093854812442895.

Vold, G., & Bernard, T. (1986). *Theoretical criminology*. New York, NY: Oxford University Press.

Wechsler, D. (1944). *Measurement of adult intelligence*. Baltimore, MD: William & Wilkins.

Wierson, M., & Forehand, R. (1995). Predicting recidivism in juvenile delinquents: The role of mental health diagnoses and the qualification of conclusions by race. *Behaviour Research and Therapy, 33*(1), 63–67. doi:10.1016/0005-7967(94)e0001-y.

Wilson, H. W., Berent, E., Donenberg, G. R., Emerson, E. M., Rodriguez, E. M., & Sandesara, A. (2013). Trauma history and PTSD symptoms in juvenile offenders on probation. *Victims & Offenders, 8*(4), 465–477. doi:10.1080/15564886.2013.835296.

Wolff, P. H., Waber, D., Bauermeister, C., Cohen, C., & Ferber, R. (1982). The neuropsychological status of adolescent delinquent boys. *Journal of Child Psychology and Psychiatry, 23*(3), 267–279. doi:10.1111/j.1469-7610.1982.tb00072.x.

Wu, B., Cernkovich, S., & Dunn, C. S. (1997). Assessing the effects of race and class on juvenile justice processing in Ohio. *Journal of Criminal Justice, 25*(4), 265–277. doi:10.1016/s0047-2352(97)00012-3.

Yeudall, L. T., & Fromm-Auch, D. (1979). Neuropsychological impairments in various psychopathological populations. In J. G. Gruzelier & P. Flor-Henry (Eds.), *Hemisphere asymmetries of function in psychopathology* (pp. 401–428). Maryland Heights, MO: Elsevier Science.

Yeudall, L. T., Fromm-Auch, D., & Davies, P. (1982). Neuropsychological impairment of persistent delinquency. *The Journal of Nervous and Mental Disease, 170*(5), 257–265. doi:10.1097/00005053-198205000-00001.

Ysseldyke, J. E., Algozzine, B., & Thurlow, M. L. (1992). *Critical issues in special education*. Boston, MA: Houghton Mifflin.

Zahn, M.A., Agnew, R., Fishbein, D., Miller, S., Winn, D.M. Dakoff, G., ... Chesney-Lind, M. (2010). *Causes and correlates of girls' delinquency*. Office of Juvenile Justice and Delinquency Prevention: U.S. Department of Justice.

Zamora, D. (2005). Levels of academic achievement and further delinquency among detained youth. *The Southwestern Journal of Criminal Justice, 2*(1), 42–53.

Zhang, D., Barrett, D. E., Katsiyannis, A., & Yoon, M. (2011). Juvenile offenders with and without disabilities: Risks and patterns of recidivism. *Learning and Individual Differences, 21*(1), 12–18. doi:10.1016/j.lindif.2010.09.006.

Zillmer, E., & Spiers, M. (2001). *Principles of neuropsychology*. Belmont, CA: Wadsworth.

Chapter 3
Juvenile Delinquency and Disability

Over the past few decades, both the adult and juvenile justice system have been increasingly cognizant of the rights and needs of offenders with disabilities. For example, in the 1990s, the Civil Rights Division of the US Department of Justice conducted a series of investigations that identified gross negligence in many juvenile delinquency facilities in the provision of support and care for juvenile offenders with disabilities (Butterfield, 1998). Around this time, the US Department of Health and Human Services' Center for Mental Health Services also initiated the first survey of juvenile delinquency facilities to identify which mental health services were available (Center for Mental Health Services, 1998), while during this same time period, the US Congress reviewed and/or adopted bills and amendments that mandated mental health and substance abuse screening and treatment programs for juvenile delinquents (Manisses Communications Group Incorporated, 1999). Subsequently, since the early 2000s, policies, laws, and other mandates have been put into place to better protect the rights of juvenile offenders with disabilities, as well as to better serve this population of youth.

The urgent need for courts to acknowledge and address the problems of juvenile offenders with disabilities has been highlighted as research has continually demonstrated the prevalence of disabilities among child and adolescent offenders in the juvenile justice system, as well as the difficulties that such youth have when they are processed within the system. Some researchers have attributed these difficulties to the "get tough" movement in the 1990s, during which the juvenile justice system shifted from a treatment or rehabilitative model to a punishment-oriented system (Puzzanchera, 2014). As noted previously, the 1990s saw a large increase of juveniles treated more similarly to adult criminals, which resulted in more juveniles being involved in the legal system and subsequently more juveniles with disabilities involved in the legal system. This has been a contributing factor to the increased need for the juvenile justice system to respond to issues previously more prevalent in the adult system, such as the increasing need to determine a youth's competency and ability to stand trial. While progress over the past two decades has been slow in providing special services to those juveniles having a disability, we are finding an increase in these services across the nation. For example, over the past decade, there has been an increase in specialized courts such as a substance abuse court or mental health court, in which all personnel involved with the processing of youth offenders have specialized training in the disability being addressed. While these types of changes are encouraging, the increasing number of youth offenders with disabilities being detained, adjudicated, and retained in both detention and long-term correctional facilities suggests that additional resources and further understanding of youth with disabilities are needed.

What Is a Disability?

A disability diagnosis is typically based on the distinguishing features of the disability, such as significantly low IQ and low adaptive behavior scores; significantly low math, reading, and/or written language scores; a significant delay in language or emotional development; or significant depressed mood and anxiety. In this regard, in order for a youth to be considered as having a disability versus having a "difficulty" or "challenge," a specific set of primary symptoms must be present, and the symptoms must cause *significant impairment* in the youth's functioning in comparison to his or her typically developing peers in such areas as the school or work environment, education/academics, cognition, language develoment, and/or social/emotional development. The primary classificatory systems for diagnosing youth as having a disability are the *Diagnostic and Statistical Manual of Mental Disorders Fifth Edition* (DSM-5) published by the American Psychiatric Association ([APA] 2013), *Individuals with Disabilities Education Improvement Act* ([IDEA], 2004), and the *International Classification of Diseases* (ICD; World Health Organization, 2012).

In addition to the significant impairments that are required for a diagnosis, most disabilities have a variety of secondary symptoms that contribute to the negative impact that the disability has on the individual's functioning. For example, while depression is primarily characterized by depressed mood, secondary symptoms often include attention and concentration difficulties, as well as memory impairments. Therefore, when understanding the impact that a specific disability can have on one's functioning, it is important to consider the primary *and* secondary symptoms. Moreover, as research in cognitive neuroscience continues to advance, researchers have increasingly identified structural and functional abnormalities in the brain to be associated with many disabilities (APA, 2013). These abnormalities may contribute to thinking impairments or atypical behaviors, and understanding this can better help us understand the reason that individuals act or think in antisocial, atypical, or other maladaptive ways. In addition, knowledge of neurological or neuropsychological impairments related to certain disorders can help professionals in the field to better differentiate between youth who act in a purposeful way versus those having less control over their behaviors and actions. For example, just as science has helped courts understand the implications that brain development has on functioning (Kolb & Winshaw 2008), science can also help us understand if a particular youth was likely acting with premeditated intent or if his or her actions may have been an impulsive response related to a disability. It is both the primary symptoms of a disability, as well as the secondary features associated with the disability, that may have consequences on how a particular youth offender will function once he or she comes into contact with the juvenile justice system. The level of functioning of a youth having a disability within the juvenile justice system will be discussed in subsequent chapters.

Prevalence and Incidence of Juveniles with Disabilities

The juvenile delinquency research literature clearly suggests that there is an overrepresentation of youth having a disability within the juvenile justice system, with studies finding prevalence values ranging from 20 to 75 % (e.g., Bullis & Yovanoff, 2005; Bullock & McArthur, 1994; Morgan, 1979; Morris & Morris, 2006). The wide range in prevalence values may be due to a variety of factors, such as the definition of disability used in particular studies, the classification system used to determine whether a delinquent has a disability, and/or the evaluation procedures and methodology used by researchers in gathering the data (Morris & Morris, 2006). Prevalence studies have further suggested that many youth have gone through the juvenile justice system with undiagnosed disabilities (e.g., Schumacher & Kurz, 2000; Shelton, 2001).

The reasons and theories related to the overrepresentation of youth with disabilities in the juvenile justice system have varied considerably. Some have argued that children or adolescents with disabilities are more likely to engage in delinquent behaviors, while others have suggested that these youth are disproportionately identified as having behavioral or related problems, which in turn increases their interaction with the juvenile justice system. A variety of other theories exist which attempt to explain the overrepresentation of youth with disabilities in correctional and detention facilities, such as school failure theory, susceptibility theory, and differential treatment theory.

School failure theory maintains that disabilities lead either directly or indirectly to school failure and, consequently, school dropout and delinquency (Murray, 1977). *Susceptibility theory* supposes that a disability indicates a predisposition to criminal behavior because of characteristics such as poor impulse control or poor problem-solving ability (Keilitz & Dunivant, 1987). *Differential treatment theory* hypothesizes that disabled students engage in comparable behaviors to nondisabled students but that the police, courts, and/or corrections respond differently to youth with disabilities (e.g., Keilitz & Dunivant, 1987; Leone & Meisel, 1997; Osher, Woodruff, & Sims, 2002).

In addition to these latter theories, there are a variety of other reasons suggested for why youth with disabilities are overrepresented in the juvenile justice system. For instance, over the past few decades, every state in the United States has passed legislation related to implementing a *zero tolerance policy* in the school setting in hopes of decreasing violence among youth and improving school safety (Glanzer, 2005). These zero tolerance policies have subsequently been associated with lower academic achievement and school failure in students (Skiba & Rausch, 2006), higher rates of suspension and expulsion (Boccanfuso & Kuhfeld, 2011), and what researchers describe as a "school-to-prison pipeline" (Cregor & Hewitt, 2011; Gonsoulin, Zablocki, & Leone, 2012). Specifically, zero tolerance policies seem to increase the number of risk factors for disruptive students and their subsequent interaction with the juvenile justice system. Those with disabilities are at a greater risk of having contact with school administrators and school disciplinarians as studies have shown that students who receive special education services are also more likely to violate school rules and to be suspended than are those students who do not receive these services. For instance, despite approximately 10 % of students in public education receiving special education services, one study found that approximately 20 % of all suspended students received special education services (Leone, Mayer, Malmgren, & Meisel, 2000). In addition, students having an emotional disability and/or conduct problems had even higher rates of suspension than students with other disorders or special education diagnoses (Zhang, Katsiyannis, & Herbst, 2004). In addition, many zero tolerance policies require police referral and legal involvement for school-related offenses that previously would have been taken care of within the school system.

In addition to increased discipline, the impaired social skills and decision-making abilities often identified in youth with disabilities may increase their negative involvement in the juvenile justice system, reduce their ability to avoid apprehension by school and police authorities, and interfere with a youth's performance of appropriate responses to school discipline practices or juvenile justice policies and/or ability to successfully respond to psychological or educational interventions, particularly if an intervention does not take the individual's disability into consideration. In addition to increasing their initial involvement with the juvenile justice system, the impairments associated with many disabilities may further increase negative involvement after an arrest has occurred.

There are several steps involved in processing a youth through the juvenile justice system, and many of these steps permit some discretion on the part of individual court personnel. For example, there is often some discretion in whether to allow a youth to receive diversion or community service instead of having a formal adjudication hearing. Individual discretion from a judge or other court personnel can also determine, in some cases, whether a youth is detained, returned home, sent to a group home, or sent to a long-term juvenile facility (Snyder & Sickmund, 1999). A youth's demeanor, social perception, social communication style, and overall ability to interact positively with court personnel and other authority figures may very well affect the likelihood of individual discretion being implemented to work in a more lenient or positive manner for the juvenile. Finally, cognitive and other thinking impairments could affect a juvenile's competency to stand trial, his or her ability to understand and waive Miranda rights, or the ability to fully recall and express details of the incident that resulted in his or her arrest (i.e., recalling what specifically occurred that led to the arrest and/or manifesting the ability to identify witnesses). These impairments, in turn, may affect the decisions regarding a youth that are made by court personnel during the processing of that youth (National Council on Disability, 2003).

As mentioned earlier, it is clear from the literature that youth with educational, cognitive, developmental, and/or mental health disabilities are significantly over-represented in the juvenile justice system. In this regard, a national survey was conducted by the Center for Effective Collaboration and Practice and the National Center of Education Disability (Quinn, Rutherford, Leone, Osher, & Poirier, 2005) to determine the number of students in juvenile correctional and detention facilities who were eligible for special education services under the IDEA (2004). The results showed that prevalence values varied widely between states, with values ranging from as low as 9.1 up to 77.5 %, with a median prevalence rate of 33.4 %. The results also revealed that a high percentage of juveniles with a special education label were identified as having an emotional disability (47.7 %) with 38.6 % having a specific learning disability, 9.7 % with an intellectual disability (previously referred to as "mental retardation"), and 0.8 % identified as having multiple disabilities. These percentages differ markedly from those students involved in the general public education system during the equivalent school year in terms of the types of IDEA categories represented. For example, 47.7 % of delinquents were identified with an emotional disturbance, compared to only 8.2 % in the general population during that same time period (US Department of Education, 2005). Appreciable differences were also found in other IDEA diagnostic categories.

In addition to a high prevalence of educational disabilities among delinquents, there is a significant representation of mental health disabilities in youth within the juvenile justice system. Although the actual number is unknown, it is estimated that as many as 75 % of juvenile delinquents have diagnosable mental disorders (e.g., Skowyra & Cocozza, 2007; Teplin, Abram, McClelland, Dulcan, & Mericle, 2002). In this regard, a multi-state study of over 1400 youth involved with the juvenile justice system indicated that the most common mental health disorders among juvenile delinquents are disruptive behavior disorders (e.g., attention-deficit/hyperactivity disorder, conduct disorder, and oppositional defiant disorder), followed by substance use disorders, anxiety disorders, and mood disorders. Given that many youth qualify for a diagnosis of conduct disorder based solely on their involvement in the juvenile justice system, these researchers controlled for this factor and found that over 63 % of the youth still qualified for a mental health diagnosis. Moreover, after controlling for substance use disorder, the researchers found that over 61 % still qualified for a mental health diagnosis. Lastly, after controlling for both conduct disorder and substance use disorder, over 45 % of youth still qualified for a mental health diagnosis. In addition, over 60 % of the youth in this study had a comorbid mental health disorder (Skowyra & Cocozza, 2007).

Though it is evident that mental health disorders are quite prevalent among juvenile offenders, the actual causal relationship between such disorders and juvenile delinquency is not understood at this time. There are some writers who maintain that certain types of mental health disorders may be a causal or contributing factor to delinquency, while others have suggested that some mental health disorders do not contribute to delinquency but rather are exacerbated as a juvenile is processed through the various phases of the juvenile justice system. For example, Defoe, Farrington, and Loeber (2013) examined the relationship between depression and juvenile delinquency and failed to find that depression was a causal factor of delinquency. Rather, the results of their study indicated that engaging in illegal acts was a causal factor of depression, suggesting that participation in such acts, whether it involved addressing the legal ramifications of such acts or responding to stressors that were related to the illegal acts, contributed to the development of depression versus the depression contributing to committing the illegal acts.

In addition to educational and mental health disabilities, cognitive disabilities such as intellectual disabilities have long been shown to be overrepresented in the juvenile delinquency and adult criminal population. Early theorists attempted to find a link between intellectual disability and adult criminal behavior and between intellectual disability and juvenile offenders (e.g., Kauffman, 1997). While there is research that demonstrates a relationship between lower IQ and delinquency, contemporary research has failed to find a *causal* relationship between intellectual disability and delinquency. Interestingly, however, it is evident from the research literature that youth with intellectual disabilities are overrepresented in the juvenile justice system, with studies suggesting that the prevalence of youth in juvenile corrections facilities who have a mild to moderate intellectual disability is as high as three times that found in the general education public school population (e.g., Casey & Keilitz, 1990; Morgan, 1979; Stahlberg, Anckarsater, & Nilsson, 2010).

An important consideration when examining statistical data related to the prevalence of juvenile offenders with disabilities is that these data typically include only those youth who have already been identified and diagnosed with a specific disability. Disruptive behaviors are common among many youth having a disability, and many writers have suggested that these latter behaviors may become the primary focus of school and/or court personnel, with the accompanying educational, cognitive, developmental, or mental health disability never being properly identified. This would mean that while disabilities are already known to be overrepresented in the juvenile justice system, current statistics may actually underestimate the actual prevalence rates among youth offenders.

Conclusion

Given the complexity of the legal system, the heterogeneous nature of the juvenile delinquency population, and the variability in the presentation of disabilities in youth, it is important that those working with youth offenders have an understanding of the relationship between juvenile delinquency and disability. In particular, those working with youth offenders having a disability should have an awareness and understanding of the impact that the disability can have on a youth's functioning as he or she progresses through the juvenile justice system, as well as issues that may occur when determining the youth's risk to reoffend or competency to stand trial. Disabilities are often as complex as the juvenile offenders, so having an understanding of symptoms of the various disabilities and the implications these disabilities can have on a youth's cognitive, social, and behavioral functioning will be critical in better serving juvenile delinquents with disabilities.

References

American Psychiatric Association. (2013). *Diagnostic and statistical manual of mental disorders* (4th ed.). Washington, DC: Author.

Boccanfuso, C., & Kuhfeld, M. (2011). *Multiple responses, promising results: Evidence based, nonpunitive alternatives to zero tolerance.* Washington, DC: Child Trends.

Bullis, M., & Yovanoff, P. (2005). More alike than different? Comparison of formerly incarcerated youth with and without disabilities. *Journal of Child and Family Studies, 14*(1), 127–139. doi:10.1007/s10826-005-1127-7.

Bullock, L. M., & McArthur, P. (1994). Correctional special education: Disability prevalence estimates and teachers' preparation programs. *Education and Treatment of Children, 17*, 347–355.

Butterfield, F. (1998). Prisons replace hospitals for the nation's mentally ill. *New York Times, A1.*

Cregor, M., & Hewitt, D. (2011). Dismantling the school-to-prison pipeline: A survey from the field. *Poverty & Race, 20*(1), 5–7.

Casey, P., & Keilitz, I. (1990). Estimating the prevalence of learning disabled and mentally retarded juvenile offenders: A meta-analysis. In P. E. Leone (Ed.), *Understanding trouble and troubling youth* (pp. 82–101). Newbury Park, CA: Sage.

Center for Mental Health Services. (1998). *1998 Inventory of mental health services in juvenile justice facilities, halfway houses, and group homes.* Rockville, MD: U.S. Department of Health and Human Services.

Defoe, I. N., Farrington, D. P., & Loeber, R. (2013). Disentangling the relationship between delinquency and hyperactivity, low achievement, depression, and low socioeconomic status: Analysis of repeated longitudinal data. *Journal of Criminal Justice, 41*(2), 100–107. doi:10.1016/j.jcrimjus.2012.12.002.

Glanzer, P. L. (2005). The limited character education of zero tolerance policies: An alternative moral vision for discipline. *Journal of Research in Character Education, 3*(2), 97–108.

Gonsoulin, S., Zablocki, M., & Leone, P. E. (2012). Safe schools, staff development, and the school-to-prison pipeline. *Teacher Education and Special Education: The Journal of the*

Teacher Education Division of the Council for Exceptional Children, 35(4), 309–319. doi:10.1177/0888406412453470.

Individuals With Disabilities Education Act, 20 U.S.C. § 1400 (2004).

Kauffman, J. M. (1997). *Characteristics of emotional and behavioral disorders of children and youth.* Upper Saddle River, NJ: Merrill/Prentice Hall.

Keilitz, I., & Dunivant, N. (1987). The learning disabled offender. In C. M. Nelson, R. B. Rutherford, & B. I. Wolford (Eds.), *Special education in the criminal justice system* (pp. 120–137). Columbus, OH: Merrill.

Kolb, B., & Winshaw, I. Q. (2008). *Fundamentals of human neuropsychology* (6th ed.). New York, NY: Macmillan.

Leone, P. E., Mayer, M. J., Malmgren, K., & Meisel, S. M. (2000). School violence and disruption: Rhetoric, reality, and reasonable balance. *Focus on Exceptional Children, 33*(1), 1–20.

Leone, P. E., & Meisel, S. (1997). Improving education services for students in detention and confinement facilities. *Children's Legal Rights Journal, 17*, 1–12.

Morgan, D. I. (1979). Prevalence and types of handicapping conditions found in juvenile correctional institutions: A national survey. *Journal of Special Education, 13*(3), 283–295. doi:10.1177/002246697901300307.

Morris, K., & Morris, R. J. (2006). Disability and juvenile delinquency: Issues and trends. *Disability and Society, 21*(6), 613–627. doi:10.1080/09687590600918339.

Murray, C. A. (1977). *The link between learning disabilities and juvenile delinquency: Current theory and knowledge.* Washington, DC: U.S. Government Printing Office.

National Council on Disability. (2003). *Addressing the needs of youth with disabilities in the juvenile justice system: The current status of evidence-based research.* Washington, DC: National Council on Disability.

Osher, D., Woodruff, D., & Sims, A. (2002). Schools make a difference: The relationship between education services for African American children and youth and their overrepresentation in the juvenile justice system. In D. Losen (Ed.), *Minority issues in special education* (pp. 93–116). Cambridge, MA: The Civil Rights Project, Harvard University and the Harvard Education.

Puzzanchera, C. (2014). *Juvenile offenders and victims: National report series, juvenile arrests 2012.* Washington, DC: Office of Juvenile Justice and Delinquency Prevention, U.S. Department of Justice.

Quinn, M. M., Rutherford, R. B., Leone, P. E., Osher, D. M., & Poirier, J. M. (2005). Youth with disabilities in juvenile corrections: A national survey. *Exceptional Children, 71*(3), 339–345. doi:10.1177/001440290507100308.

Schumacher, M., & Kurz, G. A. (2000). *The 8% solution: Preventing serious, repeat juvenile crime.* Thousand Oaks, CA: Sage.

Shelton, D. (2001). Emotional disorders in young offenders. *Journal of Nursing Scholarship, 33*(3), 259–263. doi:10.1111/j.1547-5069.2001.00259.x.

Skiba, R. J., & Rausch, M. K. (2006). Zero tolerance, suspension, and expulsion: Questions of equity and effectiveness. In C. M. Evertson & C. S. Weinsten (Eds.), *Handbook of classroom management: Research, practice, and contemporary issues* (pp. 1063–1089). New York, NY: Routledge.

Skowyra, K. R., & Cocozza, J. J. (2007). *A blueprint for change: Improving the system response to youth with mental health needs involved with the juvenile justice system.* Delmar, NY: National Center for Mental Health and Juvenile Justice.

Snyder, H. N., & Sickmund, M. (1999). *Juvenile offenders and victims: 1999 national report.* Washington, DC: Office of Juvenile Justice and Delinquency Prevention.

Stahlberg, O., Anckarsater, H., & Nilsson, T. (2010). Mental health problems in youth committed to juvenile institutions: Prevalence and treatment needs. *European Child & Adolescent Psychiatry, 19*(12), 893–903. doi:10.1007/s00787-010-0137-1.

References

Teplin, L. A., Abram, K. M., McClelland, G. M., Dulcan, M. K., & Mericle, A. A. (2002). Psychiatric disorders in youth in juvenile detention. *Archives of General Psychiatry, 59*(12), 1133–1143. doi:10.1001/archpsyc.59.12.1133.

World Health Organization. (2012). *The ICD-10 classification of mental and behavioural disorders: Clinical descriptions and diagnostic guidelines, 10th Revision.* Geneva, Switzerland: World Health Organization.

Zhang, D., Katsiyannis, A., & Herbst, M. (2004). Disciplinary exclusions in special education: A 4-year analysis. *Behavioral Disorders, 29*(4), 337–347.

Chapter 4
Theories of Juvenile Delinquency

Philosophers and researchers have attempted to explain the etiology of juvenile delinquency since early Greek and Roman times. In past centuries, for example, philosophers developed subjective explanations based on what they observed first-hand, while in more recent times, researchers have attempted to develop and expand theories based on findings from empirical research. Most causal theories of juvenile delinquency have attempted to integrate within one conceptual position a series of factors or variables that have been identified through research, or have been hypothesized based on research data, to be causing delinquency. As a function of integrating this information, theorists provide us with their best guess as to what are the cause(s) of juvenile delinquency. Caution must be taken, however, in presuming that these latter "best guess" positions are, in fact, causal statements since most theoretical positions are based largely on correlational research findings and other non-causal research findings and, as such, do not imply causality (Borowski, 2003). In this regard, given the complexity of the study of juvenile delinquency, as well as the characteristics and risk factors that have been found to be associated with delinquency, it is unlikely that any one current theory can explain what causes youth to become juvenile offenders. This is especially the case when one adds to this area of study the findings from the research literature since the mid-1990s on the relationship between cognitive, developmental, educational, and/or mental health disabilities and the performing of illegal acts by youth, as few theorists have incorporated into their theoretical positions the fact that there is a significant overrepresentation of disabilities among delinquents.

Another important consideration when examining theoretical perspectives in regard to juvenile delinquency is that many theories have little or insufficient empirical validation. While some theories have been shown empirically to have more predictive and statistical power than others, few, if any, are able to account for all the variation in risk factors associated with juvenile delinquency (Borowski, 2003). These theories, however, remain in various discussions of the etiology of juvenile delinquency since they provide an historical perspective on the progress that society and the social and behavioral sciences, as well as the biological sciences and neurosciences, have made in the understanding of the factors that contribute to delinquency. In addition, these theories collectively provide researchers with a wealth of knowledge concerning potential hypotheses needing further investigation in regard to the origin(s) of juvenile delinquency. In our discussion below, we present an overview of the major theories of juvenile delinquency and provide a perspective on how these theories fare in relation to the contemporary research literature in developmental and cognitive psychology, child clinical and school psychology, and child and adolescent neuropsychology. Although certain disabilities found to be associated with juvenile delinquency are briefly mentioned in our analysis of each theory, a more detailed account of each disability and its impact on juvenile delinquency is discussed in subsequent chapters.

Theories of Juvenile Delinquency

Classical Theories

Classical theory of crime dates back to the eighteenth century and the work on crime and punishment by Cesare Beccaria, a philosopher and early advocate for reforming the criminal justice system (Beccaria, 1764/1963). This theory is based on the premise that behavior is the result of conscious, calculated thought, and it argues that individuals act on *free will* and make *rational choices* with the intent of achieving a goal (Shoemaker, 2005). Beccaria stated that individuals commit crimes voluntarily and do so because they derive pleasure and gratification from the acts. A juvenile delinquent, therefore, differs from a nondelinquent in the way that he or she goes about achieving goals: the nondelinquent abides by society's laws in his or her various pursuits, whereas the delinquent does not (Gottfredson & Hirschi, 1990). For example, according to this theory, a juvenile may steal because he or she wants to steal a car, with the youth making a rational, independent choice to steal the car. Although this is a frequently referenced theoretical perspective, it is also often critiqued for many reasons, including that the theory (1) assumes all individuals have the ability to reason and act rationally, (2) fails to take into account individual differences such as age or cognitive ability, and (3) does not account for mitigating factors that may influence one's decision(s) to engage in criminal behavior, such as environmental stressors (Curran & Renzetti, 1994; Vold & Bernard, 1986).

Neoclassical theory is a close relative of classical theory in that it argues that individuals behave to gain pleasure and gratification; however, this theory does allow for environmental or individual factors that may influence the person's decision to commit a certain act or behavior (Vold & Bernard, 1986). Neoclassical theory takes classical theory a step further by acknowledging that there are individual differences between those youth who choose to commit a crime.

Another theory related to classical theory is *rational choice theory*, which takes the position that individuals commit crimes using reasoning and rational approaches to their behavior (Cornish & Clarke, 1986). Similar to neoclassical theory, it also allows for mitigating factors that may influence an individual's choice to commit a crime. Rational choice theory continues the classical thought that a crime is committed out of self-interest, but it argues that the decision to commit a criminal act is reasoned out and based on a "rational choice" (Onwudiwe, 2004). For example, an individual who decides to steal a car may decide that the benefits of having the car outweigh the risks associated with stealing the car. The primary criticism of this theory, however, is that it assumes that the individual has the ability to make a reasoned, calculated decision (Paternoster, 1989).

Classical theories assume that abstract thinking and behavioral regulation are inherent in an individual. While many individuals do have these abilities, the expectation that higher-level thinking, reasoning, and self-regulation are inherent in youth directly conflicts with current findings in cognitive neuroscience. In this regard, contemporary studies have demonstrated that children and adolescents lack the brain maturation to think and reason at the same level as that of adults (Kolb & Winshaw, 2008). This, therefore, calls into question some of the assumptions upon which classical theories were formulated, namely, that an illegal act is conducted only after a calculated decision has been made. For example, rational choice theory posits that individuals make a rational decision in whether to engage in a specific act, whereas a hallmark symptom of the mental health disorder attention-deficit/hyperactivity disorder (ADHD) is impulsivity, or the tendency to act *without* thinking of the consequences (American Psychiatric Association [APA], 2013). Moreover, behavioral and emotional *dysregulation* are symptoms associated with the mental health disorder bipolar disorder (APA, 2013); therefore, in the case of youth offenders having bipolar disorder, their symptoms would be inconsistent with the assumptions surrounding classical theories. A similar argument can be made for those youth offenders having an intellectual disability, since these youth do not have the intellectual capacity to logically reason at the same level presumed in classical theories.

Psychological Theories

Psychological theories assume that while environmental factors may influence an individual, the cause of juvenile delinquency is internal to the youth and, therefore, the individual is directly responsible for his or her behavior and actions (Shoemaker, 2005). This theoretical approach also assumes that the psychological disturbance in the youth began in early childhood. Types of psychological theories include psychoanalytic and psychodynamic theories, as well as personality trait theory, social learning theory, and labeling theory.

Psychoanalytic and psychodynamic theories assume that individuals develop in stages, at which point abnormalities may occur and, consequently, the development of their personality is hindered. This, in turn, leads to conflicts between an individual's personal desires and restraints placed on him or her by society, which may lead to delinquent behaviors (Shoemaker, 2005). The psychodynamic approach to juvenile delinquency can be traced back to Sigmund Freud (1900/1953). Psychodynamic theory assumes that delinquency is a manifestation of underlying constructs comprising a person's psychological framework, including Freud's conceptualizations of the "conscious" and "unconscious" and the interactions between the *id*, *ego*, and *superego*. This theory, therefore, assumes that delinquency is the result of psychic conflict between the mainly unconscious ego and conscious superego (Vold & Bernard, 1986).

Personality trait theory, as related to juvenile delinquency, is similar to psychodynamic theories in that it assumes that traits develop primarily from childhood and are internal mechanisms controlling the individual's behavior (Shoemaker, 2005). Most research supporting personality trait theory describes general personality traits exhibited by juvenile delinquents. Eysenck (1977), for example, constructed a theory that specifically studied personality and delinquency. He stated that juvenile delinquents differ from nondelinquents on three dimensions of personality: psychoticism, extraversion, and neuroticism. Eysenck (1977) argued that delinquents score high on all three of these traits. More recent studies, however, have failed to confirm Eysenck's position or hypotheses (e.g., van Dam, De Bruyn, & Janssens, 2007).

Other research has also attempted to discern personality traits specific to juvenile delinquents, using such measures as the *Minnesota Multiphasic Personality Inventory-Adolescent* and the *Millon Adolescent Clinical Inventory* (Oxnam & Vess, 2006; Sorenson & Johnson, 1996; Taylor, Kemper, Loney, & Kistner, 2006). Although studies using these latter assessment instruments have yielded significant results, many of the findings have yielded poor predictive power (Shoemaker, 2005).

Social learning theory is based on the work of Albert Bandura and maintains that individuals learn to behave through their social interactions with others (Bandura, 1977). As applied to delinquent behavior, social learning theory suggests that individuals learn social behaviors such as delinquent behavior through modeling (Akers, 1977). It supposes that because social behavior is learned through modeling or imitating the behavior of others, criminal behavior will thus begin or continue when it is seen in others with whom the delinquent strongly identifies or when the youth observes that others are rewarded by engaging in the criminal behavior(s). If an individual observes others reinforced for a crime (e.g., peer support or attention, monetary gains), then she or he develops positive attributions and beliefs regarding engaging in similar illegal acts (Akers, 1977). In this regard, a study by Elliot and Menard (1996) investigated the relationship between delinquent peer group association and delinquent behavior and found numerous results that support social learning theory, such as: (1) the onset of exposure to delinquent friends typically preceded the onset of a juvenile's own illegal behavior; (2) adolescents tend to gradually become involved with delinquent friends and gradually become involved in delinquent behavior in early to middle adolescence and become less involved with delinquent friends and engaging in delinquent behavior as the person enters young adulthood; and (3) there is some association with delinquent peers by youth before they begin engaging in minor delinquent acts. Other studies have also found support for social learning theory, with many focused on the influence that family members, friends, and gangs may have on the youth's behavior (Caputo, 2004; Winfree & Backstrom, 1994).

Labeling theory assumes that the initial delinquent act is caused by a number of factors, with the primary reason for repeat offending being the label "delinquent" appended becomes incorporated into the youth's cognition of himself or herself. This theory argues that the label alters the adolescent's self-image so that she or he construes herself or himself as a "delinquent" and, therefore, will act accordingly (Shoemaker, 2005). Labeling theory can be traced back to Lemert (1951), who focused on the impact of both formal and informal labeling on behavior. He identified formal labels as those which social agencies place on youth, and informal labels as those placed on youth by teachers, parents, friends, or peers (Adams, Robertson, Gray-Ray, & Ray, 2003). In this regard, Becker (1963) argued that peer social groups may also impact the affect of labeling, because many serve as social support systems for the youth in which their delinquent behaviors are accepted and supported.

Although many psychological theories tend to take into account the impact that a disability, particularly a mental health disability, may have on a youth's conduct, these theories typically focus on psychological variables or concepts that are internal to the individual. In addition, these theories appear to assume that a youth has responsibility over the acts in which he or she engages; a presumption that we indicated above in regard to classical theories has increasingly been questioned as a function of the findings from more contemporary research (Kolb & Winshaw, 2008). More specifically, these psychological theories do not take into consideration the increased presence of cognitive, developmental, educational, and/or mental health disabilities that have been found in juvenile offenders, which can subsequently have a negative effect on a juvenile's ability to engage in rational thinking and related decision-making. In addition, these theories do not account for the impact that a disability often has on a youth's social functioning which, in turn, may subsequently influence the youth's behavior choices and contribute to his or her negative social interactions.

Sociological Theories

Sociological theories posit that delinquent behavior is caused primarily by the environment. Personal and situational influences may be taken into consideration with these theories, but ultimately, it is assumed that delinquency is caused primarily by social factors in the environment (Shoemaker, 2005).

Social disorganization theory links social and demographic characteristics associated with those juveniles who commit crimes and is a frequently referenced social theory of crime. The theory proposes that juvenile delinquency is the result of a breakdown of institutional structures in the youth offender's environment (Lander, 1954). This theory hypothesizes that social disorganization in an area leads to a community's inability to maintain social order and exert informal social control. This disorganization, in turn, leads to the development of criminal values and traditions which replace conventional values and traditions, with the process then becoming a self-perpetuating revolving door (Bursik, 1988; Kornhauser, 1978). This theory argues that the disorganization occurs more readily in urban areas because of rapid industrialization and urbanization, and it is often used to understand social conditions associated with crime rates (Jacob, 2006). Shaw and McKay (1942, 1969) were the first to apply this theory to juvenile delinquency. They studied delinquency rates in Chicago and found that in addition to juvenile crime rates being substantially higher in the central city, areas with low rates of juvenile delinquency were characterized by "uniformity, conformity, and universality of conventional values and attitudes with respect to child care, conformity to laws, and related matters..." (Shaw & McKay, 1969, p. 88). Relative to other theories of delinquency, social disorganization theory has had a substantial amount of empirical research to support its claim that juvenile delinquency is greater in an unstructured social environment (Bernburg & Thorlindsson, 2007; Lowenkam, Cullen, & Pratt, 2003; Osgood & Anderson, 2004; Rice & Smith, 2002; Sampson & Groves, 1989; Veysey & Messner, 1999).

Anomie theory is similar to social disorganization theory; however, a primary difference between these two theories is that anomie generally refers to larger societal conditions than does social disorganization theory, and it refers mostly to the inconsistency between societal conditions and individual opportunities for growth, fulfillment, and productivity within a society (Shoemaker, 2005). Anomie theory's primary assumption in the etiology of juvenile delinquency is that youth who find themselves at an economic disadvantage are more motivated to engage in delinquent behaviors. The theory argues that if these individuals were allowed the same opportunities as others, they would not engage in delinquent behaviors. When these youth are not allowed these same opportunities, they become frustrated with society and engage in criminal activities or engage in crime acts out of economic necessity. Emile Durkheim first coined the term *anomie* in his work conducted in the late 1800s (Durkheim, 1893/1933). Although originally applied to labor and financial crises, this theory was applied to criminal behavior in Durkheim's later work (Durkheim, 1893/1933). Durkheim's work on anomie theory and its association with criminal behavior was continued by Merton (1957). He expanded on anomie, maintaining that it is a relatively permanent feature of society rather than one that only occurs during economic change. Merton suggested that criminal behavior results after one's inability to obtain his or her desired goal(s). More recently, this theory was expanded upon and is now generally referred to as strain theory (2006, Agnew, 1992; Agnew & White, 1992).

Strain theory posits that it is strains or stressors in the individual's environment that increase the likelihood of criminal behavior occurring. General strain theory is an extension of Durkheim's (1893/1933) and Merton's (1957) work on anomie work and states that individuals try to obtain certain goals as well as avoid painful situations. The attempt at avoiding painful situations may become frustrating for the individual and consequently produces strain (Agnew, 1992). Attempts to escape this strain may include criminal activities. Agnew described likely situations under which criminal behavior would occur in response to strain, including the strain (1) being severe or high in magnitude, (2) seen as unjust, (3) associated with low social control, and (4) creating some pressure or incentive for violent or criminal behavior (Agnew, 2007). Agnew explained the cycle of violence with this theory and has related it to the effect that victimization of adolescents can have on subsequent delinquency. Agnew (1992) noted in his theory that not all juveniles who experience strain become delinquents, arguing that there are constraints, such as values, goals, self-esteem, intelligence, interpersonal skills, social support, or societal values, which may support the individual. Therefore, delinquency is less likely to occur if the costs of the delinquent acts exceed the benefits. Although available research is limited and in many cases methodologically flawed, empirical evidence does exist to support a general strain theory of crime (Broidy, 2001; Froggio, 2007; Ostrowsky & Messner, 2005; Perez, Jennings, & Gover, 2008). In addition, while strain theory does not specifically mention the impact of disability on juvenile delinquency, it does attempt to account to some extent for individual differences that may impact a youth's participation in delinquent behavior, such as intelligence, social skills, or internalizing difficulties. However, similar to the comments made regarding classical and psychological theories, sociological theories do not appear to take into consideration more contemporary research findings regarding the presence of poor impulse control, emotional dysregulation, or cognitive immaturity common in many youth having a cognitive, developmental, educational, or mental health disability.

Control Theories

Control theories of criminal behavior assume that the motivation an individual has to commit a crime is similar to the motivation for all other behaviors. Similar to social learning theories, control theories assume that behavior is motivated by the pursuit of pleasure and the avoidance of pain. Control theories, therefore, seek to explain what drives the majority of society to refrain, in general, from engaging in criminal behavior. Types of control theory include social control and self-control theories.

Social control theory was developed by Hirschi (1969) and argues that when an individual's relationships with family, friends, and society are broken, they are more likely to engage in delinquent behavior. According to Hirschi, individuals abide by society's rules and values because they fear having bonds broken with other individuals in society. Once these are broken, the individual has less motivation to abide by society's laws and, consequently, is more likely to engage in criminal behavior.

Self-control theory assumes that the basis for the development of conforming behavior is the attachments that children form early in life with parents or other caregivers. This theory argues that it is these early attachments and bonds that aid in the tendency of the child to regulate his or her conduct by developing an ability to delay instant or near gratification and avoid long-term negative consequences (Gottfredson & Hirschi, 1990). Specifically, self-control theory is the ability to delay short-term personal gain for long-term personal rewards and interests, and it focuses on socialization as a primary means for an individual to develop self-control (Gottfredson, 2007). In regard to delinquency, this theory maintains that while many delinquent acts provide for immediate satisfaction and serve desires, they do so only at the risk of long-term goals. Therefore, those with lower levels of self-control are more likely to engage in delinquent behavior than those with higher levels of self-control (Gottfredson, 2007).

Unlike the theories discussed in previous sections, control theories do account for the impact of impulsivity and behavioral dysregulation that are often found in juvenile offenders having a disability, suggesting that youth having less self-control are more likely to engage in delinquent behavior. Control theories also appear to be able to explain why social difficulties may be related to delinquency, which is an important consideration when understanding the relationship between juvenile offending and disability. Although control theories do not directly discuss the interaction of disability and delinquency, they do provide researchers with a foundation for further exploring hypotheses focusing on the relationship between juvenile delinquency and disability.

Biological Theory

A *biological* approach to juvenile delinquency assumes that criminal behavior, whether it is genetically or biologically influenced, is caused by a mechanism internal to the individual (Hoge, 2001; Shoemaker, 2005). Classical biological theories assume that there is a biological basis within an individual that *causes* the criminal behavior, while more contemporary biological theories of crime maintain that the biological basis of an individual leaves one *predisposed* to commit a crime, implying that not all persons with a biological predisposition for crime will engage in illegal acts. Recently, researchers have identified certain physiological measures such as low resting heart rate, abnormalities or lesions in different areas of the brain, and slow EEG wave activity as being related to juvenile delinquency and antisocial behavior (e.g., Lorber, 2004; Ortiz & Raine, 2004; Patrick & Verona, 2007; Raine, 2002). Consequently, some researchers have posited that juvenile delinquency may be the result of hypoarousal, as these individuals have a need for sensation-seeking behavior (Eysenck, 1977; Raine, 2002).

A genetic theory of juvenile delinquency posits that delinquency is determined by factors passed biologically from the parent to child. The exploration for a genetic link associated with crime has existed for centuries, with early studies using a "family tree" method to explain the continuation of criminal behavior between generations of families (Fink, 1938; Shoemaker, 2005). A major criticism of this theory, however, is that it fails to account for any social learning that may be occurring. Twin studies are a commonly used method for supporting a biological link to criminal behavior. One of the earliest twin studies published was by Newman, Freeman, and Holzinger (1937). These researchers evaluated the concordance of juvenile delinquency in 42 pairs of identical twins and 25 pairs of fraternal twins. Results indicated that 93 % of identical twins were both adjudicated while only 20 % of fraternal twins were both adjudicated, strongly supporting a genetic link to criminal behavior. More recent studies have also supported the findings that identical twins exhibit higher rates of concordance on delinquency than fraternal twins (Reid, 1979; Vold & Bernard, 1986). A meta-analysis of twin and adoptee studies by Rhee and Waldman (2007) examined five studies focusing on criminal behavior and

14 studies focusing on aggression and concluded that there was a significant link between genetics and criminal behavior.

With regard to a neuropsychological basis to delinquency, research has consistently found that juvenile delinquents display a variety of neuropsychological deficits in the areas of verbal processing, executive functioning, and verbal memory (e.g., Linz, Hooper, Hynd, Isaac, & Gibson, 1990; Ross, Benning, & Adams, 2007; Teichner & Golden, 2000; Wolff, Waber, Bauermeister, Cohen, & Ferber, 1982). There are a variety of explanations regarding the etiology of the neuropsychological impairment, including natural brain abnormalities, illicit drug use by adolescents, or brain damage (Lewis, Shanock, Pincus, & Glaser, 1979; Millsaps, Azrin, & Mittenberg, 1994; Rosselli & Ardila, 1996).

Despite the evidence suggesting a biological and genetic link to juvenile crime, the majority of available research focuses on adults. Given that many youth offenders cease delinquent behavior as they enter into adulthood, generalization of available studies should be done with caution. Moreover, in regard to the nature versus nurture debate, some contemporary biological theories do acknowledge the contribution that the environment may also have (e.g., Burt, McGue, Krueger, & Iacono, 2007, Dodge & Pettit, 2003). Dodge and Pettit (2003), for example, argue for a biopsychosocial model of the development of conduct problems. This model suggests that youth with conduct problems have a biological disposition toward certain cognitive and emotional processes, as well as sociocultural factors that place them at risk for conduct problems. These risk factors are then exacerbated and exploited or mediated by life events and environmental risk factors.

From our perspective, biological theories of delinquency provide a more thorough explanation of the relationship between juvenile delinquency and disability than do the other theories discussed in this chapter. As research in the field progresses, we are increasingly becoming aware of the cognitive factors associated with many disabilities in children and adolescents and how these factors contribute to the behaviors manifested by these youth. Biological theories presume that there is a brain-behavior relationship and that neuropsychological variables, such as emotional and behavioral dysregulation, are associated with various types of cognitive, developmental, educational, and mental health disabilities. As we stated in regard to control theories, we believe that biologically based theories provide researchers with a foundation for further exploring hypotheses focusing on the relationship between juvenile delinquency and disability

Conclusion

As was discussed in Chap. 2, juvenile delinquents are a heterogeneous group, with a number of risk factors being identified as being related to delinquency. While there is some empirical support for many of the theories of juvenile delinquency described above, few, if any, are able to account for the complex behaviors observed in juvenile delinquents. In addition, some theories assume a degree of rational thinking or decision-making in these youth, which research findings have shown is actually a common impairment in many youth having a disability. These theories assume rational thinking, therefore, they do not appear to be applicable to those juvenile delinquents having a disability. Other theories, however, do appear to be more relevant to our understanding of the relationship between juvenile delinquency and disability, especially the control theories and the biological theories emphasizing a brain-behavior relationship. Moreover, the biopsychosocial model appears to address both the biological and social/environmental influences that may contribute to juvenile delinquency.

While no theory may explain the cause of juvenile delinquency, theoretical explanations are nevertheless important to consider, since they provide further scientific and professional discussion, as well as research hypotheses, on the possible factors that contribute to delinquency. An understanding of contributing risk factors is particularly important when trying to assess a youth offender's risk to reoffend, as well as when developing effective intervention programs for these youth. While these theories still cannot explain why, for example, many at-risk youth do not offend of help us identify those who will continue to engage in illegal activity through adulthood, they do provide professionals who work in this field with some direction regarding developing more effective intervention programs and better measures for identifying at-risk youth.

References

Adams, M. S., Robertson, C. T., Gray-Ray, P., & Ray, M. C. (2003). Labeling and delinquency. *Adolescence, 38*, 171–186.
Agnew, R. (1992). Foundation for a general strain theory of crime and delinquency. *Criminology, 30*, 47–87.
Agnew, R. (2006). *Pressured into crime: An overview of general strain theory*. Los Angeles, CA: Roxbury.
Agnew, R. (2007). Strain theory and violent behavior. In D. J. Flannery, A. T. Vazsonyi, & I. D. Waldman (Eds.), *The Cambridge handbook of violent behavior and aggression* (pp. 519–532). New York, NY: Cambridge University Press.
Agnew, R., & White, H. R. (1992). An empirical test of general strain theory. *Criminology, 30*, 475–499.
Akers, R. L. (1977). *Deviant behavior: A social learning approach* (2nd ed.). Belmont, MA: Wadsworth.
American Psychiatric Association. (2013). *Diagnostic and statistical manual of mental disorders* (4th ed.). Washington, DC: Author.
Bandura, A. (1977). *Social learning theory*. Englewood Cliffs, NJ: Prentice-Hall.
Beccaria, C. (1963). *On crimes and punishments* (H. Paolucci, Trans.). New York, NY: Bobbs-Merrill. (Original work published 1764).
Becker, H. (1963). *Outsiders: Studies in the sociology of deviance*. New York, NY: Free Press.
Bernburg, J. G., & Thorlindsson, T. (2007). Community structure and adolescent delinquency in Iceland: A contextual analysis. *Criminology, 45*, 415–444.
Borowski, A. (2003). Danger of strong causal reasoning in juvenile justice policy and practice. *Australian Social Work, 56*, 340–351.

References

Broidy, L. M. (2001). A test of general strain theory. *Criminology, 39*, 9–36.
Bursik, R. (1988). Social disorganization and theories of crime. *Criminology, 26*, 519–551.
Burt, S. A., McGue, M., Krueger, R. F., & Iacono, W. G. (2007). Environmental contributions to adolescent delinquency: A fresh look at the shared environment. *Journal of Abnormal Child Psychology, 35*, 787–800.
Caputo, R. K. (2004). The effects of parent religiosity, family processes, and peer influences on adolescent outcomes by race/ethnicity. *American Journal of Pastoral Counseling, 7*, 23–49.
Cornish, D. B., & Clarke, R. V. (1986). *The reasoning criminal*. New York, NY: Springer.
Curran, D. J., & Renzetti, C. M. (1994). *Theories of crime*. Needham Heights, MA: Allyn & Bacon.
Dodge, K. A., & Pettit, G. S. (2003). A biopsychosocial model of the development of chronic conduct problems in adolescence. *Developmental Psychology, 39*, 349–371.
Durkheim, E. (1933). *The division of labor in society* (G. Simpson, Trans.) London, England: The Free Press of Glenco. (Original work published 1893).
Elliot, D. S., & Menard, S. (1996). Delinquent friends and delinquent behavior: Temporal and developmental patterns. In J. D. Hawkins (Ed.), *Delinquency and crime: Current theories* (pp. 28–67). Cambridge, England: Cambridge University Press.
Eysenck, H. J. (1977). *The biological basis of personality*. Springfield, IL: Charles C. Thomas.
Fink, A. E. (1938). *Causes of Crime*. New York, NY: A.S. Barnes.
Freud, S. (1953). *The standard edition of the complete psychological works of Sigmund Freud* (J. Strachey, Trans.). London, England: The Hogarth Press. (Original work published 1900).
Froggio, G. (2007). Strain and juvenile delinquency: A critical review of Agnew's general strain theory. *Journal of Loss and Trauma, 12*, 383–418.
Gottfredson, M. R. (2007). Self-control theory and criminal violence. In D. J. Flannery, A. T. Vazsonyi, & I. D. Waldman (Eds.), *The Cambridge handbook of violent behavior and aggression* (p. 533). New York, NY: Cambridge University Press.
Gottfredson, M. R., & Hirschi, T. (1990). *A general theory of crime*. Palo Alto, CA: Stanford University Press.
Hirschi, T. (1969). *Causes of delinquency*. Berkley, CA: University of California Press.
Hoge, R. (2001). *The juvenile offender: Theory, research, and applications*. Norwell, MA: Kluwer Academic.
Jacob, J. C. (2006). Male and female youth crime in Canadian communities: Assessing the applicability of social disorganization theory. *Canadian Journal of Criminology and Criminal Justice, 48*, 31–60.
Kolb, B., & Winshaw, I. Q. (2008). *Fundamentals of human neuropsychology* (6th ed.). New York, NY: Macmillan.
Kornhauser, R. (1978). *Social sources of delinquency*. Chicago, IL: University of Chicago Press.
Lander, B. (1954). *Toward an understanding of juvenile delinquency*. New York, NY: Columbia University.
Lemert, E. M. (1951). *Social pathology*. New York, NY: McGraw-Hill.
Lewis, D. O., Shanock, S., Pincus, J., & Glaser, G. (1979). Violent juvenile delinquents: Psychiatric, neurological, psychological and abuse factors. *Journal of the American Academy of Child Psychiatry, 136*, 419–423.
Linz, T. D., Hooper, S. R., Hynd, G. W., Isaac, W., & Gibson, L. J. (1990). Frontal lobe functioning in conduct disordered juveniles: Preliminary findings. *Archives of Clinical Neuropsychology, 5*, 411–416.
Lorber, M. F. (2004). Psychophysiology of aggression, psychopathy, and conduct problems: A meta-analysis. *Psychological Bulletin, 130*, 531–552.
Lowenkam, C. T., Cullen, F. T., & Pratt, T. C. (2003). Replicating Sampson and Groves's test of social disorganization theory: Revisiting a criminological classic. *Journal of Research in Crime and Delinquency, 40*, 351–373.
Merton, R. K. (1957). *Social theory and social structure*. London, England: The Free Press of Glencoe.

Millsaps, C. L., Azrin, R. L., & Mittenberg, W. (1994). Neuropsychological effects of chronic cannabis use on the memory and intelligence of adolescents. *Journal of Child and Adolescent Substance Abuse, 3*, 47–55.

Newman, H. H., Freeman, F. N., & Holzinger, K. J. (1937). *Twins: A study of heredity and environment.* Chicago, IL: University of Chicago Press.

Onwudiwe, I. (2004). Theoretical perspectives on juvenile delinquency: Root causes and control. *Corrections Today, 66*, 153–156.

Ortiz, J., & Raine, A. (2004). Heart rate level and antisocial behavior in children and adolescents: A meta-analysis. *Journal of the American Academy of Child and Adolescent Psychiatry, 43*, 154–162.

Osgood, D. W., & Anderson, A. L. (2004). Unstructured socializing and rates of delinquency. *Criminology, 42*, 519–549.

Ostrowsky, M. K., & Messner, S. F. (2005). Explaining crime for a young adult population: An application of general strain theory. *Journal of Criminal Justice, 33*, 463–476.

Oxnam, P., & Vess, J. (2006). A personality-based typology of adolescent sexual offenders using the Millon Adolescent Clinical Inventory. *New Zealand Journal of Psychology, 35*, 36–44.

Paternoster, R. (1989). Decisions to participate in and resist from four types of common delinquency: Deterrence and the rational choice perspective. *Law and Society Review, 23*, 7–40.

Patrick, C. J., & Verona, E. (2007). The psychophysiology of aggression: Autonomic, electrocortical, and neuro-imaging findings. In D. J. Flannery, A. T. Vazsonyi, & I. D. Waldman (Eds.), *The Cambridge handbook of violent behavior and aggression* (pp. 111–150). New York, NY: Cambridge University Press.

Perez, D. M., Jennings, W. G., & Gover, A. R. (2008). Specifying general strain theory: An ethnically relevant approach. *Deviant Behavior, 29*, 544–578.

Raine, A. (2002). Biosocial studies of antisocial and violent behavior in children and adults: A review. *Journal of Abnormal Child Psychology, 30*, 311–326.

Reid, S. T. (1979). *Crime and criminology* (2nd ed.). New York, NY: Holt, Rinehart and Winston.

Rhee, S. H., & Waldman, I. D. (2007). Behavior-genetics of criminality and aggression. In D. J. Flannery, A. T. Vazsonyi, & I. D. Waldman (Eds.), *The Cambridge handbook of violent behavior and aggression* (pp. 77–90). New York, NY: Cambridge University Press.

Rice, K. J., & Smith, W. R. (2002). Sociological models of automotive theft: Integrating routine activity and social disorganization approaches. *Journal of Research in Crime and Delinquency, 39*, 304–336.

Ross, S. R., Benning, S. D., & Adams, Z. (2007). Symptoms of executive dysfunction are endemic to secondary psychopathy: An examination in criminal offenders and noninstitutionalized young adults. *Journal of Personality Disorders, 21*, 384–399.

Rosselli, M., & Ardila, A. (1996). Cognitive effects of cocaine and polydrug abuse. *Journal of Clinical and Experimental Neuropsychology, 18*, 122–135.

Sampson, R., & Groves, W. B. (1989). Community structure and crime: Testing social disorganization theories. *American Journal of Sociology, 94*, 774–802.

Shaw, C. R., & McKay, H. D. (1942). *Juvenile delinquency and urban areas.* Chicago, IL: University of Chicago Press.

Shaw, C. R., & McKay, H. D. (1969). *Juvenile delinquency and urban areas, Revised edition.* Chicago, IL: University of Chicago Press.

Shoemaker, D. (2005). *Theories of delinquency: An examination of explanations of delinquent behavior* (5th ed.). New York, NY: Oxford University Press.

Sorenson, E., & Johnson, E. (1996). Subtypes of incarcerated delinquents constructed via cluster analysis. *Journal of Child Psychology and Psychiatry, 37*, 293–303.

Taylor, J., Kemper, T. S., Loney, B. R., & Kistner, J. A. (2006). Classification of severe male juvenile offenders using the MACI clinical and personality scales. *Journal of Clinical Child and Adolescent Psychology, 35*, 90–102.

Teichner, G., & Golden, C. J. (2000). The relationship of neuropsychological impairment to conduct disorder in adolescence: A conceptual review. *Aggression and Violent Behavior, 5*, 509–528.

References

van Dam, C., De Bruyn, E. J., & Janssens, J. A. M. (2007). Personality, delinquency, and criminal recidivism. *Adolescence, 42*, 763–777.

Veysey, B. M., & Messner, S. F. (1999). Further testing of social disorganization theory: An elaboration of Sampson and Groves's 'community structure and crime.'. *Journal of Research in Crime and Delinquency, 36*, 156–175.

Vold, G., & Bernard, T. (1986). *Theoretical criminology*. New York, NY: Oxford University Press.

Winfree, T. L., & Backstrom, T. V. (1994). Social learning theory, self-reported delinquency, and youth gangs. *Youth and Society, 26*, 147–177.

Wolff, P. H., Waber, D., Bauermeister, C., Cohen, C., & Ferber, R. (1982). The neuropsychological status of adolescent delinquent boys. *Journal of Child Psychology and Psychiatry, 23*, 267–279.

Chapter 5
History of the Juvenile Justice System

As discussed briefly in Chapter 2, after reaching an all-time high in the late 1980s and early 1990s, juvenile crime rates have slowly declined over the past decade. In fact, there was a 32 % decrease in juvenile arrests from 1980 to 2011 according to the Office of Juvenile Justice and Delinquency Prevention (Puzzanchera, 2013). Despite this considerable decline, in 2011 there were still more than 1.5 million arrests of juveniles. In fact, despite the data showing that children and adolescents between 5 and 18 years of age comprise approximately 18 % of the national population, youth between the ages of 12 and 18 comprise 16 % of all arrests nationwide (Puzzanchera, 2013).

While most people refer to any individual who commits a crime as a "criminal," this label is *not* used for individuals under 18 years of age who commit offenses. Rather, the term "juvenile delinquent" is considered a more appropriate label as the legal system assumes that children and adolescents are not mature enough to be held responsible for a criminal act. In general, the term "juvenile delinquent" refers to a youth between 10 and 17 years of age who commits an illegal act (National Council on Disability, 2003; Shoemaker, 2005). There is, however, some lack of clarity in this definition across states in the United States, with many states having varying definitions of what constitutes delinquency and how certain juvenile offenses are accepted within the juvenile court system. For example, although individuals under age 18 are typically considered juveniles and treated accordingly, most states allow juveniles to be treated and prosecuted as adult offenders if they commit crimes such as murder or rape. This determination may be modified based on the youth's age at the time of the offense. In addition, across most states children below the age of 7 are usually exempt from being adjudicated as a juvenile delinquent as they are presumed to be incapable of criminal intent (Snyder & Sickmund, 2006).

In regard to the definition of an "illegal act," what is considered "illegal" for juveniles also varies across states. In addition, what is considered "illegal" for a juvenile may not be considered an "illegal act" if the same individual is above the age of 18. For example, the category of "status offense" is reserved for those offenses that are considered illegal merely because of an individual's age. Status offenses include actions such as running away from home, truancy, possession or

© Springer International Publishing Switzerland 2016
K.C. Thompson, R.J. Morris, *Juvenile Delinquency and Disability*, Advancing Responsible Adolescent Development, DOI 10.1007/978-3-319-29343-1_5

consumption of alcohol, and possession or consumption of tobacco products. Most of these latter offenses would not be considered a criminal or illegal act if the individual engaging in the action(s) was 18 years of age or older and, therefore, presumed to be of legal adult status. This variability in the definition of juvenile delinquency has led some writers to suggest that a delinquent criminal act is any action which violates a law or ordinance of the jurisdiction in which the action is performed (Hoge, 2001).

Development of the Juvenile Justice System

Before the inception of the juvenile justice system over a century ago, juvenile offenders were commonly referred to as "little adults" and punished accordingly. In the infancy of the United States, laws were heavily influenced by the common law of England, as it governed many of the American colonies. William Blackstone, who was a prominent English lawyer in the mid-1700s, wrote *Commentaries on the Laws of England* (Sprague, 1915), which was essentially a commentary on the laws of England and served as a guide for the founding fathers of the United States. Blackstone made reference to juvenile crime when discussing individuals who were incapable of committing crimes. For example, he described children under seven years of age as being incapable of committing crimes, as they were too young to fully understand their actions. Children below 7 were also presumed to be incapable of criminal intent and, consequently, were immune from the justice system. Blackstone described those between 7 and 10 years of age as being in an undefined, gray area of what was considered criminality, with society and the legal system wavering, in some cases, in the belief of whether a child of this age could have criminal intent as well as an understanding of the illegal act that was committed. On the other hand, according to Blackstone's commentaries, children above the age of 14 were considered to be capable of understanding the consequences of their actions and were often required to stand trial in a manner that was similar to adults. If found guilty, these children received punishments similar to those of adults—including imprisonment, harsh corporal punishment, or even death depending on the crime (Sprague, 1915).

Although Blackstone does not specifically address intellectual or mental health disabilities in "infancy"–the term he used for children and adolescents–he does indicate that those people having a "deficiency in will," such as in the case of an "idiot" or a "lunatic," should not be charged for their criminal acts if such crimes were directly related to what he terms their "incapacity" (Sprague, 1915). With respect to youth 7 years of age and older, Blackstone states, "…that the capacity of doing ill, or contracting guilt, is not so much measured by years and days as by the strength of the delinquent's understanding and judgment. For one lad of eleven years old may have as much cunning as another of fourteen…." (Sprague, 1915, p. 432). The deciding factor, therefore, whether a youth was guilty of a crime, especially a capital crime, often centered on whether the youth had intent. In this regard, Blackstone reports on children as young as 9 years of age being sentenced to death after the courts determined that their intent when they committed the criminal act was, in fact, to murder the victim. For example, Blackstone made reference to a 10-year-old boy being hung after he and another 9-year-old peer killed a friend and hid the body. It was determined that hiding the body indicated that the child had "conscious guilt" and hence was punished appropriately. Blackstone also described the case of a second 10-year-old boy who murdered his "bedfellow" and tried to cover up the incident. Blackstone acknowledged the young age of the boy but argued that providing impunity for the child's act could put the public in danger as it would set a precedent that children could freely commit such serious crimes without punishment (Sprague, 1915). The boy was determined to have had intent and an understanding of the implications of his actions, as evidenced by his attempt at covering up his misbehavior, and was sentenced to capital punishment.

These cases in England, as discussed by Blackstone, were also consistent with practices in the United States during the 1700s, with society viewing children, in many cases, as "little adults" and punishing them accordingly. Because few alternatives existed, children of all ages had the potential of being punished as adults by the courts and confined with adults in jails or prisons. Not surprisingly, given that little consideration was given to adult offenders with disabilities and the mitigating influence that a disability may have on a person's behavior, there was also little to no consideration given to juvenile offenders who had a disability. As the decades progressed through the 1700s and into the 1800s, society began to consider the notion that children were cognitively and developmentally different from adults. This developmental perspective led to various movements that encouraged the use of alternative methods of dealing with youth offenders. Such reform movements led to the establishment in the 1820s of the Society for the Reformation of Juvenile Delinquents, which was instrumental in successfully lobbying the New York State Assembly to pass legislation in 1824 to establish the New York House of Refuge. The resulting correctional institution or "reformatory" opened on January 1, 1825 and was the first correctional institution for youth in the United States. Within a few years, other "reform schools" were built in various states and became a popular way of disciplining and treating juveniles (Picket, 1969).

Therapeutic programs were also implemented in the early 1800s. One example was the cottage system, which served to make reform schools and institutions more like family units through the creation of small cottage-type buildings. A system referred to as "placing out" was also used, in which children from high poverty urban areas who engaged in delinquent behavior were placed with rural families to work and learn with a different family. The utilization of facilities such as the House of Refuge was a forward movement in working with delinquents in that society began understanding that juveniles needed to be treated differently than adults; however, these institution-like facilities also began facing many of the same difficulties that were prevalent within adult prisons or institutions, including deteriorating conditions, overcrowding, and abuse (Pickett, 1969; Zimring, 2005). Practices such as "placing out" appear to have relied on theoretical positions regarding delinquency in which a change in environment for youth was believed to be capable of changing their behavior, with such beliefs excluding the contribution that biological influences, such as a developmental disability, might have on committing delinquent acts.

The reform movements of the 1800s contributed to changes in public policy and practices in regard to youth offenders, as well as to increased public interest in the fact that delinquent youth needed a different punishment system for their crimes compared to adult offenders. As a result, in 1899 the first juvenile court was established in the United States in Chicago (Cook County), Illinois. This, in turn, led to a new stance on the part of society regarding the punishment of youth committing illegal acts. This new stance focused on *protecting and rehabilitating* youth within the juvenile justice system versus the previous punitive approach (Zimring, 2005). By 1925, nearly all states had established some type of juvenile court system, with the primary focus of this court being the rehabilitation of youth who had engaged in delinquent behavior. Julian Mack (1909), one of the first judges to preside over Cook County Juvenile Court, described juvenile courts in the following manner:

> The child who must be brought into court should, of course, be made to know that he is face to face with the power of the state, but he should at the same time, and more emphatically, be made to feel that he is the object of its care and solicitude. The ordinary trappings of the courtroom are out of place in such hearings. The judge on a bench, looking down upon the boy standing at the bar, can never evoke a proper sympathetic spirit. Seated at a desk, with the child at his side, where he can on occasion put his arm around the shoulder and draw the lad to him, the judge, while losing none of his judicial dignity, will gain immensely in the effectiveness of his work. (p. 120)

Relevant Case Law and Statutes

In addition to having the authority to decide on alternative interventions for juveniles rather than relying only on punishments traditionally used with adults, early juvenile courts operated under the concept of *parens patriae* (*Prince v Massachusetts*, 1944). *Parens patriae* gave states the responsibility of protecting and supervising children whose legal guardians were not providing the appropriate level of supervision, consequently allowing courts to supervise juvenile offenders. Both this and dispositional flexibility were large contributing factors toward the development of a rehabilitative model for the juvenile justice system. However, a number of legal decisions, cases, and laws have also contributed to advancing the rehabilitative model as a procedure for addressing juvenile offenders. These have helped ensure that the courts had flexibility in dealing with the juveniles while, at the same time, making sure that juveniles have many of the same constitutional rights as those granted to adult offenders (Snyder & Sickmund, 1999). For example, in the early phases of the juvenile justice system, juveniles were not provided with due process rights; however, due process rights were guaranteed by a US Supreme Court decision, *In re Gault* (1967). As a result, juveniles were provided the right to legal counsel, the right against self-incrimination, the right to timely notification of the charges, and the right to confront witnesses. *In re Gault* (1967) involved a 15-year-old boy, Gerald Francis Gault, who was accused of making an indecent phone call to his neighbor while the boy was on probation for theft. Police apprehended the juvenile from his home, giving no notice to parents, and before the hearings neither the juvenile nor his parents received any notice of the specific charges against him. At the hearing, there was no record of the proceedings, and no witnesses (including the neighbor who made the complaint) were present. Because of a variety of extenuating circumstances in the child's background, the judge in the case sentenced the juvenile to Arizona's State Industrial School until he was 21 years old, despite the fact that an adult accused of using vulgar language toward a neighbor would have likely received a maximum penalty of a $50 fine and imprisonment for no more than 2 months.

In 1968, the *Juvenile Delinquency Prevention and Control Act* was passed. This act indicated that children charged with status offenses (i.e., those offenses deemed illegal only because of the child's age, such as running away) be handled outside of the court system. Subsequently, this limited the level of court involvement for juveniles who were committing relatively minor delinquent acts. In 1974, the US Congress passed the *Juvenile Justice and Delinquency Prevention (JJDP) Act*, which set additional standards for the manner in which state and local juvenile justice systems can deal with youth offenders. Specifically, this act consisted of four core protections for juveniles, including the following: (1) deinstitutionalization of status offenders, which specified that juveniles charged with status offenses should not be placed in detention or other secure facilities; (2) juveniles found delinquent should not be placed in a secure settings with adult offenders; (3) juveniles should not be detained in adult jails (though there were several exceptions to this); and (4) states must work to reduce disproportionate confinement of minority youth.

There have also been several US Supreme Court decisions that have contributed to the protection of the rights of juveniles who are arrested. These include, but are not limited to, the following major decisions:

- *Kent v. United States* (1966)—The 1960s were witness to several cases before the Supreme Court that drastically changed juvenile court proceedings. The case of *Kent v. United States* examined the complex interaction of *parens patriae* and due process. The case essentially decided that delinquents have a right to a formal hearing before having their cases transferred to adult criminal court, and the formal hearing must meet the provisions of due process and fair treatment. In this case, Morris A. Kent, Jr., first began having interaction with the legal system at age 14 after a series of thefts, which included breaking into houses. At age 16 he was charged with rape and robbery after his fingerprints were found in the apartment of a woman who had been robbed and raped. He confessed to this charge, as well as admitted to several similar acts. A psychiatric evaluation was conducted, at which time it was concluded that the youth suffered from "severe psychopathology," and it was recommended that he receive inpatient psychiatric care. Given the serious nature of the crime and charges of the crime, Kent's case was to be transferred to criminal court, where he would be tried as an adult. His lawyer, however, filed a motion for the youth to remain in juvenile court, including the argument that if he received proper psychiatric care, he may be able to be rehabilitated. Despite this, the court did not conduct a full investigative hearing. The court instead entered an order stating that the investigation had been made, with no verbal or written explanation of what was found, and the case was transferred to adult criminal court. Kent was subsequently found guilty and sentenced to 30–90 years in prison. His lawyer filed an appeal that the waiver to adult court was invalid as a full investigation had not, in fact, been made and the juvenile's constitutional rights were violated merely because of his status as a minor. The case ultimately went to the US Supreme Court, at which time the waiver to adult court was deemed invalid. A key point in this case was that while it serves to protect them in many capacities, juveniles may be provided less due process because of *parens patriae*. Due process is essentially the right for every person involved in a legal proceeding to have certain safeguards to ensure that the legal proceeding is fair and impartial. *Parens patriae* is supposed to ensure that the court's primary concern is the juvenile's best interest, but this case showed that it could also put juveniles in a position where their loss of constitutional rights may actually put them in a worse position, such as being transferred to a different jurisdiction (i.e., adult court) without the same due process (e.g., hearing) that would typically be granted to adults.

- *In re Winship* (1970)—This case established that juvenile courts must operate on the same standards of adult courts, particularly within the context of a "reasonable doubt" standard. In this case, a 12-year-old boy, Samuel Winship, was charged with stealing $112 from a woman's purse in a store. A store employee claimed to have seen the boy running from the scene, with other employees stating that the store employee was not in a position to have seen the act. The boy was adjudicated and sent to a training school. The New York courts argued that they were not required to operate similarly to the standards of adult court and could rely on a preponderance of evidence to determine guilt, which is a lower standard of burden of proof than is required for adult criminal cases. The boy's family appealed, and the case eventually reached the Supreme Court which decided that juvenile courts must hold to the stricter "beyond a reasonable doubt" burden of proof (used in adult criminal cases) than the lower "preponderance of the evidence" standard (which is commonly used in adult civil cases), as not doing so is a violation of the Fourteenth Amendment. Consequently, the court found that when establishing guilt for criminal charges, the reasonable doubt standard must be applied to both adult and juveniles alike, as both juveniles and adults alike faced the possible loss of liberty if sentenced.
- *Breed v. Jones* (1975)—This case mandated that a waiver of a juvenile to criminal court following adjudication in juvenile court constitutes double jeopardy. In this case, a 17-year-old, Gary Steven Jones, was charged with armed robbery in juvenile court and adjudicated. At the disposition, the judge waived jurisdiction to adult court. The youth's counsel argued that doing so violated the double jeopardy clause, which the court denied, saying that an adjudication hearing is not a trial. The US Supreme Court ruled that adjudication in juvenile court, which stipulates that a juvenile was found to have committed a crime, is equivalent to a

trial in adult court and, therefore, waiving jurisdiction to adult court was placing the youth in double jeopardy.
- *Eddings v. Oklahoma* (1982) — It was ruled here that a defendant's youthful age should be considered a mitigating factor in deciding whether to apply the death penalty. In this case, a 16-year-old male, Monty Lee Eddings, was transferred to adult court and charged with first-degree murder. He was found guilty under Oklahoma statutes and found eligible for the death penalty; however, the Supreme Court decision ruled that age should be a mitigating factor when deciding whether an individual should be put to death, and the youth's death sentence was reversed.
- *Schall v. Martin* (1984) — In *Schall v. Martin*, it was decided that pretrial juveniles who pose a serious risk of committing another crime may be detained until their trial. In this case, a 14-year-old boy, Gregory Martin, was charged with robbery, assault, and possession of a weapon. Before his adjudication hearing, the juvenile was held in detention as the court found that he posed a serious risk of committing another crime. His lawyer challenged this, to no avail. The case was heard by the US Supreme Court, which decided that pretrial detention is allowed as it protects both the juvenile and society from pretrial crime, and it is not intended to punish the juvenile.
- *Thompson v. Oklahoma* (1988) — It was ruled here that imposing the death penalty on an individual who was 15 years old at the time of the offense violated the Eighth Amendment, which protects against cruel and unusual punishment. In this case, a 15-year-old, William Wayne Thompson, along with three other adult males, kidnapped and beat a man to death. The man, who was married to the juvenile's sister and was alleged to have engaged in domestic violence, was found in a river, his body gashed and bruised, with gunshot wounds. All men involved in the crime were arrested. Thompson went through a psychiatric evaluation and was found eligible to stand trial as an adult and was subsequently sentenced to death by a jury trial. An appeal was filed with the Supreme Court under the notion that executing a juvenile violated the Eighth Amendment's prohibition of cruel and unusual punishment.
- *Roper v. Simmons* (2005) — This case held that juveniles could not be sentenced to death for crimes they committed before they reached 18 years old. In this case, a 17-year-old, Christopher Simmons, admitted that he and another individual had premeditated a murder and broken into a woman's home, bound her hands, and threw her off a bridge. The juvenile was found guilty in a jury trial and sentenced to death. His lawyers appealed and the US Supreme Court ultimately heard the case. The court cited evidence from cognitive neuroscience, developmental psychology, and social science fields that adolescents' brains are not fully developed, which affects cognitive abilities such as self-control and the ability to take responsibility for their actions. Specifically, the court acknowledged that juveniles have a lesser capacity for mature judgment than adults, are more vulnerable to negative external influences, and are more likely to be reformed than adults. In addition, the court held that there is a consensus in society that juveniles lack culpability for their crimes, and hence execution of crimes committed by individuals under 18 would be cruel and unusual punishment, a violation of the Eighth Amendment.

- *Graham v. Florida* (2010) — This case found that juvenile delinquents cannot be sentenced to life imprisonment without parole for non-homicide offenses. A 16-year-old, Terrance Jamar Graham, had been arrested for armed robbery and pled guilty to the first-degree felony, a crime that is punishable by life. Six months later, while still on probation, he was again arrested for robbery. He did not admit guilt to this latter offense, but he did acknowledge he was in violation of his plea agreement from his previous felony. Subsequently, he was sentenced to life in prison. Because Florida abolished parole, it essentially became a life sentence at the age of 16, without the possibility of parole. The US Supreme Court decided that this was a violation of the Eighth Amendment prohibiting cruel and unusual punishment.
- *Miller v. Alabama* (2012) — It was determined here that proportionality, or the idea that the punishment must be appropriate to the crime committed, must take into account juvenile status. In this case, two youth committed crimes that had mandatory minimum sentencing, which disallowed the judges from considering other factors, such as the youths' age, that could make the sentence disproportionate to the crime. Consequently, the court ruled that the mandatory life sentence without parole was a violation of the Eighth Amendment and purported that judges must take a defendant's age into consideration when determining sentencing for a crime.

Many of these court decisions have served to protect the rights of juveniles. As will be discussed in Chap. 6, there have also been other decisions and laws over the years that have further contributed to protecting the rights of juveniles with disabilities. While these court decisions and related laws have served to protect the rights of juveniles, they have also contributed to having juvenile courts function in a manner that is similar to the adult criminal court, with formal hearings and decisions. Specifically, although the juvenile justice system was created as a way to encourage a more informal, rehabilitative model of dealing with youth engaging in illegal acts, it has become more formal over time as it begins to mirror the adult justice system.

In addition, in response to rising rates of juvenile delinquency in the 1980s and 1990s, the juvenile court system has become increasingly more punitive, with many states making it easier for a juvenile to be prosecuted and treated as an adult offender (Snyder & Sickmund, 1999). A movement toward a more punitive approach within the juvenile court system emerged in 1984 through the National Advisory Committee for Juvenile Justice and Delinquency Prevention, which began encouraging state legislators to pass laws that allowed more juvenile delinquents to be transferred to adult court (Sacks & Reader, 1992). This movement led several states across the country to automatically charge juveniles as adults when they committed certain violent crimes that involved, for example, the use of deadly weapons or engaging in violent offenses against persons (Heilbrun, Leheny, Thomas, & Huneycutt, 1997). Other changes in the 1990s included giving states expanded sentencing options for juveniles, removing confidentiality provisions for juvenile courts, making proceedings more open to the public, and promoting victims' rights (Snyder & Sickmund, 1999).

Processing of Youth and Adults Within the Justice System

Although the similarities between the adult and juvenile justice systems are increasing, there are differences between the two systems. The discussion below describes, in general, the processing of youth in the juvenile justice system (see Fig. 5.1) versus the processing of adults through the criminal justice system (see Fig. 5.2).

Processing of a Youth Within the Juvenile Justice System

1. Upon arrest, an initial decision is made by the police as to whether to pursue the matter further within the juvenile court system or to divert the case to an alternative program.
2. If the case is referred to the juvenile court, there are a variety of options. For example, many cases are dismissed or may be handled through a "consent decree" specifying certain conditions the juvenile must follow, such as drug counseling, curfew, or victim restitution. Juveniles may also be offered an informal disposition of their case—referred to as "diversion"—if the offense is relatively minor and nonviolent (such as driving without a license) and the youth agrees to plead guilty. Such a disposition might include the youth completing a specified number of hours of community service and having his or her diversion requirements monitored by a probation officer. This type of diversion program allows a case to be handled without the juvenile incurring formal charges. However, if the juvenile fails to comply with the consent decree or informal disposition or if it is decided that the case should be handled formally in juvenile court, an adjudicatory hearing may be requested (Snyder & Sickmund, 2006).
3. At a formal hearing, the decision as to whether to adjudicate the juvenile—that is, determine that the youth is guilty of the charges filed against him/her—will be made by a judge.
4. If the juvenile is adjudicated—found guilty—at the formal hearing, a variety of options are available as to consequences and placement. For example, the youth may be allowed to continue living with his or her family, while being placed on probation. Probation requirements typically entail following up with the youth probation officer weekly as well as complying with other provisions such as curfew, community services, random drug testing, and/or counseling. The judge could also order the juvenile to be on intensive probation or house arrest, which requires daily check-ins with a probation officer and a very rigid, structured schedule with little free time. If it is decided that circumstances at home are not adequate and/or the juvenile presents a more serious risk to the community and needs more intensive supervision, the judge could also order out-of-home placement, such as in a group home, inpatient residential setting, inpatient substance abuse setting, or more secure, environment such as a youth boot camp. The juvenile may also be sentenced to a state department's juvenile

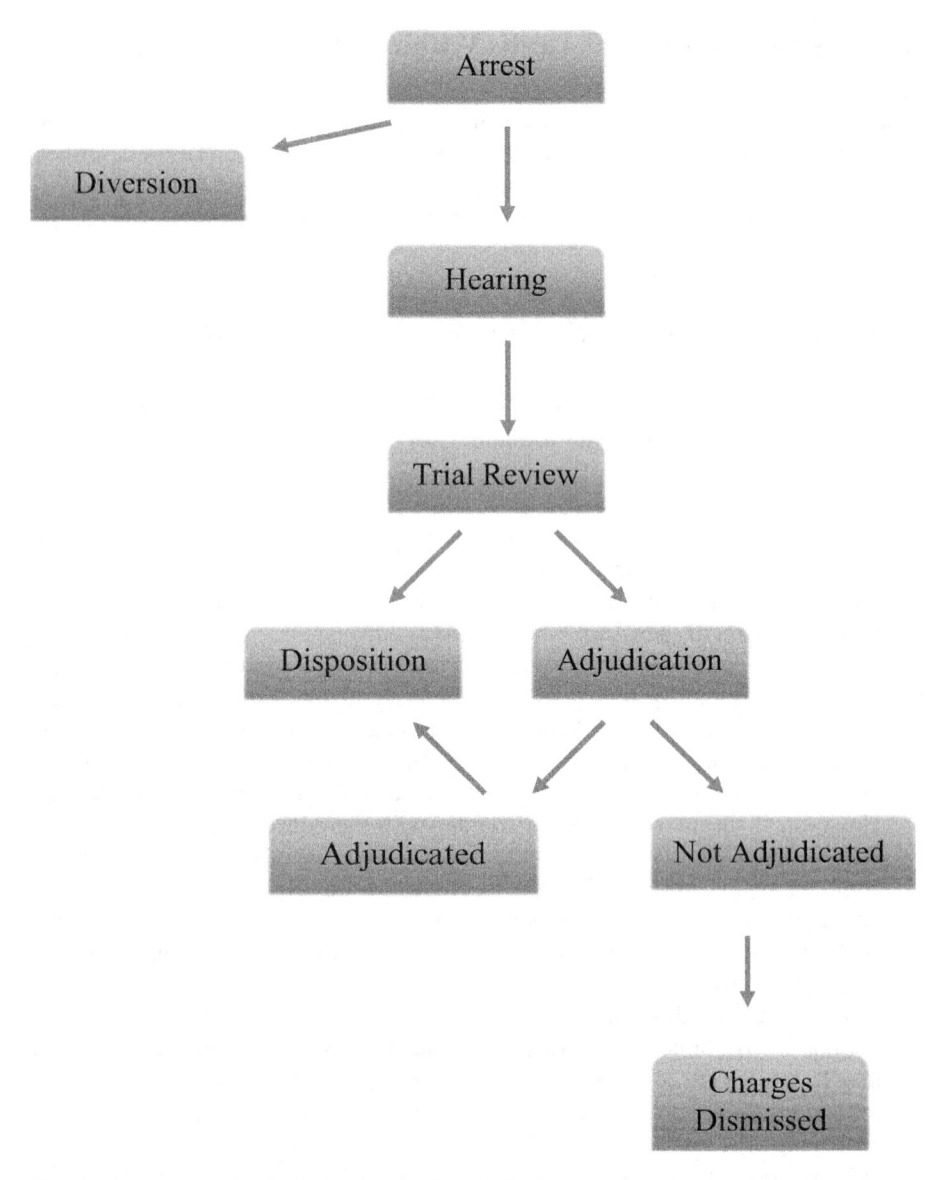

Fig. 5.1 Processing of a youth through the juvenile justice system

corrections residential facility (Snyder & Sickmund, 2006) should the judge warrant it necessary. It is also not uncommon for juveniles to remain detained between the trial/adjudication hearings and the placement hearing.

A variety of factors are typically considered prior to determining whether a formal adjudication hearing will take place or whether the juvenile will be allowed an informal resolution. Often, law enforcement officials make the decision to refer juveniles to the juvenile justice system only after speaking with the victim, the juvenile, and the youth's guardians and after reviewing the juvenile's offense history. Other factors that may impact the referral determination include whether the prosecutor determines there is sufficient evidence to support the allegation against the juvenile, the type of offense committed by the juvenile, and the juvenile's adjudication history (Snyder & Sickmund, 2006).

Processing of an Adult Within the Criminal Justice System

The adult criminal justice system is described in general below (Bureau of Justice Statistics, 2015). As can be seen, there are many similarities between the juvenile and adult judicial systems:

1. Initial police contact—an individual is arrested or a citation is issued to appear in court at a specific time.
2. The prosecutor considers the evidence and decides whether to file written charges or release the accused without prosecution.
3. If formal charges are filed, a court hearing occurs, and the judge decides whether there is enough evidence to hold the accused individual in jail or release the individual.
4. Either a grand jury or preliminary hearing occurs. In many states in the United States, an accused has a right to have the case heard by a grand jury, which decides whether there is enough evidence to indict the individual of the crime. Otherwise, the judge hears evidence to determine if the individual will be formally indicted.
5. An arraignment hearing occurs in which the individual can plead guilty, not guilty, or no contest. If the individual pleads guilty or no contest, then no trial is held.
6. Adjudication occurs either through a plea agreement between the defense and prosecuting attorneys with the endorsement of the trial judge or through a judicial court trial.
7. If the individual is found guilty, the judge typically determines sentencing, which can include restitution, fines, probation, jail, prison, or the death penalty. It should be noted that while a judge determines sentencing in most cases, in many states a jury is used to determine if the death sentence will be issued.

Diversion may also be a pretrial option for some adults who have little or no arrest history and are accused of a relatively minor offense, with diversion programs often involving nonpunitive measures such as mental health services, vocational training, or community service. Diversion for adults is more commonly used for substance use or first-time domestic violence offenses.

In general, the primary difference between juvenile justice and adult justice court processing of cases is the fact that juveniles are *not* prosecuted for committing

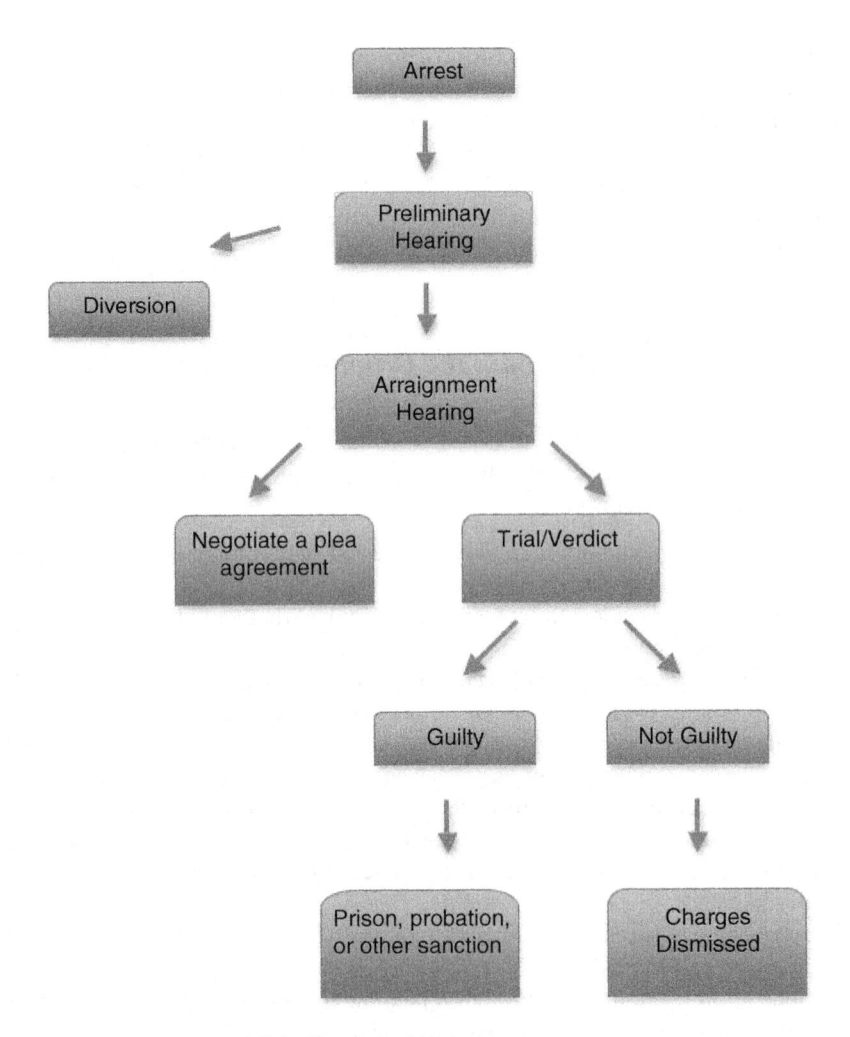

Fig. 5.2 Processing of an adult in the criminal justice system

crimes, but, rather, they are prosecuted for committing juvenile acts. Juvenile court hearings, therefore, are often more informal than adult court hearings, and juveniles do not have a public trial by jury, but rather the trial involves a judge hearing evidence and making the decision whether the youth is adjudicated (guilty) or non-adjudicated (not guilty). Moreover, in the case where the juvenile has been adjudicated and/or found guilty, the sentencing decisions are based on a variety of factors. These include issues unique to the youth and/or the youth's family or environment, offense severity, and the youth's offense history. In contrast, sentencing for adults is typically based on the offense severity, offense history, and/or cognitive and psychological functioning (Bureau of Justice Statistics, 2015).

There are also many similarities between juvenile and adult courts, including the right to an attorney, the right to confront witnesses, the privilege against self-incrimination, the right to notice of charges, and the need for the state prosecution to prove beyond a reasonable doubt that the individual is guilty. In addition, although juveniles do not have a parole system like adults, upon release from an out-of-home placement, the juvenile is typically required to complete some type of aftercare or probation program. If the juvenile does not follow the conditions, he or she may be committed to a facility once again. This process, while semantically different, is similar to adult parole. Beyond the court proceedings, there are other differences between juvenile and adult courts. For example, although most states allow the names of juveniles to be released to the media or public, this is done less commonly than in adult trials and typically requires a court order or is allowed only in cases involving certain crimes.

As previously mentioned, all states have provisions that allow juveniles to be transferred to adult courts. This phenomenon has actually been in existence since the early 1900s in some states. Criteria considered when determining transfer to adult court differ among states, but they typically include offense severity, offense type, offense history, and/or the age of the juvenile offender. For example, while Alabama allows a waiver to adult court for any juvenile over the age of 14, Arizona only allows juveniles to be waived to adult court if they are charged with a felony offense. New Jersey, on the other hand, allows any juvenile over the age of 14 who has prior adjudications for specific offenses to be waived to adult court, regardless of the most current offense. Interestingly, many states also require that juveniles who have been tried as an adult for one case must subsequently always be tried in adult court, regardless of the severity of the subsequent offenses.

Impact of Having a Disability in the Processing of Youth Within the Juvenile Justice System

Aside from overt implications such as financial considerations, staffing issues, and other logistical considerations of working with juveniles with disabilities, there are a variety of areas in which a disability may impact a youth offender's processing and interaction within the juvenile justice system. As will be discussed in later chapters, a disability can have negative implications as early as the initial point of police contact. Many disabilities are concurrent with social difficulties, impulsivity, or emotional reactivity, which may lead to misbehavior and poor communication with police officers and the potential for additional charges if, for example, a youth becomes argumentative, combative, or uncooperative at the time of arrest. Similarly, upon being detained these issues may persist and result in negative interactions with other detained youth, detention staff, court personnel, or even a juvenile court judge. Moreover, the presence of these latter behaviors will not reflect well on a youth in a court setting when a judge is using past and current behaviors when deciding placement, punitive actions, and treatment considerations. In regard to treatment, issues related to a disability could also contribute to a juvenile having difficulties successfully participating in, completing, or benefiting from many common treatment modalities. For example, a youth with an intellectual disability is likely to have considerable difficulty understanding and participating in a cognitively based individual or group therapy program. It may appear that this particular youth is uninterested in changing his or her behaviors or addressing his or her thoughts and feelings when, in fact, he or she does not have the ability to fully access and benefit from the treatment being provided.

As is discussed below, the presence of a disability can also have significant implications on how the courts determine the level of risk a juvenile presents to the community, as well as his or her competency to stand trial.

Risk Assessment

A common part of the processing of a youth within the juvenile justice system is the identification of the immediate and long-term level of risk the youth poses to the community. Courts typically want an estimate of the youth's level of risk if he or she is placed back into the community, and they also want a measure of risk of future offending when deciding consequences or placement after a youth commits an illegal act. Most court systems have formalized risk assessment instruments and processes that attempt to assess risk in an objective manner. These instruments attempt to classify delinquents' likelihood of reoffending by examining the presence of various risk factors associated with delinquency, such as age of first offense, number and types of offenses, family problems, substance use, and school achievement (e.g., Hoge, 2002; Schwalbe, 2007), and the results can have substantial weight in the determination of which sanctions or placements are mandated for a youth offender (e.g., standard probation, intensive probation, detention, long-term correctional facility).

There are two main approaches used when determining one's level of risk, including the actuarial approach and the structured professional judgment approach. *Actuarial assessment* relies primarily on statistical calculations of which risk factors are present, and a formula determines if a particular youth is at a low, moderate, or high risk to reoffend. *Structured professional judgment* approaches, on the other hand, allow a rater to consider risk factors on a case-by-case basis and then render a professional opinion on the level of risk a youth presents (Vincent, Guy, & Grisso, 2012). Professionals differ in their respective beliefs regarding which risk assessment method is most appropriate, with some advocating for a statistical-only model (Grove & Meehl, 1996; Quinsey, Harris, Rice, & Cormier, 2006), while others emphasize the importance of professional clinical judgment and individualization and still others advocating for a combined approach (e.g., Olver, Stockdale, & Wormith, 2009; Vincent et al., 2012).

While risk assessment instruments may be useful in helping court personnel more strategically classify the risk posed by a particular juvenile offender, studies examining the predictive validity of these assessments are sparse. In addition, the impact that cognitive, developmental, mental health, and/or learning disabilities may have on a juvenile offender's real or perceived risk is relatively unknown and often not taken into consideration. This leaves for the possibility that many symptoms or behaviors related to a disability may be misperceived as being related to antisocial thinking or other serious risk factors. For example, *risk of dangerousness* is typically assessed. This is usually based on variables such as the youth's history and potential for violent or aggressive acts, the presence of psychopathic features (e.g., lacking remorse or empathy, being manipulative or overly egocentric), and the extent of planned and criminally associated acts in which the youth has participated. Youth with social communication disorders (e.g., autism spectrum disorder), those with impulse control disorders (e.g., intermittent explosive disorder or ADHD), or even some with mood disorders (e.g., bipolar disorder) may appear as lacking empathy and being highly aggressive when, in fact, these latter behaviors are related to symptoms of their particular mental health disorders. Risk assessments also typically assess for features of *sophistication and maturity* in thinking and juvenile offending, as well as *treatment amenability*, with those responding to treatment typically appearing to be at a lower risk.

Competency

Another component in the processing of a youth through the juvenile justice system involves "competency," which could be significantly affected by the presence of a disability in the youth. The legal definition of competency was established as a result of a decision in *Dusky v. United States* (1960). In this case, a 33-year-old man with schizophrenia had been found guilty for assisting in a kidnapping and rape. It was argued that despite being found competent to stand trial through the use of a brief mental status exam, he was experiencing active symptoms of schizophrenia at the time of the trial and, therefore, was not able to fully understand the charges against him or actively participate in his defense during the trial. This was a landmark case in that the US Supreme Court affirmed that the defendant did have a right to a competency evaluation before trial (rather than the brief mental status exam). Competency was described in *Dusky* as meaning that the defendant had "…sufficient present ability to consult with his lawyer with a reasonable degree of rational understanding…" and "…a rational as well as factual understanding of proceedings against him" (*Dusky v. United States*, 1960, p. 402). Competence to stand trial does not suggest that an individual is or is not responsible for their delinquent behavior or criminal behavior; rather, it serves to ensure that a disability does not impair an offender's ability to defend him- or herself (Grisso, 2005).

While the decision made in *Dusky v. United States* did not directly involve juvenile delinquents, the case did set the precedent for assessing juvenile competence. Early in the juvenile justice system, *competency to stand trial* was not a consideration, as the courts were viewed as a governing body whose purpose was to act in the best interest of the child (*parens patriae*), and, therefore, formal hearings were unnecessary. As the juvenile justice system has continued to evolve, the concept of juvenile competency has become increasingly important in regard to delineating the juvenile court system from the adult criminal court system.

While each state is allowed to determine its specific requirements for competency, in general the concept of juvenile competence is similar to that for adult offenders and consistent across the states. Being competent purports that a juvenile has both a *reasonable degree of understanding of the court process* and an *ability to sufficiently participate in the trial*. Although a competency evaluation does not objectively measure cognitive abilities, determining competency essentially relies on determining whether a youth has the cognitive capacity to understand and reason, which are higher-level thinking abilities. The immaturity displayed by many youth alone may be sufficient to restrict their ability to demonstrate competence (e.g., Grisso, 1998; Grisso & Quinlan, 2005; Warren, Aaron, Ryan, Chauhan, & DuVal 2003), but the higher-level thinking, language, and social skills needed to be competent may also be negatively impacted by the presence of certain disabilities. This may be relatively obvious for youth having a particular disability such as an intellectual disability in which thinking is directly impaired, but the level of thinking and social skills needed regarding competency may be more covert or obscured in youth having, for example, mental health disorders. Consideration, therefore, needs to be given to all youth having a mental health, educational, developmental, or cognitive disability in terms of their competence, particularly for high-stress cases (Grisso, 1998).

Finally, those not found competent are typically considered for a *remediation program* to "restore" competency. Remediation programs are individual or small group programs that help educate individuals on the court system and their role in the judicial process. Determining whether competency can be restored for juvenile delinquents with disabilities includes consideration of several factors, such as whether an intervention is actually available that could improve the youth's deficit in functioning, what the likelihood is that change could occur, and the amount of time likely to be required for change and competency to occur (Grisso, 1998). In general, the type and severity of the disability will be important considerations as some disabilities have a more significant impact on functioning than others (e.g., bipolar disorder versus mild depression), others may be more long term (e.g., schizophrenia), and others may be difficult to treat or relatively "incurable" (e.g., intellectual or other developmental disabilities).

Conclusion

As is evident by the history presented, the way that society deals with juvenile offenders has wavered over time. In colonial times, society treated child and adolescent offenders similar to how they treated adult offenders, namely, within the context of a punishment-oriented system that placed children as young as 10 years of age in prison if it could be determined that the youth had willful intent to commit and an understanding of the crime committed. The creation of a separate juvenile justice system led to a more rehabilitative approach that took into consideration a child or adolescent's moral, intellectual, social, and emotional development. Over the past 30–40 years, however, the juvenile justice system has begun to mirror the adult system, both in terms of court processes, rights provided, and consequences subsumed.

While early movements focused on rational and moral understanding of the differences between children and adult thinking, more recently the contributions of psychological science and neuroscience have helped society better understand the biological and functional differences between the brains of children and adolescents to that of adults and how the undeveloped brain impacts cognitive and emotional functioning, including facets such as reasoning, planning, judgment, and impulse control. This science has slowly been playing a role in legal cases, providing support for the need for juveniles to be treated differently than adults. Scientific research has also helped society become more aware of other factors, independent of age, which can have an impact on brain development and an individual's functioning. While this area of science is relatively young in the volume of research that has been published, emerging evidence does suggest that developmental, learning, and mental health disabilities can significantly impact functioning and one's ability to reason, plan, and judge. This increase in scientific knowledge purports that a better understanding of these implications will be important to continue ensuring that juveniles are treated appropriately and effectively within the juvenile justice system, particularly given the high prevalence of disabilities among the juvenile delinquency population.

References

Dusky v. United States. (1960). 362 U.S. 402.
Breed v. Jones, 421 U.S. 519 (1975).
Bureau of Justice Statistics. (2015). *What is the sequence of events in the criminal justice system?* Retrieved from http://www.bjs.gov/content/justsys.cfm.
Eddings v. Oklahoma, 455 U.S. 104 (1982).
Graham v. Florida, 560 U.S. 48 (2010).
Grisso, T. (1998). *Forensic evaluation of juveniles*. Sarasota, FL: Professional Resource Press.
Grisso, T. (2005). *Evaluating juveniles' adjudicative competence: A guide for clinical practice*. Sarasota, FL: Professional Resource Press.
Grisso, T., & Quinlan, J. (2005). *Juvenile court clinical services: A national description*. Worcester, MA: Law and Psychiatry Program, University of Massachusetts Medical School.
Grove, W. M., & Meehl, P. E. (1996). Comparative efficiency of information (subjective, impressionistic) and formal (mechanical, algorithmic) prediction procedures: The clinical-statistical controversy. *Psychology, Public Policy, and Law, 2*(2), 293–323. doi:10.1037//1076-8971.2.2.293.
In re Gault, 387, U.S. 1 (1967).
In re Winship, 397 U.S. 358 (1970).
Heilbrun, K., Leheny, C., Thomas, L., & Huneycutt, D. (1997). A national survey of U.S. statutes on juvenile transfer: Implications for policy and practice. *Behavioral Sciences and the Law, 15*, 125–149.
Hoge, R. (2001). *The juvenile offender: Theory, research, and applications*. Norwell, MA: Kluwer Academic.

Hoge, R. D. (2002). Standardized instruments for assessing risk and need in youthful offenders. *Criminal Justice and Behavior, 29*(4), 380–395.

Kent v. United States, 383 U.S. 541 (1966).

Mack, J. (1909). The juvenile court. *Harvard Law Review, 23*, 120.

Miller v. Alabama, 567 U.S. (2012)

National Council on Disability. (2003). *Addressing the needs of youth with disabilities in the juvenile justice system: The current status of evidence-based research*. Washington, DC: National Council on Disability.

Olver, M. E., Stockdale, K. C., & Wormith, J. S. (2009). Risk assessment with young offenders: A meta-analysis of three assessment measures. *Criminal Justice and Behavior, 36*, 329–353. doi:10.1177/0093854809331457.

Prince v. Massachusetts, 321 U.S. 158 (1944).

Puzzanchera, C. (2013). *Juvenile arrests 2011*. Washington, DC: Office of Juvenile Justice and Delinquency Prevention.

Quinsey, V., Harris, G., Rice, M., & Cormier, C. (2006). *Violent offenders: Appraising and managing risk* (2nd ed.). Washington, DC: American Psychological Association.

Roper v. Simmons, 543 U.S. 551 (2005).

Sacks, H., & Reader, W. (1992). History of the juvenile court. In M. G. Kalogerakis (Ed.), *Handbook of psychiatric practice in the juvenile court* (pp. 5–11). Washington, DC: American Psychiatric Association.

Schall v. Martin, 467 U.S. 253 (1984).

Shoemaker, D. (2005). *Theories of delinquency: An examination of explanations of delinquent behavior* (5th ed.). New York, NY: Oxford University Press.

Snyder, H. N., & Sickmund, M. (1999). *Juvenile offenders and victims: 1999 National report*. Washington, DC: Office of Juvenile Justice and Delinquency Prevention, Office of Justice Programs, U.S. Department of Justice.

Snyder, H. N., & Sickmund, M. (2006). *Juvenile offenders and victims national report*. Washington, DC: Office of Juvenile Justice and Delinquency Prevention, Office of Justice Programs, U.S. Department of Justice.

Sprague, W. (1915). *Blackstone commentaries, abridged* (9th ed.). Chicago, IL: Caloghan.

Thompson v. Oklahoma, 487 U.S. 815 (1988).

Vincent, G. M., Guy, L. S., & Grisso, T. (2012). *Risk assessment in juvenile justice: A guidebook for implementation*. Chicago, IL: MacArthur Foundation.

Warren, J., Aaron, J., Ryan, E., Chauhan, P., & DuVal, J. (2003). Correlates of adjudicative competence among psychiatrically impaired juveniles. *Journal of the American Academy of Psychiatry and the Law, 31*(3), 299–309.

Zimring, R. E. (2005). *American juvenile justice*. New York, NY: Oxford University Press.

Chapter 6
Disability Law

Although the criminal justice system has made accommodations to deal with youth offenders differently than their adult counterparts under the presumption that they are unable to understand and control their environment in the same way as adults, society has been less responsive to dealing with juvenile offenders with mental health, educational, developmental, and/or cognitive disabilities. Despite evidence suggesting that between 30 and 70 % of youth involved in the juvenile justice system have a disability that may affect their ability to participate in their trial as well as respond to, understand, and participate in treatment, little advocacy or case law exists which protects the rights of these youth. Although there have been court decisions rendered that protect the rights of incarcerated delinquents with disabilities (e.g., *Green v. Johnson*, 1981; *Paul Y. by Kathy Y. v. Singletary*, 1997), those that exist focus primarily on protecting the rights of juvenile delinquents who have already been adjudicated. Little, if any, decisions exist to protect the rights of those juveniles with disabilities who are arrested and being processed through the juvenile justice system.

On the other hand, there is some case law for adult offenders that addresses how disability may relate to competency and punishment. For example, in the case of *Atkins v. Virginia* (2002), the US Supreme Court issued a landmark ruling that prohibited the execution of individuals with an intellectual disability who have committed a capital offense, with the court stating that it is a violation of the Eighth Amendment that bans cruel and unusual punishment (Duvall & Morris, 2006). Other case laws or state statutes exist within the adult criminal justice system that also protect the rights of individuals with disabilities, such as when an adult defendant commits an illegal act under "diminished capacity (diminished responsibility)" or the person did not have "the necessary culpable mental state" when he or she committed the act (Sales, Miller, & Hall, 2005, p. 175, 177). Given the history of the development of the juvenile justice system, it is likely that decisions and related state statutes like those rendered within the adult criminal justice system will eventually be included in the juvenile justice system.

Disability Law

The Fourteenth Amendment was ratified in response to the end of the civil war, and it primarily served to guarantee individual rights to recently freed slaves by providing the basis for the *Equal Protection Doctrine* that guarantees equal rights to all, stating:

> All persons born or naturalized in the United States and subject to the jurisdiction thereof, are citizens of the United States and of the state wherein they reside. No state shall make or enforce any law which shall abridge the privileges or immunities of citizens of the United States; nor shall any state deprive any person of life, liberty, or property, without due process of law; nor deny to any person within its jurisdiction the equal protection of the laws. (U.S. Const. amend. XIV)

While this amendment was originally added in response to slavery, it has subsequently been utilized to protect the rights of individuals and protect them from discrimination based, for example, on their race, ethnicity, religion, sexual orientation, or disability. The case of *Yick Wo v. Hopkins* (1886), in which Chinese shopkeepers were fighting for their rights, was an early example of the US Supreme Court applying the Fourteenth Amendment to protect individuals in the United States against discrimination. There has since been subsequent litigation, as well as the development of policy and law, that has further protected against the discrimination of minority groups, with substantial gains being observed in the past century.

In addition to further protection of minority races, ethnicities, and religious groups, the Fourteenth Amendment has helped to protect the rights of individuals with mental health disabilities. For example, during the twentieth century, there was a gradual but steady disappearance of "insane asylums," which had become popular in the nineteenth century as a way of dealing with individuals having psychiatric or mental health issues. In addition, in 1999, the US Supreme Court held that individuals with mental health disabilities have the right to the *least restrictive setting* (*Olmstead v. L.C.*, 1999). Specifically, the court found that, when it can be reasonably accommodated, individuals with mental health disabilities such as schizophrenia or intellectual impairments should receive community-based treatment programming versus being placed in institutional treatment facilities. While landmark legal decisions such as *Olmstead v. L.C.* and an associated societal shift toward *deinstitutionalization* led to increased rights for individuals with mental health and related disabilities, deinstitutionalization has also led to an increase in homelessness of individuals with some types of mental health disabilities such as schizophrenia, as well as an increase in the incarceration of individuals with these disabilities. For example, a national survey found that while in 1983 approximately 6 % of inmates in correctional settings had been diagnosed with a mental illness, by the early 2000s this was up to 16 % (Torrey, Kennard, Eslinger, Lamb, & Pavle, 2010). This survey also found that by 2005 there were three times more individuals with severe mental illness in jails and prisons than in psychiatric hospitals or institutions. In addition, in some states there were as many as ten times more people with severe mental health problems in prisons and jails than there were in hospitals. This dramatic increase in the rate of incarceration for individuals with disabilities has been referred by some as *shifting institutionalization*, as many individuals with disabilities who would have been sent to an insane asylum in the early twentieth century are now housed in an equally restrictive, nontherapeutic prison or correctional facility.

Constitutional amendments have also supported various case laws that provide additional interpretation of laws and further protect the rights of individuals with disabilities in correctional settings. For example, in the case of *Atkins v. Virginia* (2002) that was mentioned earlier, the US Supreme Court ruled 6-3 that executing individuals with an intellectual disability was a violation of the Eighth Amendment, which bans cruel and unusual punishment. In this case, 18-year-old Daryl Atkins was convicted of capital murder after he and an accomplice robbed a man and then shot him eight times. During the penalty phase of the trial, Atkins' school records were shown to reveal that he had a documented IQ of 59, which indicated a mild intellectual disability (referred to in the penalty phase of the trial as the then more typically used term of "mildly mentally retarded"). He was nevertheless sentenced to death. The sentence was appealed and ultimately went to the US Supreme Court which ruled that it was a violation of the Eighth Amendment to execute an individual with an intellectual disability. A subsequent case in Texas, *Tennard v. Dretke* (2004), also supported that an individual's IQ must be considered a mitigating factor when determining an appropriate penalty. In this case, a court accepted that the defendant's IQ was 67, which is in the mildly impaired range; however, it found that the defendant deliberately committed the crime and was likely to be dangerous in the future, so he was sentenced to death. The US Supreme Court, however, held that all relevant mitigating factors must be considered in the penalty phase of a death penalty case and that it was a violation of the cruel and unusual punishment clause of the Eighth Amendment. In this case, the defendant's death sentence was reduced to life in prison.

As discussed in subsequent sections of this chapter, there are several federal laws that provide protections for individuals with disabilities, including those with educational, developmental, cognitive, and mental health disabilities. These include the *Individuals with Disabilities Education Improvement Act* ([IDEIA], 2004), *Americans with Disabilities Act* ([ADA], 1990), and Section 504 of the *Rehabilitation Act* (Section 504; 1973). The IDEIA applies directly to the education of individuals with disabilities and is the only federal mandate that applies directly to children and adolescents since it focuses exclusively on the education of individuals under 22 years of age. The ADA and Section 504 apply to youth and adults and maintain that individuals with disabilities cannot be denied access to or services from public agencies. There are no federal disability laws specific to correctional settings; however, IDEIA, Section 504, and ADA have each been applied by the courts to correctional settings given that these are all public agencies. Nevertheless, the implementation in correctional settings of the individual rights that are established under these federal statutes can be difficult given the responsibility of correctional facilities in maintaining a secure, restricted environment and the limited resources that are often available in juvenile correctional facilities (Morris & Thompson, 2008).

Individuals with Disabilities Education Improvement Act

As mentioned earlier, IDEIA applies directly to children and adolescents having a disability, as it is a federal mandate that was passed to ensure that all individuals are afforded the right to a free and appropriate public education (FAPE). Specifically, IDEIA ensures that all students are provided an education without charge (**Free**); an education that meets the standards of the state educational agency (**Appropriate**); and an education that includes appropriate preschool, elementary school, or secondary school services (**Public** Education; *Board of Education v. Rowley*, 1982). IDEIA was first enacted by congress in 1997 as the *Individuals with Disabilities Education Act* (IDEA) and then amended and reauthorized again in 2004 as the *Individuals with Disabilities Education Improvement Act* (IDEIA). The 1997 IDEA was based on the *Education for All Handicapped Children Act* ([EHA], 1975), which was enacted by US Congress to ensure that all children in public schools received an appropriate education by providing special education services to all children in need. Prior to the EHA, children and adolescents with disabilities were often transferred from public schools to "specialized" public or private schools or institutions that only focused on providing services to handicapped children and which were often understaffed and underfunded and where minimal education or no educational services were provided (Murdick, Gartin, & Crabtree, 2007). Eventually, litigation ensued that determined that if states were going to enforce compulsory school attendance laws for all citizens under a certain age, then they must also assume responsibility for all citizens, not just those who can be successful in the traditional public school environment. The EHA also provided that all public schools receiving federal funds must provide equal access to all children, including those with disabilities. The EHA had several other provisions, such as requiring that disabled students be placed in the *least restrictive environment* for their education, that their educational experience emulate that of nondisabled students to the largest extent possible, and that parents be allowed to have direct involvement in the educational decision-making process for their children.

Each IDEA and IDEIA reauthorization further delineated the types of special education programs and services that must be made available for all eligible students (regardless of their placement) in order to ensure a FAPE. These subsequent reauthorizations have also helped shift the original focus of ensuring that all students with a disability receive special education services, to ensuring that all students with a disability receive *quality* special education services. Under IDEIA, each state must provide FAPE to any child between the ages of 3 and 21 years who has an eligible disability that impacts his or her ability to learn in the general classroom. According to the federal statute, a FAPE includes the following components:

1. *Zero reject*. This principle is based on the belief that all children can learn, and it ensures that regardless of the type or severity of a person's disability, all children are entitled to receive a free and appropriate public education.
2. *Nondiscriminatory assessment*. This principle provides that when assessing students to provide a diagnosis or educational plan, fair and culturally sensitive

procedures are used, a variety of assessment tools are used, and technically sound instruments that are administered by a trained professional serve as the basis for the assessment.
3. *Procedural due process.* Due process provides safeguards for parents and school districts to ensure that IDEIA is implemented fairly.
4. *Parental participation.* This provision of IDEIA ensures that parents or guardians have a pivotal role in the special education services provided to their student.
5. *Least restrictive environment.* This principle is based on the assumption that the preferred educational placement for a student with a disability is the general education classroom. If the general education classroom is deemed inappropriate, even with medications, then the next least restrictive environment should be used. Ultimately, this provision ensures that students with disabilities are not immediately removed from the general education classroom but rather are given a chance to be educated with their peers.
6. *Individualized education program* (IEP). The IEP serves as a written statement for the child receiving special education services, and it identifies the child's current levels of performance, goals for special education, and other information that helps ensure that the appropriate interventions are being utilized and monitored.

In addition to these provisions of FAPE, IDEIA also mandates a variety of other services that an educational agency must provide. For example, the school is responsible for identifying those students who may need special education services. Specifically, any child or adolescent who is suspected of having a learning disability must be referred for an evaluation to determine if he or she is eligible for special education services [34 CFR § 300.343(b)(1)]. Once identified as possibly needing services, the educational agency must then provide a comprehension evaluation that is individually tailored to the specific educational needs of the child (34 CFR §300.532). If a student qualifies for special education services because of a disability, IDEIA also requires that the school must provide the appropriate related services, such as physical therapy, speech therapy, occupational therapy, or counseling (34 CFR §300.24), as well as appropriate transition services, when moving from the school setting to a post-high school setting (34 CFR §300.29). IDEIA also provides guidelines for discipline procedures that must be used when dealing with students with disabilities, primarily related to suspensions and expulsions (34 CFR §300.519).

There are several types of disabilities that make one eligible for special education services under the IDEIA. Eligible disability categories include:

1. Autism
   Autism is a developmental disability that affects verbal and nonverbal communication and social interaction. Individuals with autism often engage in stereotyped movements, restricted patterns of interest, a need for sameness and difficulties with transition and change, and sensory sensitivities to sound, lights, fabrics, or other stimuli (see Chap. 7 for a more thorough description of autism and how it may impact a juvenile's interaction with the juvenile justice system).

2. Deaf-Blindness
   This category implies simultaneous hearing and visual impairments, which cause severe communication difficulties as well as developmental and educational needs that cannot be accommodated for in a program solely for children with deafness or a program solely for children with blindness.
3. Deafness
   Under IDEIA, deafness implies that the child has a hearing impairment so severe that he or she is impaired in his or her ability to process auditory information, which adversely affects the child's educational performance.
4. Developmental Delay (Ages 3–9)
   Children between 3 and 9 years of age (inclusive) can qualify for special education services under the category of developmental delay if they experience developmental delays in at least one of the five following areas: (a) physical development, (b) cognitive development, (c) communication development, (d) social or emotional development, or (e) adaptive development.
5. Emotional Disturbance
   Emotional disturbance (ED) is a category used when a child exhibits one or more of the following characteristics over a long period of time, which adversely affects his or her educational performance. The characteristics of ED can include the following: (a) an inability to learn that cannot be explained by intellectual, sensory, or health factors; (b) an inability to build or maintain satisfactory interpersonal relationships with peers and teachers; (c) inappropriate types of behavior or feelings under normal circumstances; (d) a general pervasive mood of unhappiness or depression; or (e) a tendency to develop physical symptoms or fears associated with personal or school problems. The classification of ED does include children with schizophrenia, but it purports to rule out children who are "socially maladjusted" unless it is determined that they also have an emotional disturbance. Children who qualify for special education under the category of ED often display significant social difficulties and behavioral difficulties in the classroom. Many delinquent children who are in special education fall under this category, while many others who have educational deficits do not, as it is presumed that their academic and behavioral difficulties at school are related to "social maladjustment" rather than an ED (see Chap. 8 for a more detailed description on mental health or emotional disabilities, the prevalence of delinquents with mental health or emotional disabilities, and how it may impact their functioning in the juvenile just system).
6. Hearing Impairment
   This category indicates that a child has impairment in hearing that adversely affects his or her educational performance. This hearing impairment can be permanent or fluctuating and is not at the level of deafness.
7. Intellectual Disability
   An intellectual disability is a condition in which a child displays significantly below average intelligence (IQ), as well as significant deficits in adaptive behavior. These deficits adversely affect the child's educational performance (see Chap. 6 for a more thorough discussion of intellectual disabilities and the relationship between intellectual disability and delinquency).

8. Multiple Disabilities

    This category covers children who display simultaneous impairments in which the combination of disabilities requires educational programming that cannot be accommodated by a special education program designed for just one of the disabilities. For example, this category may include a child with an intellectual disability as well as an orthopedic impairment or an intellectual disability as well as blindness and deafness.

9. Orthopedic Impairment

    To qualify for this category, a student must display a severe bodily impairment that adversely affects the child's educational performance. Impairments may include those caused by congenital abnormalities, disease, or other causes such as amputation or burns. One example may be a child with cerebral palsy who has severe orthopedic impairments that require him or her to have individualized instruction to learn how to adequately read or write.

10. Other Health Impairment (OHI)

    A child who qualifies for special education under OHI may have limited strength, vitality, or alertness that limits his or her ability to focus and be successful in the educational environment. Conditions that may qualify a child for the diagnosis of OHI include asthma, attention deficit hyperactivity disorder, diabetes, epilepsy, leukemia, or Tourette syndrome. Similar to other categories, it must be shown that the condition adversely affects the child's educational performance.

11. Specific Learning Disability (SLD)

    An SLD is a disorder in one or more of the basic psychological processes involved in understanding or in using language (spoken or written) that may manifest itself in difficulty with the ability to listen, think, speak, read, write, or do math. SLD does not include learning problems that are primarily the result of visual, hearing, motor, or intellectual disabilities or emotional disability. Examples of specific learning disabilities include deficits in basic reading skills, reading fluency, reading comprehension, written expression, oral expression, listening comprehension, math calculation, or math problem solving (see Chap. 7 for a more detailed description of SLD, their prevalence among juvenile delinquents, and how SLD may impact a youth offender's interaction with the juvenile justice system).

12. Speech or Language Impairment (SLI)

    A SLI is a category for children with communication disorders that adversely affects their educational performance. Examples include stuttering or poor articulation. Chapter 6 provides background on communication disorders, including a discussion on language disorders and other issues related to SLI.

13. Traumatic Brain Injury (TBI)

    The category of TBI covers individuals who have had an acquired injury to the brain that was caused by an external physical force, which resulted in total or partial functioning disability or psychosocial impairment (or both), which adversely affects a child's educational performance. Impairments are often observed in areas such as cognition, language, memory, attention, reasoning, abstract thinking, judgment, problem solving, motor abilities, perceptual abilities,

psychosocial behavior, physical functions, or information processing. The category of TBI does not include brain injuries that were induced by birth trauma or those which are congenital or degenerative.
14. Visual Impairment (Including Blindness)
    This is an impairment in vision that, even with correction, adversely affects a child's educational performance. This can include both partial sight and full blindness.

Under IDEIA, a child may not be considered as having a disability if the educational impairment is a result of being an English language learner (e.g., he or she has a primary language other than English and does not speak English well) or if the child has not had appropriate instruction in English. IDEIA has led to significant improvements in education for students with disabilities. More students with disabilities are identified as having special needs, more students are given access to appropriate educational services, and the majority of students with disabilities are now educated in regular public schools rather than separate facilities or institutions (American Youth Policy Forum and Center for Education Policy, 2002).

IDEIA in Juvenile Correctional Settings. While IDEIA has brought significant improvements to students with disabilities in the public school system, it has not come without difficulties and policy implementation issues. A study by the National Council on Disability (2012), for example, found that every state in the United States was out of compliance with IDEIA requirements. Similarly, the implementation of EHA, IDEA, or IDEIA in juvenile correctional settings has met various roadblocks, considerably more than those within public school settings. For example, in 1979, a juvenile inmate incarcerated in the Commonwealth of Massachusetts filed a lawsuit against the state for failure to provide him and other eligible students with special education services (*Green v. Johnson*, 1981). The court decided that although the incarcerated status of an inmate may require adjustments in the special education programs available to him or her as compared to programs available to students who were not incarcerated, all students having a disability—regardless of their incarceration status—are entitled to special education services. This ruling was especially timely given that research over the past 35–40 years has repeatedly shown that a history of academic failure and the presence of an educational disability are among the most prevalent characteristics of juveniles who reside in short-term detention settings or long-term correctional settings (e.g., Morris & Morris, 2006; Ollendick, 1979; Waldie & Spreen, 1993; Wang, Blomberg, & Li, 2005; Zabel & Nigro, 1999).

Implementing the provisions of IDEIA into juvenile detention and long-term correctional settings can be difficult for a variety of reasons. There is a high number of youth eligible for special education services in these facilities, yet these settings often have limited resources. In addition, these youth often move frequently between facilities, making it difficult to have continuity of services. Other difficulties in implementing IDEIA include obtaining a youth offender's previous school records, particularly for those who have not been in school for an extended period of time or for those who have attended several schools and/or a school outside of their current juvenile court jurisdiction. Nevertheless, a number of legal cases have arisen over the years, which ultimately mandated that juveniles with educational disabilities are to be provided the same special education services as their nondelinquent peers (e.g., Morris & Thompson, 2008). For example, case law has provided that juveniles, even those who are incarcerated or in short-term detention facilities, must be identified and provided comprehensive evaluations. Specifically, in the cases of *Alexander S. v. Boyd* (1995) and *Smith v. Wheaton* (1998), it was found that state correctional facilities had failed to adequately identify, locate, and evaluate juvenile offenders in need of special education services. These cases also required that a juvenile offender's IEP be implemented. Additional case law has further addressed the need for the provision of related services (e.g., *New Hampshire Department of Education v. City of Manchester, NH School District*, 1996) and due process (e.g., *Paul Y. by Katy Y. v. Singletary*, 1997) (see Morris & Thompson, 2008 for a detailed description of additional case law and related policy implementation issues regarding policy issues surrounding IDEA and IDEIA in juvenile correctional facilities).

Section 504 of the Rehabilitation Act

Section 504 of the *Rehabilitation Act* (1973) was the first civil rights law that prohibited discrimination against individuals with disabilities, and it was one of the first laws that viewed individuals with disabilities as a minority group and a distinct class of individuals who shall not experience discrimination in public settings (National Council on Disabilities, 2003). Specifically, Section 504 prohibits any federally funded agency from discriminating against an individual with a disability, stating that no otherwise qualified individual can be subjected to discrimination or exclusion from the participation in, or be denied the benefits of, any program receiving federal financial assistance. Section 504 defines an individual with a disability as one who has a physical or mental impairment which significantly limits one or more major life activities. While this federal law was not developed originally for educational purposes, it directly applies to schools because nearly all public schools receive federal funding, and Section 504 considers learning to be a major life activity; therefore, public schools may not discriminate against or prevent a student from attending or participating in a school-related activity merely because of the student's disability.

In the school setting, children and adolescents with disabilities who do not otherwise qualify for special education services may qualify for educational accommodations under Section 504. To qualify for services under IDEIA, a student's disability must substantially affect his or her academic functioning or ability to learn without specialized instruction. Under Section 504, any individual who has a physical or mental impairment that limits a major life activity — such as learning — qualifies for protection under Section 504, and, therefore, the school must provide the student with an educational accommodation in order that his or her disability does not interfere with his or her ability to learn in the school environment. While a mental health disability such as attention deficit hyperactivity disorder may qualify a student for services under IDEIA because his or her attention deficit leads to difficulties in learning to read or write or learn math, this disability may not qualify a student under IDEIA if he or she is able to learn and progress in these latter academic areas, but struggles in other ways in school such as remaining focused and staying on task during class assignments, completing class exams within the allotted time period, or disrupting other students in class during regular seat work time. In this case, if the student's attention deficit and/or hyperactivity interferes with his or her ability to fully participate in the latter classroom work, then the student may qualify for school accommodations under Section 504. A common 504 accommodation plan for a student having attention deficit hyperactivity disorder may involve permitting him or her to take a class test in a quiet testing room and for an extended period of time in order to limit distractions so that the student's attention difficulties or distractibility does not prohibit him or her from being successful on the test.

Americans with Disabilities Act

In addition to IDEIA and Section 504, the *Americans with Disabilities Act* (ADA, 1990) protects individuals with disabilities from being discriminated against based on their disability. Similar to Section 504, the ADA defines an individual with a disability as one who has a physical or mental impairment that substantially limits major life activities. As is the case with Section 504, the ADA was not designed specifically to protect the rights of students with disabilities but rather to apply to any individual with a disability. Unlike Section 504, however, the ADA does not apply only to those agencies receiving federal funding. Rather, this act is much broader in scope than Section 504, in that it prevents any public agency, regardless of whether it receives federal funding, to discriminate against an individual on the basis of disability. This includes, for example, restaurants, hotels, shopping centers, private schools, hospitals, or movie theaters. ADA provides that these and other public agencies must provide *reasonable* changes in policy, practice, or procedure to avoid discrimination against an individual with a disability. Accommodations that may be provided include sign language interpreters for those with hearing impairments, ramps for people using wheelchairs, or handicapped accessible drinking fountains and restrooms.

Section 504 and ADA in Juvenile Correctional Settings

Similar to the difficulties in implementing IDEIA in juvenile correctional settings, there have been considerable difficulties associated with implementing and enforcing Section 504 and ADA, as noted in various lawsuits filed against juvenile correctional facilities. For example, a class action lawsuit was filed against the

California Youth Authority (*Stevens v. California Youth Authority. 213 F.R.D. 358*, 2001). This lawsuit alleged that the conditions provided to juveniles were in violation of the ADA. Specifically, among other complaints, the plaintiffs argued that those with educational disabilities were not provided with the appropriate academic accommodations, those with mental health disabilities were not provided with appropriate resources and accommodations, and there were other inhumane conditions present in violation of ADA. Although this specific case was dismissed without prejudice, subsequent cases have been filed against various juvenile justice systems, again using violations of ADA as a supporting claim. For example, in the case of *United States v. State of Ohio* (2008), juvenile correctional facilities were found to have provided unconstitutional conditions and not following provisions required by laws such as IDEA and ADA. In 2015 there was a settlement agreement with the LeFlore County Juvenile Detention Center in Missouri after they were found to be violating IDEIA and not providing appropriate mental healthcare and physical care.

Conclusion

As the prevalence data regarding juveniles with disabilities increases, the laws affecting individuals with disabilities and their impact on the juvenile correctional system become increasingly important. Federal disability laws exist to protect the rights of individuals with disabilities, and IDEIA and other federal laws, as well as litigation involving incarcerated youth, have all helped to clarify that the guarantee of a FAPE applies to all eligible youth, independent of their educational setting (Morris & Thompson, 2008). However, there continues to be confusion, inconsistencies, and a lack of clarity regarding the way in which these federal mandates apply to the juvenile justice system. There is increasing case law related to the rights of adult criminals with disabilities, but there is less available case law that specifically focuses on the rights of juvenile delinquents with disabilities. As has been noted by various writers in the area of juvenile delinquency and disability, one of the most significant barriers to appropriate implementation of disability laws and related policies is that the primary purpose of juvenile corrections is *not* educational in nature. For example, Eggleston (1996) states:

…the agencies that adjudicate and incarcerate are not educational entities. Their purpose is the determination of guilt and innocence and the provision of security and custody (p. 199).

Therefore, while it certainly appears that the juvenile justice system differs from the adult criminal justice system in that it aligns itself as more rehabilitative in nature, this rehabilitative approach does not necessarily include an educational or schooling component. In addition, there is limited evidence to suggest that juvenile correctional facilities routinely consider youth who have a disability as different from those youth who have committed similar illegal acts but who have no apparent disability or that youth having a disability have special needs that require special remediation efforts in order to assist them in becoming productive citizens.

References

Alexander S. v. Boyd, 22 IDELR 139 (D.S.C. 1995).
American Youth Policy Forum & Center on Education Policy. (2002). *Educating children with disabilities*. Washington, DC: Author.
Atkins v. Virginia, 536 U.S. 304 (2002).
Americans With Disabilities Act of 1990, Pub. L. No. 101-336, § 2, 104 Stat. 328 (1991).
Board of Education of the Hendrick Hudson Central School District v. Rowley, 458 U.S. 176 (1982).
Education for All Handicapped Children Act of 1975, Pub. L. No. 94-142.
Eggleston, C. R. (1996). The justice system. In S. C. Cramer & W. Ellis (Eds.), *Learning disabilities: Lifelong issues* (pp. 197–201). Baltimore, MD: Paul H. Brookes.
Green v. Johnson, 3 EHLR 552:550 (D.M.A. 1981).
Individuals with Disabilities Education Improvement Act of 2004, Pub. L. No. 108-446.
Morris, K. A., & Morris, R. J. (2006). Disability and juvenile delinquency: Issues and trends. *Disability and Society, 21*, 613–627. doi:10.1080/09687590600918339.
Morris, R. J., & Thompson, K. C. (2008). Juvenile delinquency and special education laws: Policy implementation issues and directions for future research. *Journal of Correctional Education, 59*(2), 173–190.
Murdick, N. L., Gartin, B. C., & Crabtree, T. (2007). *Special education law*. Upper Saddle River, NJ: Pearson Education.
National Council on Disabilities. (2003). *Addressing the needs of youth with disabilities in the juvenile justice system: The current status of evidence-based research*. Washington, DC: Author.
National Council on Disabilities. (2012). *National disability policy: A progress report—August 2012*. Washington, DC: Author.
New Hampshire Department of Education v. City of Manchester, NH School District, 23 IDELR 1057 (D.N.H. 1996).
Ollendick, T. H. (1979). Discrepancies between verbal and performance IQs and subtest scatter on the WISC-R for juvenile delinquents. *Psychological Reports, 45*(2), 563–568. doi:10.2466/pr0.1979.45.2.563.
Olmstead v. L.C., 527 U.S. 581 (1999).
Paul Y. by Kathy Y. v. Singletary, 27 IDELR 1 (S.D. Fla. 1997).
Sales, B. D., Miller, M. O., & Hall, S. R. (2005). *Laws affecting clinical practice*. Washington, DC: American Psychological Association.
Section 504 of the Rehabilitation Act of 1977, Pub. L. No. 93-112, § 87, Stat. 394 (1973).
Smith v. Wheaton, 29 IDELR 200 (D.C.T. 1998).
Stevens v. California Youth Authority. 213 F.R.D. 358 (2001).
Tennard v. Dretke, 542 U.S. 274 (2004).
Torrey, E. F., Kennard, A. D., Eslinger, D., Lamb, R., & Pavle, J. (2010). *More mentally ill persons are in jails and prisons than hospitals: A survey of the states*. Arlington, VA: Treatment Advocacy Center.
United States v. State of Ohio (S.D. OH.). (2008).
U.S. Const. amend. VIII.
Waldie, K., & Spreen, O. (1993). The relationship between learning disabilities and persisting delinquency. *Journal of Learning Disabilities, 26*(6), 417–423. doi:10.1177/002221949302600608.
Wang, X., Blomberg, T. G., & Li, S. D. (2005). Comparison of the educational deficiencies of delinquent and nondelinquent students. *Evaluation Review, 29*(4), 291–312. doi:10.1177/0193841x05275389.
Yick Wo v. Hopkins, 118 U.S. 356, 6 S. Ct. 1064, 30 L. Ed. 220 (1886).
Zabel, R. H., & Nigro, F. A. (1999). Juvenile offenders with behavior disorders, learning disabilities, and no disabilities: Self- reports of personal, family, and school characteristics. *Behavioral Disorders, 25*(1), 22–40.

Part II
Developmental and Educational Disabilities

Chapter 7
Developmental Disabilities

Developmental disabilities encompass a wide range of diagnostic categories, each of which is manifested in individuals before 22 years of age, with symptoms and impairment generally being observed early in the person's life, such as during infancy or early childhood. The presence of a developmental disability reflects the significant differences from the norm in the way a child develops cognitively and, in some instances, the manner in which the child develops early language, mobility, or emotionality, with these developmental differences affecting the child through adolescence and often into adulthood. The hallmark symptoms associated with a developmental disability usually involve the child not meeting early developmental milestones such as not walking, talking, and/or emoting within the typical developmental age range norms. Developmental disabilities cannot be cured. While some of the symptoms may wane over the individual's lifespan, they often continue to be apparent to some degree throughout his or her life. Major areas of the individual's life that may be negatively affected include language and the ability to communicate in a manner that is "typical" for the person's same-age and same-sex peers, self-care activities, social relationships, mobility, education, independent living, and/or employment.

Developmental disabilities are not as prevalent within the juvenile delinquency population as are other disabilities such as mental health disabilities or educational disabilities. Nevertheless, they are still overrepresented, and more importantly, the presence of a developmental disability can have a substantial impact on a juvenile's functioning within the justice system given the significant cognitive and social impairments commonly observed with developmental disabilities. While there are a number of developmental disability diagnostic categories that are discussed in the literature (e.g., intellectual disability, cerebral palsy, epilepsy and other types of seizure disorder, communication disorder, and autism spectrum disorder (ASD)), the present chapter will focus only on the three that appear most commonly within the juvenile justice system, namely, intellectual disability (previously referred to in the literature as "mental retardation"), ASD, and communication disorders (e.g., Quinn, Rutherford, Leone, Osher, & Poirier, 2005).

Intellectual Disability

Intellectual disability is primarily characterized by impairment in cognitive functioning with concurrent deficits in adaptive functioning. Such impairments can be in intellectual functioning as well as problem solving, abstract thinking and reasoning, planning, and the ability to learn from experience. These deficits must be great enough to lead to impairments in one's ability to function independently (American Psychiatric Association [APA], 2013). In addition to having deficits present during the developmental period, which is identified by the American Association of Intellectual and Developmental Disabilities (AAIDD) as being before 18 years of age (Schalock et al., 2010), specific criteria are required to be present in order to qualify for a diagnosis of an intellectual disability. These include the following:

(a) *Deficits in intellectual functioning* (APA, 2013)
This criterion is primarily related to intelligence, which is measured by an IQ test. The average IQ is 100, and approximately 95 % of the population has an IQ between 70 and 130. A person is typically considered for an intellectual disability if he or she has an IQ around or below 70 (less than the second percentile). Previous editions of the DSM mandated that an intellectual disability could not be considered if IQ was not below 70 (e.g., APA, 1980, 2000); however, this strict criterion is no longer used in the DSM-5. Rather, cognitive deficits are determined by impaired intelligence, as well as deficits such as impaired problem solving, abstract thinking, reasoning, or inability to remember and learn.

(b) *Deficits in adaptive functioning* (APA, 2013)
Adaptive functions are essentially those skills one needs to live independently, adapt to changes in the environment, and carry on everyday life activities at a level expected for one's age. Adaptive functioning is typically categorized into three main areas, including conceptual skills, social skills, and practical skills. *Conceptual skills* include an understanding of more abstract concepts such as finances and money management, time, and generally planning and self-direction of activities. *Social skills* include interpersonal skills, social problem solving, ability to follow rules, or ability to make up one's own mind. *Practical skills* are those skills needed to complete basic daily activities, such as personal care and hygiene, managing money or finances, staying safe and healthy, traveling from place to place, being employable, and otherwise being able to follow schedules and routines and manage daily life safely. Adaptive skills are assessed relative to one's age (i.e., the skills expected for a 16-year-old boy are clearly different from those adaptive skills that are considered typical for a 4-year-old boy). Assessment of adaptive functioning is an important consideration for determining if one has an intellectual disability, since low IQ alone would not be sufficient for a child to qualify as having an intellectual disability. For example, if a 17-year-old male scores in the second percentile on an IQ test (IQ of 70) but is otherwise functioning independently (e.g., can be left alone during the day, cook, perform regular housekeeping chores, communicate needs, or otherwise

complete tasks at a level expected for a "typical" person his age), then he would *not* meet the criteria for an intellectual disability.

An intellectual disability is identified as being *mild, moderate, severe,* or *profound*. While deficits in both intellectual and adaptive functioning have long been required to qualify for a diagnosis of intellectual disability (APA, 1980), in the past, the level of *severity* of the diagnosis was determined by the level of impairment observed in an individual's intelligence. However, as of 2013 professional guidelines changed so that severity is determined based on the deficits in one's adaptive functioning and level of support required (APA, 2013). Mild intellectual disabilities are the most common, with research suggesting that as many as 85 % of those diagnosed with an intellectual disability are classified as mild, approximately 10 % classified as having a moderate intellectual disability, 3–4 % diagnosed with a severe intellectual disability, and approximately 1–2 % being diagnosed as having a profound intellectual disability (APA, 2013).

Since an intellectual disability is a developmental disability, the symptoms occur in early development and continue across an individual's lifespan. There are many signs and symptoms of intellectual disability, but in young children the symptoms may first be observed with the infant being delayed in rolling over, sitting up, crawling, or walking. The child may also be slow to start talking and may take additional time to be toilet trained or perform such self-help skills as dressing, tying shoes, or feeding himself or herself. While delays must be observed during a child's normal developmental period in order for the person to qualify for a diagnosis of intellectual disability, for those children with mild intellectual disability, it is not uncommon for parents or guardians not to notice any significant cognitive, motoric, or language impairments until the child begins school as this is when children frequently engage in more higher-level thinking (APA, 2013).

Impact on Functioning

Based on the nature of this disability, we would expect that children and adolescents will take appreciably longer than their same-age typical peers to learn and advance academically in school and have difficulty in the following areas: abstract reasoning, performing tasks involving higher-order thinking, remembering facts and events, connecting actions with consequences, learning from experience, adapting to new environments and changes in old environments, and logical thinking and problem solving (Mervis & John, 2010). That being said, the level of impact that an intellectual disability has on a person's functioning varies considerably depending on the level of impairment that is present (i.e., mild, moderate, or profound).

In those cases involving a person having a mild intellectual disability, it would be expected that delays in language development would be observed during adolescence and that advancement in academic skills relative to same-age typical peers in the regular classroom setting would be increasingly difficult after approximately the sixth grade. Therefore, while a child with a mild intellectual disability could learn, it would be expected that such learning would occur at a slower rate than it would for their typically developing peers in the classroom. On the other hand, most individuals with a mild intellectual disability would also be expected to live independently as adults, with only minimal support from social service agencies and/or guardians. For individuals having a moderate intellectual disability, we would expect that as a child, he or she would probably develop functional language skills by adolescence but would probably not be fluent in his or her language and that academic skills would typically develop through the second-grade level. In terms of independent living, we would expect a person with this level of intellectual disability to need support and supervision throughout adulthood. Lastly, for those persons having a severe or profound intellectual disability, we would expect both language and academic skills to be extremely limited and that close supervision and intensive support would be likely required throughout the lifespan of these individuals (e.g., see APA, 2013; World Health Organization [WHO], 1996).

Etiology and Treatment

Intellectual disability has been estimated to be present in approximately 1 % of the United States population (APA, 2013). While some people associate intellectual disability with the genetic condition known as "Down Syndrome," this disorder only accounts for a very small portion of those people having an intellectual disability (Winnepenninckx, Rooms, & Kooy, 2003). Rather, there are a variety of causes of intellectual disability, such as genetic conditions other than the one that causes Down Syndrome (e.g., Angelman syndrome), problems during pregnancy that may interrupt normal brain development in utero (e.g., preeclampsia, infections, malnutrition, fetal alcohol syndrome, drug use), problems during childbirth (e.g., being deprived of oxygen for an extended period of time), and early childhood infections (e.g., meningitis). It has been estimated that approximately 50 % of the cases involving intellectual disability are due to genetic causes and the rest are due to environmental impacts (Winnepenninckx et al., 2003). Despite the variety of factors that can contribute to the development of intellectual disability, the actual cause is often identified in less than half of all reported cases (McDermott, Durkin, Schupt, & Stein, 2007).

Diagnosis of an intellectual disability often occurs during early or middle childhood after delays in functioning and difficulties learning have been noticed. A psychologist or psychiatrist typically diagnoses an intellectual disability after conducting a formal evaluation. This evaluation typically includes a review of background history, administration of a standardized intelligence test, and use of history and standardized rating scales to assess adaptive functioning. There is not a cure for an intellectual disability and no treatments exist that can reduce the primary cognitive deficit and adaptive behavior symptoms. Rather, interventions typically focus on providing children and adolescents special educational, vocational and other support services at school to help them maximize their learning potential and subsequent independent living potential. In addition to special education services, a range of support services are generally offered and can include such programs as case management, vocational programs, day programs, and residential treatment options (Schalock, Borthwick-Duffy, Buntinx, Coulter, & Craig, 2009). The types of intervention and support systems provided typically depend on the presumed etiology and level of severity of the intellectual disability (see, for example, Matson, Terlonge, & Minshawi, 2008).

Juvenile Delinquents with Intellectual Disabilities

The case of Alex that was presented in the introduction to this book was an example of a juvenile offender who presented with a mild intellectual disability. Alex had participated in serious juvenile offenses yet lacked the cognitive ability to fully participate in treatment programming. While it is impossible to know the degree to which low motivation contributed to Alex's lack of participation, it is possible to know that inherent in an intellectual disability is an impairment in one's ability to communicate needs and ideas, to learn from experience, to problem solve in novel situations, and to otherwise reason and learn at the same level as expected for same-age typical children or adolescents. With an IQ of 61 it will be difficult for Alex to hold a job that requires more than rote memorization of a simple skill. It will be difficult for him to plan for himself financially, and to live independently on his own and take care of all of the associated activities that are necessary for such living unless there is daily supervision is provided by a social services agency.

A considerable amount of research exists that has examined the relationship between intellectual functioning and juvenile delinquency (e.g., Fergusson & Horwood, 2002; Hirschi & Hindelang, 1977; Koolhof, Loeber, Wei, Pardini, & D'Escury, 2007). These and other studies suggest that there is a relationship between intellectual functioning and juvenile delinquency, and that while the frequency of intellectual disability is lower in the juvenile delinquency population relative to other forms of disability, there is an overrepresentation of youth having an intellectual disability in the juvenile offender population than in the general child and adolescent population. The findings from these studies have varied considerably in their estimates, however. For example, Bullock and McArthur (1994) reported a prevalence rate of 2 % regarding the prevalence of intellectual disability in detained juveniles, while a meta-analysis conducted by Casey and Keilitz (1990) estimated that upwards of 12.6 % of youth offenders had an intellectual disability. In addition, a Swedish study that examined the prevalence of mental health disabilities in juvenile delinquents found that of the 73 % who had a mental health diagnosis, 10 % also had a diagnosis of an intellectual disability (Stahlberg, Anckarsater, & Nilsson, 2010). Similarly, a study by Quinn et al. (2005) surveyed juvenile correctional institutions across the United States and found that of the 33.4 % of delinquents who were classified as having a disability under the IDEA or IDEIA, 9.7 % were diagnosed as having an intellectual disability.

Various theories exist to help explain why these youth may be more likely to become involved in the justice system. For example, the *school failure theory* suggests that disabilities such as intellectual disability negatively impact school achievement which, in turn, leads to other problems such as dropout and juvenile delinquency (Osher, Woodruff, & Sims, 2002). The *susceptibility theory* posits that youth with intellectual and other disabilities have cognitive deficits that predispose them to delinquent behavior, with these deficits including poor impulse control, suggestibility, inability to anticipate consequences of behavior, and poor perception of social cues (Keilitz & Dunivant, 1987). The *differential treatment hypothesis* suggests that youth with disabilities respond differently to interactions with law enforcement and others in authority and, therefore, are more likely to be arrested despite being involved in comparable levels of delinquency as their nondisabled peers (Keilitz & Dunivant, 1987). Finally, the *metacognitive deficits hypothesis* asserts that the problem-solving strategies of delinquent youth are less developed than their typically developing peers; therefore, youth with disabilities would be at an increased risk of offending (Larson, 1988).

Youth offenders having an intellectual disability may also have difficulties once they come into contact with the juvenile justice system. For example, given the deficits in thinking skills inherent in the diagnosis of an intellectual disability, it is to be expected that youth with an intellectual disability will have difficulty with communication skills, abstract thinking, higher-level reasoning, and learning from consequences. Therefore, these youth may struggle to fully participate in their treatment programming while they are detained, incarcerated, placed in a group home setting or even returned to their own home under their parents' supervision. In this regard, youth offenders are often required to participate in group substance abuse treatment, anger management training, or other therapeutic interventions. These programs rely heavily on verbal skills and comprehension, which will be difficult for those youth having an intellectual disability. It may appear that these youth are refusing to cooperate or are not actively participating in the treatment sessions when, in fact, they actually lack the necessary communication skills to participate. Similar patterns of behavior will also likely be observed in any individual therapy that is cognitively-based, as cognitive therapies rely heavily on abstract thinking in order to be successful. Other forms of treatment that are not cognitively-based may be more successful for these youth, such as the use of behavioral rehearsal and modeling procedures based on social learning theory (Bandura, 1969), as well as positive reinforcement procedures that are based on operant conditioning (Skinner, 1938, 1953).

Youth offenders with intellectual disabilities may also struggle with many common diversion or probation requirements, such as composing and writing a letter of apology, since having an intellectual disability also means that the reading and/or writing levels of these youth will be significantly below that of their same-age typical peers. In addition to difficulty complying with certain court probation requirements or participating in particular treatment programs, juveniles having an intellectual disability may struggle to fully understand the implications of the illegal acts in which they engaged or fully understand the intricacies associated with breaking the law. For example, they may not fully understand that while they received diversion for their initial offense, this is not the typical court response for chronic offenders. Therefore, they may not comprehend the magnitude of re-offending and impact it may have on future consequences and punishments.

Finally, in addition to difficulties associated with actively completing common court-requirements after being adjudicated, youth having an intellectual disability may also have negative interactions with authorities following their arrest and as they are being processed through the juvenile justice system. As presented in Chap. 5, the processing of a youth offender through the juvenile justice system allows for greater subjectivity and flexibility in comparison to the adult criminal court system. While this can be advantageous for many youth, it may serve as a disadvantage for some youth having an intellectual disability, as their social interaction skills are typically not as well developed as they are for their same-age peers (APA, 2013). This may put them at a greater risk for negative interactions with court personnel, as well as having probation violations and additional arrests, which could lead to increased involvement with the juvenile justice system and decreased chances for becoming productive citizens.

Impact on Risk and Risk Assessment. As discussed in the introduction to this chapter, assessment of risk involves reviewing a variety of factors. In regard to determining *risk of dangerousness*, because these youth often do not fully understand the implications that their actions have had on others (Leffert, Siperstein, & Widaman, 2010), they may be viewed as having limited empathy or remorse for their behaviors (antisocial traits). In addition, while any youth can present as a risk for dangerousness if there is a history of cruelty or aggressiveness toward others, it is highly unlikely that a youth with an intellectual disability has the cognitive capacity to execute planned and extensive illegal acts because of their significant intellectual impairments or to fully understand the implications and consequences for such acts. Moreover, while the total number of offenses committed by a youth is often a predictor of risk, in the case of a juvenile with an intellectual disability it would be important to examine the types of repeated acts in which the youth has engaged to determine whether the youth with an intellectual disability fully understood the requirements/consequences associated with probation. This is not to imply that the apparent risk of individuals with intellectual disabilities should be disregarded or explained away by the presence of their disability.

In the case of Alex, the fact that he was a repeat sex offender highlights that he is a risk to the community; therefore, this fact should be taken into consideration in determining how to best intervene and balance community protection and Alex's treatment. Sending him to a long-term correctional facility removes any immediate risk that he may pose to the community; however, this does not address the difficulties posed by his intellectual disability or address the fact that he has (and will) remain relatively "untreated" in terms of sexual offending given that he does not have the ability to participate in traditional forms of intervention. Therefore, his long-term risk remains unknown.

Competency. Although one might hypothesize that a youth's level of cognitive and intellectual abilities would have an effect on his or her *competency to stand trial* and participate in his or her own defense, a standardized intelligence test is not required when a clinician is completing a competency evaluation (Grisso, 2013). As discussed earlier in this book, juvenile competency is determined by evaluating two different capacities: the degree of reasonable understanding a juvenile has in regard to the court process, as well as the juvenile's ability to sufficiently participate in the court trial and collaborate with him or her attorney. Competency to stand trial assumes that a youth has both a factual *and* rational understanding of the juvenile justice system and court process. For a youth with an intellectual disability, both of these facets may be difficult to meet.

Significant intellectual impairments make learning difficult. Youth with mild intellectual disabilities rarely exceed the 6th grade equivalency for academic skills and, therefore, higher-level skills are difficult for these youth to learn. Currently, no literature is available that identifies what specific grade-level or intellectual ability is necessary for an individual to have a complete factual understanding of court proceedings. Regardless, even if a juvenile with an intellectual disability could express an understanding of the court proceedings and the roles of those involved in the trial, one might question whether this individual would fully understand the charges against him or her, as well as the seriousness of the charges and the likely outcomes of the trial. In addition, we believe that the level of communication difficulties that are often observed in youth having an intellectual disability would make it difficult for these youth to fully collaborate and communicate with their attorney and actively participate in the numerous decisions that need to be made in their own defense prior to and during their trial.

When determining whether competency can be restored, the amount of time likely to be required for change is given consideration (Grisso, 2013). Even if an individually-based restoration program was utilized resulting in a youth with an intellectual disability being able to memorize factual knowledge of court proceedings and processes, it is questionable whether a reasonable understanding could ever be obtained by that youth of the court process given the youth's limitations in higher-order thinking. Because an intellectual disability is a lifelong disorder, the amount of time needed for the youth to obtain a factual and rational understanding may be indeterminable (and possibly indefinite).

Autism Spectrum Disorder

The Case of Andrew

When Andrew was 11-years-old, he was allegedly "dared" by his 15-year-old male neighbor to take explicit photos of Andrew's 6 year-old sister and share them with the neighbor. Before Andrew could share the photos with the neighbor, his sister reported the incident to their parents and they immediately talked to Andrew about what was wrong with the incident. They also established "family rules" for Andrew, which included rules that he was not allowed to take pictures of his sister, be alone with her in a room, or have the neighbor at their house. Despite his parents setting of these rules, 2 years later it was discovered that Andrew and the male neighbor had been sexually abusing his sister for the past 2 years. His parents called the police and Andrew and the neighbor were arrested. Although Andrew did not have any previous arrests or involvement with law enforcement agencies, he was placed in detention throughout his adjudication process because of the seriousness of the charges against him. Andrew and the neighbor were each charged with sexual molestation of a child. Andrew adamantly denied any wrong doing in this case. He admitted that both he and his neighbor had sexual contact with his sister; however, he said that he did not break the rules established by his parents. He did not engage in sexual acts with his sister at his own house; he did not take pictures of his sister; he was not alone with her in her room; and the neighbor boy was not at their house. Instead, Andrew and his sister were at the neighbor's house when the incidents occurred.

Andrew was evaluated for competency and found competent to stand trial. This was based both on two independent competency evaluations conducted by a psychologist and a psychiatrist, as well as a review of educational records that indicated Andrew's IQ was in the "Above Average" range. Although Andrew had been found competent to stand trial despite his age, his public defender remained concerned about his capacity to fully participate in his trial. Andrew's attorney stated that Andrew often had difficulty talking with her about the case and what took place over the past 2–3 years, with her describing Andrew as becoming very anxious anytime the case was mentioned. She stated that he would fidget, rub his hands on his pants over and over again, pull on his hair, and ask her to stop talking about the charges against him. He refused to speak with her on most occasions, and when he would meet with her, his involvement in the discussion of the charges was minimal.

The attorney also reported that while Andrew was able to verbalize a definition of her role as his attorney, she often felt that he did not trust her and did not fully understand that her role was to help him rather than punish him. She stated that he would not look at her when they were talking, he often did not respond to even informal questions she asked (e.g., "How has your day gone?"), and she perceived him as not quite understanding the serious nature of his offense and the possible implications if he would be found guilty. She stated, for example, that at his pretrial hearing he appeared relaxed, unengaged, and spent the trial coloring and drawing on scratch paper despite having been told in advance the purpose of the hearing and the importance of him using pencil and paper to write down questions he had or concerns that he had about comments that were made during the hearing. His attorney also expressed the view that she did not feel that Andrew clearly understood the seriousness of the child molestation charges against him and was concerned that he did not accept blame for his acts. She, therefore, maintained that Andrew could not participate in his trial to the same extent as other same-age typical youth.

Andrew's attorney sought outside consultation from a psychologist, as she was concerned that despite Andrew having above average intelligence, Andrew did not appear to fully understand the serious nature of his illegal act and the upcoming trial. She also knew that Andrew had been diagnosed with autism at his school and received special education services because of this disability, and she wanted to know if the autism could be a contributing factor to his inability to interact with her and fully participate in his own defense. Moreover, because of the serious nature of his offense, Andrew was also being evaluated for an out-of-home placement, and she was concerned that his difficulty cooperating with her would result in more negative behaviors if he was placed outside of his home environment.

Andrew's attorney was not familiar with what exactly autism was or the impairments it can cause in functioning, but her experience with Andrew was consistent with many of the social and communication deficits displayed by individuals who are diagnosed as having autism. Although Andrew was previously found to have above average intelligence and, presumably, had the ability to understand court proceedings, his disability also suggested that he would have a variety of other difficulties that could impact his ability to interact with his attorney, understand the intricacies of a court hearing, and rationally understand the severity of what he had done and the long-term consequences if he would be found guilty.

Diagnostic Symptoms and Characteristics of Autism Spectrum Disorder

More than 70 years ago, Leo Kanner (1943) described a group of 11 children who displayed a similar pattern of behaviors that he indicated were appreciably different from those of other childhood behavior disorders. Kanner called this form of childhood psychopathology "early infantile autism" and noted that among its characteristics were marked withdrawal; dislike of being held; unresponsiveness to people as well as to the environment; manipulation of objects in a rigid, stereotyped manner; lack of appropriate play; failure to acquire normal speech; echolalia and difficulties with pronoun use; anxious insistence on sameness in the environment; excellent rote memories; normal physical appearance; and, good cognitive potential (Morris & Morris, 2010).

Kanner's work on early infantile autism has been expanded and transformed into the study of what is now labeled "autism spectrum disorder" (ASD). This disorder is conceptualized as a developmental disability that is, in general, characterized by impairments in social functioning, communication, and behavior—many of the same impairments described by Kanner. In this regard, the DSM-5 diagnostic criteria for ASD identify two major categories of impairments that are typically found in individuals, namely: (1) "social communication and social interaction across settings" and (2) "restricted, repetitive patterns of behavior, interests, or activities" (APA, 2013, p. 50). These are described in more detail below.

1. *Deficits in social communication and social interaction across settings*
   Communication and social deficits can be observed in a variety of ways. This may be evident by the child or adolescent having delayed or limited language skills (or, in some instances, no language). Communication deficits may also be observed by the child or adolescent having difficulty participating in back-and-

forth conversation and be relatively unable to engage in "social chitchat" or side conversations. When observing a youth in conversation, it may be noticed that he or she has limited or no eye contact with the other person, and the individual may struggle to respond appropriately to a social greeting or interaction. The person may also have difficulty using or understanding nonverbal communication such as gestures, head nods, or appropriate facial expressions (e.g., smiling to show happiness). Other symptoms of poor social communication and social interaction may include difficulty forming friendships or other social relationships, or even having very limited interest in forming relationships. Finally, a key social/communication symptom of ASD that can cause significant impairment in functioning is limited perspective taking and having difficulty understanding the feelings and opinions of others. These deficits in understanding social cues and interpreting the thoughts of beliefs of others is frequently referred to as a deficit in *theory of mind*. Theory of mind is a skill that is typically learned by middle childhood and is essentially the ability to understand the state of minds of others and know that another's thoughts or beliefs may be different from one's own (APA, 2013).

The second major category of symptoms described by the DSM-5 is:

2. *Restricted, repetitive patterns of behavior, interests, or activities.*
An individual with ASD typically displays these symptoms when they engage in odd behavior movements (e.g., hand flapping), repeating what others say, or using toys in atypical ways. For example, if a child with ASD has a toy car collection, rather than use the cars to race and play games, the child may merely line up the cars and organize them by color or size. Or when the child plays with blocks, he or she may spend time organizing them by colors rather than building things. This cluster of symptoms also includes the restricted patterns of behavior often observed in individuals with ASD. Children or adolescents with ASD often demonstrate extreme rigidity in their routines, with them insisting on sameness for activities (e.g., always washing hands before touching food, even if in a movie theater or at a fair), or even sameness in the foods they eat (e.g., eating only three different foods). It is not uncommon for younger children or adolescents to have outbursts or extreme reactions when there are changes in their daily schedule, as it disrupts their desire for sameness and restricted activities. Restricted interests may also be observed in youth with ASD having an abnormally intense interest in something. These intense interests are displayed, for example, by the individual talking, reading, and researching incessantly about the same topic (e.g., rockets, a historical event, or a certain music group). It is not uncommon for younger children to have unusual interests or obsessions with random objects. For example, the child may be hyperfocused with toilet seats, wanting to collect pictures, talk, or read about toilet seats, or even touch or see toilet seats in each setting they visit (e.g., restaurants, schools, doctors' offices). Finally, this cluster of symptoms may include the child being extremely sensitive to various sensory input, such as touch, sound, light, or smell (APA, 2013).

In summary, ASD is typically characterized by impairments in social relationships, social interactions, communication, social thinking skills, and with the presence of atypical behaviors. However, as researchers and mental health professionals have increasingly begun to understand ASD over the past few decades, they have also developed a better understanding for the odd behavior and dysregulation observed in some children. For example, while anger outbursts, aggression, or temper tantrums are not symptoms required for a diagnosis of depression, they are behaviors commonly observed in younger children when these children experience interruptions in their restricted interests or schedules (Rapin, 1997).

When working with a child or adolescent who may be displaying odd or atypical behaviors, positive symptoms for ASD that are often easily recognizable include limited or bizarre language, odd motor mannerisms (e.g., hand flapping, twirling objects, odd finger movements), limited eye contact, and/or fixation on topics or odd items (e.g., rocks, light switches, thermostats). Often though, it is the symptoms defined by "the absence of the negative" that are the most defining characteristics of ASD, yet the most difficult for an untrained clinician to note or understand. For example, "limited perspective taking" is not a characteristic that is easily observable, yet when this is identified in an individual it can contribute to an appreciable impairment in the person's daily functioning. Other symptoms defined by the "absence of the negative" are explained in a child or adolescence that may have language but his or her communication style is characterized by a lack of gesture use, limited prosody in voice, and limited reciprocity. Other characteristics that may be observed include teachers or parents having difficulty getting the child or adolescent engaged in the same activity as others, the person not responding to his or her name when called, or the child or adolescence appearing to show a complete disregard for others in the room.

The symptoms of ASD all contribute to impairment in the individual's daily functioning, but the degree of impairment can vary considerably from mild to severe. For example, a "high functioning" person having ASD is one whose symptoms cause only mild impairments and, therefore, may only need limited support to function independently in society. Conversely, an individual with ASD who has severe impairments is likely to require intensive, lifelong support. An earlier edition of the DSM, the DSM-4 (APA, 2000), had a separate diagnostic category for "Asperger's disorder," which was commonly known as a type of "high functioning" or less severe form of autism (APA, 2000); however, the DSM-5 has combined autism and Asperger's disorder into one ASD diagnostic category, with the severity of ASD defined by the accompanying level of impairment in the person's daily functioning.

This recent change in the ASD classificatory system has several implications, such as being unable to compare the incidence and prevalence of autism or Asperger's disorder over time, as well as compare the findings from current versus past intervention studies for autism or Asperger's disorder. However, even prior to this classificatory change, the prevalence of autism diagnoses had been found to steadily increase over time. For example, research from the 1960s indicated that autism occurred in approximately 5 out of 10,000 people (Lotter, 1966), whereas by the 1980s it was estimated that the ratio was approximately 10 per 10,000 people

(Burd, Fisher, & Kerbesbian, 1987), with more recent studies indicating prevalence rates of approximately 60–70 per 10,000 people (Rice et al., 2007). According to the US Center for Disease Control and Prevention (CDC) it is estimated that 1 in every 68 children is diagnosed with autism (and 1 in every 42 boys), making it more common than the total combined prevalence of childhood cancer, juvenile diabetes and pediatric AIDS (Center for Disease Control and Prevention, 2014). In this regard, it is estimated that 1.5 million individuals in the U.S. and tens of millions worldwide have an autism diagnosis (CDC, 2014). This change in prevalence may be related to a variety of factors, including a broader understanding of the disorder, more accurate diagnoses and better assessment methods available, and, as described above, changes in diagnostic criteria.

Etiology

The specific cause(s) of ASD are currently unknown. However, while evidence remains unclear it is thought that genetic factors are the primary contributing factors to this disability. Popular assumption is that these genetic factors lead to abnormalities in the development of brain structures, which, in turn, affect cognitive and behavioral functioning. Abnormalities have been found at the most basic level of the brain (e.g., reduced neuronal structures or activity in certain areas of the brain and/or impaired connectivity between brain structures) to more robust structural abnormalities (e.g., more cerebral volume) (e.g., Brambilla et al., 2003). The advancement of neuroimaging techniques (e.g., functional MRIs and PET scans) has helped researchers better understand the neurological differences in individuals having ASD versus their typical same-age peers or peers having other psychiatric disorders (e.g., Allen & Courchesne, 2003). Though controversy still remains about the degree of difference that occurs in brain structure and functioning of individuals having versus not having ASD, studies have found that the brains of those with ASD are, in fact, different than those without. For example, while some studies have found minimal differences in brain region size (e.g., Haar, Berman, Behrmann, & Dinstein, 2014), other research has indicated that the brains of children with ASD are larger (e.g., Brambilla et al., 2003; Fidler, Bailey, & Smalley, 2000; Harden, Minshew, Mallikarjuhn, & Keshavan, 2001).

Research focusing on the functional differences of the brain has also identified differences in individuals with versus without ASD. For example, researchers from Cambridge, England were the first to discover that when trying to decipher facial expressions and related emotions, the amygdala (i.e., the emotional control center of the brain) is underactive in individuals with ASD (Baron-Cohen, 1995). Moreover, other research has indicated that the communication between various brain regions and the links between networks in the brain are weak in individuals with ASD (Herbert, 2005). Since it is rare to find one specific area of the brain that controls 100 % of a specific process, different regions of the brain must communicate with each other in order to fully perform a specific skill. Researchers have suggested that in individuals having ASD there may be poor synchronization between various regions, or a lack of coordination so that each area of the brain is functioning independently (e.g., Just, Cherkassky, Keller, & Minshew, 2004; Peters et al., 2013). It is posited then that this lack of integration of information leads to atypical presentation of skills and behaviors.

Impact on Cognitive Functioning

Although the "autistic savant" as portrayed in the movie classic *Rain Man* leads many to believe that despite their atypical social skills, individuals with ASD have high levels of intelligence or other exceptional abilities. ASD is actually more often associated with the presence of an intellectual disability. Specifically, research has suggested that approximately 70 % of those having ASD may have an intellectual disability (Chakrabarti & Fombonne, 2001). For those considered high functioning, evidence suggests that these youth typically struggle more in their performance on language-related intelligence tests, as well as on tests involving processing speed and working memory (e.g., Mayes & Calhoun, 2008).

Related to this, research has also found strong evidence of executive functioning deficits in youth having ASD (e.g., de Vries, Prins, Schmand, & Geurts, 2015; Geurts, deVries, & van den Bergh, 2014). In fact, a popular cognitive theory that attempts to explain many of the difficulties experienced by individuals with ASD is the *executive dysfunction hypothesis* (Russell, 1997), which suggests that ASD is directly related to deficits in executive functioning. Executive functioning skills include planning, organization, judgment, reasoning, abstract thinking, attention, impulse control, and flexible thinking. These are the higher-level skills one uses to direct control over his or her behavior, and they typically develop as an individual matures into adulthood. The first study to examine the presence of executive functioning deficits in ASD was conducted by Rumsey (1985). He administered a common neuropsychological test that measures abstract reasoning and flexible thinking and found that individuals with ASD performed significantly worse than those peers who did not have ASD. Subsequent studies have replicated these findings (Pennington & Ozonoff, 1996), leading some to suggest that executive functioning deficits in these skills could explain much of the inflexible, rigid behavior displayed by individuals having ASD, as well as certain social deficits since social communication requires flexible thinking and the ability to change based on the demands of the environment (e.g., Bennetto, Pennington, & Rogers, 1996; Geurts et al., 2014). This is further supported by the fact that some studies have found that executive functions improve when other behavioral interventions are implemented (e.g., Baltruschat et al., 2011; Kenworthy et al., 2014). What is not addressed in the executive dysfunction hypothesis, however, is the lack of explanation regarding *why* individuals with ASD struggle in the area of executive functioning, since there has not necessarily been a related neurological insult or trauma observed in these individuals to the area of the brain associated with executive functioning (i.e., the prefrontal cortex).

Attention deficits are also commonly observed in individuals with ASD, and these may be significant enough that it is not uncommon for higher functioning children to first be misdiagnosed with having attention deficit hyperactivity disorder (ADHD; APA, 2013). Recent research has even examined and found that there may be common early developmental pathways between ASD and ADHD (e.g., Johnson, Gliga, Jones, & Charman, 2015), as well as similarities in white matter structure in the brain (Cooper, Thapar, & Jones, 2014), partially explaining the similarities between these disorders. The attention deficits in children and adolescents with ASD, however, are different from those persons having ADHD. For example, while children with ADHD typically struggle to sustain attention over a long period of time, children with ASD struggle to shift their attention. Specifically, they take longer to disengage from a task and switch attention to another task than do their typically developing peers (Wainwright-Sharp & Bryson, 1993). These attention deficits are likely related to other deficits in executive functioning displayed by individuals with ASD.

As was mentioned earlier, language impairments are also inherent in the diagnosis of ASD. Language impairments are typically so significant that the disorder was once classified under the category of language disorders (Rutter, 1978). In fact, in a small proportion of those persons having ASD, language does not develop at all, while in others it develops but is delayed and impaired throughout their lifespan (APA, 2013). Communication deficits are also found in those persons with ASD who are classified as high functioning. These individuals often lack "reciprocity" (i.e., the typical back and forth flow of a conversation), and often repeat questions or comments rather than answering or do not respond at all to others who have directed a comment or question to them. In addition, they typically do not spontaneously elaborate on responses, and their conversations can be disjointed or very tangential (APA, 2013).

Although a variety of cognitive deficits are typically observed in individuals with ASD, cognitive strengths may also be observed, such as a high level of attention to visual detail and above average performance on visual-spatial tasks. This high attention to visual detail, however, has led some to hypothesize that this strength could also be a hindrance. For example, the *weak central coherence theory* (Frith & Happe, 1994) hypothesizes that those individuals with ASD struggle to process information in context, which may be partially due to their tendency to *overfocus* on insignificant visual details. This theory has led some writers to suggest that that the social communication impairments observed in people having ASD are not specifically due to structural abnormalities in the brain but rather to the connection between neural systems and how this connectivity impacts various cognitive processes (Herbert, 2005). For example, it has been found that children having ASD focus more on insignificant aspects of an individual (e.g., neck, forehead, chest) as he or she is talking instead of focusing on facial expressions and hand gestures (e.g., Joseph & Tanaka, 2003; Klin, Jones, Schultz, Volkmar, & Cohen, 2002). This, in turn, may lead the person having ASD to have difficulties reading the body language of others and interpreting various nonverbal cues and gestures.

Diagnosis and Treatment of ASD

There is no medical test for diagnosing ASD; rather, a diagnosis is typically made from a combination of behavior observations, a review of the child's background history, and psychological testing. Because of difficulties in early language, motor, and/or social development, some children are diagnosed at first as having a general developmental delay, and it is not until the child grows older and his or her deficits become more apparent that he or she will be further evaluated and subsequently receive a diagnosis of ASD. However, since the level of impairments in social functioning, thinking skills, and behavioral regulation, as well as the presence of odd or bizarre behaviors, often vary across children—especially in high functioning children—it is not uncommon for individuals not to be diagnosed as having ASD until later childhood or adolescence. In addition, some children may first be diagnosed as having another mental health disorder or disability, such as obsessive-compulsive disorder or ADHD, before they receive a diagnosis of ASD.

While distinguishing ASD from other diagnoses can be difficult, an accurate diagnosis is critical in providing effective interventions and treatment. Children with ASD often "grow out" of certain symptoms (e.g., echolalia), but many of the characteristics associated with social difficulties and related symptoms persist into adulthood (Billstedt, Gillberg, & Gillberg, 2005). In fact, studies have found that the most improvement in the impairments observed in children having ASD is during the preschool and early childhood years, with levels of functioning remaining stable in subsequent years or occasionally diminishing in adolescence and adulthood (e.g., Sigman & McGovern, 2005).

There are a variety of treatments available that focus on improving social skills and decreasing disruptive or unwanted behaviors, and intervention programs are typically intensive, long-term programs that involve teams of specialists who work together to improve language skills, social skills, and behavioral regulation (see, for example, Charlop-Christy, Malmberg, Rocha, & Schreibman, 2008).

Juvenile Delinquents with ASD

Very little research is available that has examined the prevalence of youth with ASD among the juvenile delinquency population. Research that does exist has typically used single or small group case studies or focused exclusively on those with ASD who have been adjudicated, resulting in limited confidence or generalizability of findings. In addition, because of the low prevalence of ASD in both the youth offender and general child and adolescent population, many studies that examine mental health disorders or other disabilities in the juvenile offender population have excluded those youth having ASD from the research sample. While there is slightly more research examining ASD in the adult criminal justice system, ultimately it is flawed by similar methodological problems (King & Murphy, 2014).

While the prevalence of ASD among delinquents remains unknown, one study that examined the relationship between ASD and juvenile delinquency was conducted in South Carolina and found that 5 % of youth diagnosed with autism had been charged with a delinquent offense (Cheely et al., 2012). Compared to data from studies estimating that 15–20 % of the general adolescent population will be arrested before 18 years of age (Brame, Turner, Paternoster, & Bushway, 2012), this study suggests that a smaller percentage of youth having ASD are arrested than those without ASD. However, in another study that utilized data from a stratified random sample of youth receiving community services, it was found that 11.4 % of youth with ASD had contact with the juvenile justice system (based on self-report or parent report) compared to 31 % of those without ASD (Brookman-Frazee et al., 2009). Moreover, in a study that investigated juveniles committed to a long-term correctional facility in Sweden between 2004 and 2007, it was found that almost three-quarters of the sample had received a mental health diagnosis, with 17 % of the youth having a diagnosis of ASD (Stahlberg et al., 2010). In general, although children and adolescents with ASD are more prone to dysregulated behaviors and temper outbursts, it is not believed that this places them at a high risk for delinquency. Rather, the limited studies that have addressed this have found that there is a smaller percentage of youth with ASD involved in the juvenile justice system than those with other disabilities.

Although these youth are at a lower risk of offending compared to the general juvenile delinquency population, it has been hypothesized that when youth having ASD do commit illegal acts they are more likely to be arrested or have contact with law enforcement than are other youth (Mayes, 2003). The rationale underlying this hypothesis is similar to that for youth having an intellectual disability in that youth with ASD may lack the awareness to either hide their illegal act from others and/or interact appropriately with law enforcement personnel, resulting in a greater likelihood of their arrest and adjudication. In addition, when youth with ASD do offend they are more likely to be arrested for offenses against person (e.g., assault) versus offenses against property (e.g., burglary) (King & Murphy, 2014).

Studies have also found that youth with ASD are more likely to be charged for offenses that have occurred at school, such as having more "disturbing the school environment" charges, than youth without ASD (Cheely et al., 2012). One possible explanation for this is that individuals with ASD have a tendency to overly adhere to routines and rules, and when these are disrupted they often become dysregulated. This can result in them reacting aggressively or have a temper outburst that can include aggression toward another person; therefore, rather than the illegal act being construed as, for example, a premeditated assault, this may be an impulsive act performed out of frustration or dysregulation. As described above, there is evidence that individuals with ASD have executive functioning deficits (e.g., O'Hearn, Asato, Ordaz, & Luna, 2008), which could also contribute to impulsive reactions versus manipulative, premeditated violent acts against others.

As proposed by Howlin (2004), the social naiveté of individuals with ASD may lead them to be more prone to manipulation by others and at risk for engaging in delinquent acts, and their lack of understanding of social situations can lead to maladaptive or aggressive responses. Howlin (2004) also proposes that obsessive interests common in individuals with ASD could lead them to commit an offense while in pursuit of that interest. One popular case of this occurred in the UK by Gary McKinnon, who was an adult with ASD. His obsessive interests included UFOs, and he caused over $800,000 in damage by pursuing this interest when he hacked into US. Government computer systems in search of evidence of UFOs (BBC, 2012).

Once arrested, it has been suggested that youth with ASD are more likely to receive diversion and less likely to be adjudicated or detained (Cheely et al., 2012). However, for those whose illegal acts are serious enough to involve ongoing interaction with the juvenile justice system, there are many difficulties that may arise because of the diagnosis of ASD. For example, in the case of Andrew described earlier, his level of social impairments were inhibiting his attorney's ability to interact with him when planning and organizing his defense. In addition, although he had been found competent and appeared to have good factual understanding of court processes, his attorney advocated for the courts to take into consideration Andrew's diagnosis of ASD in the court's determination regarding the extent to which he could participate in and fully understand the implications of his trial and sexual offense charges. His attorney also advocated for Andrew's diagnosis of ASD to be taken into consideration when determining placement and treatment options, particularly since Andrew was being considered for out-of-home placement. Many potential placements may not have the staff available who are knowledgeable about and trained in providing treatment services to people who have ASD. Andrew's social deficits, lack of perspective taking, and communication impairments would likely make it very difficult for him to become actively engaged in a typical treatment program that relied heavily on communication skills.

In addition to the functional impairments caused by ASD, research has also suggested that individuals with ASD are at a higher risk of comorbid mental health disorders (Vermeiren, Jespers, & Moffitt, 2006). This may further exacerbate the difficulties these youth have in both understanding and navigating their way through juvenile court proceedings. Studies have found that nearly 70 % of youth with ASD qualified for at least one additional DSM diagnosis (e.g., Leyfer et al., 2006; Simonoff et al., 2008), and as will be discussed in future chapters, mental health disabilities themselves can create difficulties for typically developing youth and, therefore, may exacerbate those difficulties already experienced by youth offenders having ASD.

Impact on Risk and Risk Assessment. In the case of Andrew, the prosecuting attorney and others working with him felt that he demonstrated many risk factors of antisocial behavior and a "severe lack of remorse" for his offense. For example, his sexual offenses were described as premeditated and thoughtful given the 2 year period of time in which they occurred and the collaboration that occurred with his neighbor prior to and during the committing of the offenses. In addition, Andrew was perceived as lacking empathy as he refused to talk about the case, apologize for his actions, admit to wrongdoing, or otherwise acknowledge what happened. The state's argument also included evidence of the fact that Andrew was a youth with above average intelligence, so he should have had a higher level of understanding, reasoning, and thinking skills compared to most boys his age. While many of these arguments appear valid at face value, particularly when examining risk of recidivism and re-offending, when placed within the context of the fact that Andrew is a person having ASD, many of these claims may actually be a misinterpretation of his presumed level of cognitive functioning. As previously discussed, risk assessment can be based entirely on actuarial or statistical methods, clinical judgment, or a combination of both methods. In the case of Andrew, it seems reasonable that actuarial methods would be largely invalid since they would predict that Andrew was at a much higher risk than he actually may be with regard to the level of intent associated with his actions.

Examining a youth's *risk of dangerousness* involves evaluating a youth for psychopathic features (lacking remorse or empathy, being manipulative or overly egocentric), the extent of planned and criminally extensive acts, and the level of cruelty and aggressiveness toward others. While Andrew's lack of involvement and refusal to discuss the case may be perceived as poor empathy, it could also be argued that this is due to his poor social skills, limited social reciprocity, and limited insight into the perspective of others, which are all common characteristics in individuals with the diagnosis of ASD. This may also explain the fact that while Andrew's offense was against another person (and, therefore, appears to be antisocial), this may not have been the result of antisocial thinking but rather related to his deficits in social communication and interaction. In addition, Andrew's refusal to discuss the case or accept wrongdoing may be related to the concrete, literal thinking inherent in people diagnosed as having ASD. Andrew maintained that he was following the "house rules" in that he did not repeat the offense at home, did not take any more pictures of his sister, and he did not have the neighbor over at the house. While Andrew's offense happened over a long period of time and to a large extent was premeditated, deficits in abstract thinking may limit the ability for a person like Andrew to adequately assess the consequences of his actions, comprehend the severe nature of what occurred, and fully understand the punishments that can result (Lord & McGee, 2001). The societal protection question that still needs to be resolved then, is what the probability is that Andrew will repeat the illegal acts given his diagnosis of ASD?

In regard to *sophistication and maturity*, Andrew did not appear to be acting impulsively but, as stated above, this does not necessarily indicate that he demonstrated sophisticated, mature offenses. Andrew acted independently to some degree, but his acts were also prompted by his typically developing neighbor rather than being initiated entirely on his own. One's level of sophistication and maturity in offending is also related to his or her understanding of the wrongfulness of offenses, of which Andrew did not fully appreciate. In addition, sophistication requires high-level thinking and decision-making, of which individuals with ASD inherently lack.

Finally, in terms of *treatment amenability* Andrew appears to be of greater risk to the community. According to staff reports he had refused to discuss the case, participate in programming, and displayed limited insight into his functioning. While this may very well indicate that he is not amenable to treatment, it is actually very difficult to determine if Andrew would respond positively to a treatment program if it was based on individuals having ASD. On the other hand, if he was to be included in an intervention that required typical communication skills and interactions with others, then one might conclude that Andrew would not be amenable to treatment.

Competency. As mentioned earlier in this chapter, juvenile competency is determined by evaluating two different capacities: the degree of reasonable understanding a youth offender manifests in regard to the court process, and the youth's ability to sufficiently participate in the court trial and collaborate with his or her attorney in the defense. Little to no research is available that examines the impact that a diagnosis of ASD may have on an individual's competency to stand trial, so the following consists of a critical discussion of how the impairments associated with ASD may affect competency.

Being diagnosed as having ASD does not prevent a child or adolescent from learning, and those persons who have ASD and are high functioning may demonstrate learning and related knowledge at a level equal to or even better than their typically developing peers. Therefore, it would be reasonable to assume that a youth with ASD could demonstrate a factual understanding of court proceedings by defining key terms, describing the key roles of various individuals (judge, defense attorney, prosecuting attorney, probation officer, etc), and listing possible outcomes of a hearing. What may be more difficult for a youth with ASD, however, is having a *rational* understanding. While competency is something that should be addressed on a case-by-case basis, it is our belief that most youth offenders having ASD do not have the capacity to fully understand court proceedings and participate fully in their own defense. They may have a rote knowledge of the juvenile justice process and related proceedings, but it is doubtful that most will have a rational understanding of these processes and proceedings and be able to rationally participate in their own defense. The presence of language and communication impairments, limited perspective taking, poor abstract thinking, and limited executive functioning skills could make it difficult for youth offenders with ASD to participate in court proceedings. Many states have recognized developmental immaturity as a contributing factor to incompetence (Grisso & Quinlan, 2005). While young age may typically initiate this finding, we believe that it is reasonable to expect that regardless of age, youth offenders with ASD may experience developmental immaturity to a greater degree given that their disability is ultimately defined by a developmental delay.

Finally, in regard to *remediation* and whether competency can be developed or restored, there are two important factors to consider. First, is the fact that ASD is a lifelong developmental disability. While there are treatment interventions to improve functioning and reduce problematic or disruptive behaviors, the social communication deficits and interpersonal skills will be chronic. The atypical thinking style will also be prominent throughout the lifespan. Whether the brain development that occurs into adulthood is enough for an adult having to be restored cannot be determined at this time based on the available research literature. While there are interventions available to improve social thinking and communication skills, evidence-based interventions are still being developed and require long-term programmatic research to assess their relative effectiveness (see, for example, Charlop-Christy et al., 2008). It, therefore, appears at this time to be low probability whether a youth offender having ASD who has been found to be incompetent can be restored through remediation programs.

Communication Disorders

Communication disorders are defined by impairment in one's ability to receive, express, process, or comprehend verbal or nonverbal communication. These disorders can take the form of hearing, language, or speech impairments. For example, they may take the form of auditory processing difficulties (e.g., difficulty accurately hearing speech sounds), they could entail greater deficits in expressing or understanding spoken language, or they could include speech impairments such as stuttering and poor articulation. In some cases, a communication impairment is secondary to another disability (e.g., ASD) or neurological problem (traumatic brain injury). In other cases, the communication difficulty may be the primary disability, with the individual struggling with expressive (speaking) or receptive (understanding what they hear) language despite no identifiable neurological, hearing, cognitive, or other impairment. It is these latter communication difficulties that encompass developmental communication disorders and are the focus of this section.

Children begin developing language early in life. Even in early infancy they are slowly learning speech sounds, the basics of communication, and the intricacies of social interaction and communication. Because of this, the most severe forms of communication disorders may show signs in infancy, with these infants delayed in cooing or babbling or generally unresponsive to communicating with their caregivers. For moderate or more mild communication disorders, delays may not be observed until the disorder impairs daily functioning when the child fails to start speaking full words or sentences and has trouble communicating needs (APA, 2013). For example, while most children begin speaking first words before age one, children with communication disorders may not speak first words until they are closer to age two. Parents may begin noticing at this time that there is also limited sophistication in word combinations. As the child ages, parents may begin to notice that their child's grammar and speech remains developmentally inappropriate (e.g., confusing verb tense or reversing pronouns). For other children, it may not be until beginning preschool or kindergarten that a communication disorder is identified, as these children may be quieter than their peers, become anxious regarding talking in the classroom, have word-finding problems, or struggle academically as language skills are critical for learning (Cook & Cook, 2008). Inaccurate grammar is typically the most impaired language skill in a child with a communication disorder (Leonard, 1998). Other observable impairments, however, may include word-finding difficulty, in which the youth is slow to retrieve words that he or she wants to use (also referred to as "tip-of-the-tongue phenomenon").

Communication disorders can range in severity from mild to profound. For example, a child may have only mild articulation difficulties or he or she may have complete *aphasia*, which is the inability to use speech and language for communication. The severity of a communication disorder will be positively correlated with the level of impairment observed in daily functioning; however, even mild communication disorders have been associated with impaired cognitive, academic, social, and behavioral functioning (e.g., Conti-Ramsden & Botting, 2008).

The prevalence of communication disorders has been estimated to range from 3 to 6 % of the population (e.g., APA, 2013; Tomblin et al., 1997), with it being estimated that nearly six million children under the age of 18 have a communication disorder that affects their daily functioning (Cook & Cook, 2008). There has been some disagreement in whether communication disorders affect males and females equally, but it is suggested that these disorders likely affect males at a greater rate than females (e.g., APA, 2013; Snowling & Hayious-Thomas, 2010).

Types of Communication Disorders

There are two main categories under which the majority of communication disorders fall: *speech disorder* and *language disorder*.

Speech Disorder. A speech disorder can largely be classified as a deficit in one's ability to articulate the various speech sounds or to speak fluently. The DSM-5 broadly defines two specific types of speech disorder, including *Speech Sound Disorder* and *Childhood-Onset Fluency Disorder (Stuttering)*. These are both defined as developmental disorders in that the onset of symptoms is in the early developmental period, and the DSM-5 differentiates a primary communication disorder from language problems that are secondary to other difficulties (e.g., ASD, traumatic brain injury, deafness, cerebral palsy). A description of symptoms for Speech Sound Disorder as described by the DSM-5 includes the following:

(a) Persistent difficulty with speech sound production that may interfere with intelligibility of speech, resulting in unclear speech. This may include distortion of words, as well as substitutions, omissions, or additions of sounds to words. Specifically, this means that the child has difficulties with speaking clearly and articulating himself or herself to a degree that it interferes with the ability to verbally communicate a thought (APA, 2013).
(b) The difficulty in speaking clearly is significant enough that it interferes with an individual's ability to fully interact socially, as well as interfere with the person's academic achievement or the ability to work or complete other tasks (APA, 2013).

Articulation difficulties are part of the normal developmental process, with approximately 50 % of speech being understandable, for example, for a 2-year-old (APA, 2013). Therefore, a speech sound disorder is not diagnosed until it is clear that the child's difficulties are not due to young age and that they continue despite the child entering preschool or kindergarten.

The second type of speech disorder described in the DSM-5 is Childhood-Onset Fluency Disorder, otherwise referred to as stuttering. Stuttering is typically described as poor flow of speaking, with the child speaking at an atypical rate or rhythm and repeating sounds, syllables, words, or phrases while speaking. In order to qualify for a diagnosis, the DSM-5 indicates that at least one of the following two criteria must be present:

(a) Sound and syllable repetitions; sound prolongations of consonants and vowels; speaking with broken words; pausing within a word; frequent pauses in speech; word-finding difficulties which results in word substitutions; words produced with an excess of physical tension; monosyllabic whole-word repetitions (APA, 2013).
(b) These difficulties with fluent speech cause anxiety about speaking or similar to speech sound disorder the difficulty in speaking clearly is significant enough that it interferes with an individual's ability to fully interact socially, as well as interferes with the person's academic achievement or ability to work or complete other tasks (APA, 2013).

Language Disorder. A language disorder is defined by having significant impairments in receptive or expressive language. Receptive language is essentially the ability to understand what is said by others, while expressive language is the ability to express thoughts verbally. The DSM-5 criteria for diagnosing a language disorder include the following:

(a) Persistent difficulties in the use of spoken, written, or other types of language that is due directly to deficits in comprehension or expression. These deficits may include reduced vocabulary and word knowledge; limited ability to structure sentences and put words together that meet basic grammatical rules; or impairments in discourse or the ability to use vocabulary and combined sentences to verbally describe things during a conversation (APA, 2013).
(b) Similar to other communication disorders, the language difficulties must be significant enough to interfere with an individual's ability to fully interact socially, as well as interfere with the person's academic achievement or ability to work or complete other tasks (APA, 2013).

A speech-language therapist typically makes the diagnosis of a communication disorder and determines the type and severity level. A variety of diagnostic procedures are used in the assessment process, including a detailed interview and collection of background information; informal observations of the child interacting with the parents, teachers, peers, or speech-language therapist; and through the administration of standardized assessment instruments such as the *Clinical Evaluation of Language Fundamentals*, which provides an objective measure of a child's grammatical and semantic skills (Wiig, Semel, & Secord, 2013).

Etiology and Treatment

There are a variety of factors that can lead to communication difficulties, with these factors ranging from hearing difficulties, physical impairments (e.g., cleft palate), intellectual disabilities, developmental disabilities, neurological disorders, or congenital disorders. While a variety of theories and factors have been identified as contributing to the etiology of communication disorders, the cause in many children is unknown. Theories have included the one posited by Gopnik (1990) that the core to language difficulties is an inherent inability to learn and understand implicit grammar rules of language, while others have suggested that such difficulties are related to processing deficits (Van der Lely, 1994) or broad deficits in cognitive processes related to language (Ullman & Pierpont, 2005).

Research has suggested that there may be a large genetic influence of communication disorders, as has been demonstrated by several studies with monozygotic and dizygotic twin sets (e.g., Bishop & Hayiou-Thomas, 2008; DeThorne et al., 2006; Vernes et al., 2008). Interestingly, although communication disorders are developmental in nature and often present from birth, there is little research to suggest that there are structural differences in the brains of children and adolescents with communication disorders. However, there is some evidence to support that there are functional differences in the brains, with the observations of there being over- or under-activation in areas related to speech and language (e.g., Broca's areas), but these are relatively limited findings (Webster & Shevell, 2004).

Research supporting the effects of environmental influences on communication disorders is limited, but studies have found that children who are in environments that allow for frequent speaking with parents, as well as exposure to a variety of experiences, have more extensive vocabularies (e.g., Hart & Risley, 1995). Other influences include medical difficulties, with children having more chronic ear infections being at risk for developing language difficulties (Bluestone & Klein, 2007).

The primary treatment intervention for communication disorders is speech therapy. Speech therapy may be conducted in individual and/or small group settings with a speech therapist, and are typically individualized based on the child's needs. Goals may include working on articulation, helping the child learn new vocabulary, helping the child learn appropriate word forms and grammar, or helping the child better organize his or her thoughts (Kuder, 2012). In the school setting, students often receive special education services to assist with their communication difficulties and in developing modifications and accommodations in their classroom settings. These may include reading test questions aloud to a student and providing additional clarification, providing instructions both verbally and visually, and giving alternative requirements for projects or assignments (Kuder, 2012). Research has been mixed regarding the long-term prognosis for communication disorders. Typically, those with mild communication disorders (e.g., articulation) have been found to have better success with interventions; however, it is thought that secondary difficulties remain, particularly in the area of academic achievement (Law, Garrett, & Nye, 2004). Regardless, early intervention is critical to long-term success as many problems (e.g., poor articulation) are difficult to treat later in life.

Implications on Functioning

Being able to speak and understand others is an essential part of learning, socializing, and functioning in society. These experiences are important aspects of a child's life and development, which is why communication disorders have been shown to have a broad impact on the life and functioning of an individual with early communication delays (Johnson et al., 1999). Specifically, communication disorders have been found to impact cognitive development, academic skills and achievement, social skill development, and behavior regulation and control (APA, 2013). Even slight delays that are remediated early in life may impact a child's early development enough that delays are also observed in other areas later in life. For example, speech articulation difficulties, though often remediated with speech therapy in preschool and early elementary school, have been found to be related to later reading difficulties, delays, or even reading disabilities (Shaywitz, 1998).

Cognitive and Academic Implications. Research examining the cognitive effects of a communication disorder has not identified specific deficits in executive functioning, memory, or general intelligence. However, deficits in verbal intelligence have been noted. For example, studies have reported that these children take longer to learn new words (Rice, Oetting, Marquis, Bode, & Pae, 1994), which can contribute to a weak vocabulary and lower verbal reasoning.

Research findings have suggested that children who experience communication delays are at a greater risk for academic difficulties. School is largely verbal, and understanding teacher instructions, participating in class discussions, and group learning largely relies on language abilities. Therefore, it is not surprising that children with communication disorders may struggle academically. In addition, it is not surprising that these children may have significant difficulty in the area of reading. In this regard, research has found that communication delays in early childhood and preschool are a risk factor for reading disabilities (Shaywitz, 1998). For example, one difficulty associated with language disorders is auditory processing deficits. An auditory processing deficit is essentially a deficit in the ability to process the sound of speech (e.g., hear the letter "d" as /d/ rather than /g/ or /k/. These deficits can create early difficulties in comprehending language, as words do not sound as they should. It has also been hypothesized that these problems perceiving, understanding, and creating speech sounds may later manifest themselves in a reading disability (Shaywitz, 1998).

Social-Emotional and Behavioral Implications. In regard to social-emotional implications, a communication disorder or delay at a young age may prevent a child from fully interacting with his or her peers and forming appropriate peer relationships. Because of this, professionals have suggested that adolescents with communication disorders are at risk for social and familial problems, and are likely to have difficulty meeting the expectations and high demands of a verbally-oriented school environment (e.g., APA, 2013; Whitmire, 2000). Being able to effectively communicate and interact with peers and adults is an important part of the developmental process, and limited interactions can lead to weak social and interpersonal skills.

These difficulties can also lead to behavioral disruptions. The relationship between communication difficulties and disruptive behaviors has been examined in the research literature since the early 1900s. For example, an early child development specialist, E. Bosworth McCready (1926), wrote of his observations in his research involving children with language and reading difficulties in which he theorized that speech and language difficulties were likely a contributing factor to the emotional difficulties and antisocial like conduct he frequently observed in language-impaired children. Samuel Torrey Orton (1937), a neurologist, also wrote on the presentation of children with communication disorders and, similar to McCready, stated that "any disorder in the normal acquisition of spoken or written language serves as a severe hindrance to academic achievement and often also lies at the root of serious emotional disturbances" (p. 12). Later research has continued to support the increase in behavior problems associated with children having communication and disorders (e.g., Benner, Nelson, & Epstein, 2002; Conti-Ramsden & Botting, 2008).

An increased risk for mental health problems has also been noted in children and adolescents with communication disorders (e.g., Conti-Ramsden & Botting, 2008; Rescorla, Ross, & McClure, 2007; Snowling, Bishop, Stothard, Chipchase, & Kaplan, 2006). These problems have been found to be significant enough that previous analyses have found that half of all referrals for psychiatric services involve children with language or communication difficulties, many of whom have never had their language difficulties diagnosed (e.g., Cohen, Barwick, Horodezky, & Vallance, 1998).

Communication Disorders and Juvenile Delinquency

When examining the functional implications of communication disorders—social skill impairments, poor academic achievement, reading difficulties, increase in risk of mental health difficulties, and the relationship between language difficulties and disruptive behaviors—it should not be surprising that there is a higher prevalence of communication disorders in the juvenile delinquency population than there is in the general population of youth. In this regard, studies have estimated that communication disorders impact approximately 3–6 % of the general population, while prevalence rates for youth offenders with communication disorders have ranged from 14 % to over 50 % (e.g., Bryan, Freer, & Furlong, 2007; Quinn et al., 2005). The reason that these latter percentages vary is likely due to the variation in methodology used across studies to determine if the youth had a communication disorder. For example, many studies use criteria such as a history of the participants receiving speech-language services, student participation in special education for speech-language impairments, or a documented clinical diagnosis of a communication disorder, while other researchers may choose to conduct an independent speech evaluation of each participant prior to initiating the research to determine the level of language skills in participants. Those studies which rely on whether it is reported in the youth's record that special education services were provided or rely on the presence in the record of a prior diagnosis of a communication disorder are likely to find lower estimates due variability across jurisdictions in placing such information in a student's records.

In this regard, a study by Quinn et al. (2005) examined samples of delinquents across the country that were receiving special education services, but these researchers did not include speech-language impairments in their reported findings since the sample sizes were small. However, when Bryan et al. (2007) conducted speech evaluations on a randomly selected sample of youth offenders, they found that nearly three-quarters of the sample had below average language skills, with over 50 % demonstrating moderate to severe impairments. Although it is not clear from the findings whether these latter youth met the criteria for a communication disorder, the results are nevertheless noteworthy in demonstrating the level of language impairment that may exist among youth offenders. In another study, Sanger, Moore-Brown, Magnuson, and Svoboda (2001) found that while only 4 % of their sample had received speech-language services in the past, 19–46 % of those evaluated would have met criteria for speech-language services.

The deficits and impairments associated with communication disorders may affect youth offenders in a variety of ways during their interaction with the juvenile justice system, depending on the type of communication disorder that is manifested by these youth. Immediate difficulties may be present upon first interaction with law enforcement personnel, if the youth are unable to answer questions fully, explain themselves and the circumstances under which they came to the attention of law enforcement personnel, or understand instructions or demands from a police officer. During court hearings, youth having communication disorders that have a negative effect on expressive language may have trouble fully participating in their defense and communicating with their attorney or the judge. Those youth who have impaired receptive language may also be misconstrued as demonstrating defiance, noncompliance, or general conduct problems when, in fact, they do not understand the requirements or demands being asked of them.

A common difficulty in youth with communication disorders is a deficit in pragmatic language (APA, 2013). An understanding of pragmatics in language is essentially an understanding of the underlying or implied meaning, and understanding pragmatics means that an individual can use context cues to understand the meaning of various phrases. For example, the response "Yeah" could be understood as a literal "Yes" or as a sarcastic way of saying "No." It also involves understanding more than what is said. For example, if a child walks into the house on a cold winter day and his mother yells, "The heat is on!" a child with good pragmatic language would interpret that his mother is really saying, "Shut the door!" Whereas a child with poor pragmatics may take the mother's statement concretely, and only answer "Ok" rather than shut the door. This impairment in pragmatic language could make it difficult for the youth offender to interact with his or her attorney or understand all the subtle nuances that may occur when he or she has contact with juvenile court personnel or during his or her judicial proceedings.

In addition to difficulties interacting with court personnel, a communication disorder may also impact treatment programming, given that many juvenile offenders with communication disorders may not have the required verbal skills that are necessary to participate in many common intervention programs. These programs rely heavily on the ability to understand and express language (Bryan et al., 2007) and, unfortunately, a lack of participation could be misconstrued as apathy or disinterest if a youth is not participating.

Impact on Risk and Risk Assessment. Overall, there do not appear to be any significant characteristics associated with communication disorders that would specifically increase the level of risk that a youth offender presents to the community. While youth with communication disorders are at a greater risk for social–emotional and behavioral problems, there is no evidence to suggest that these impairments directly lead to antisocial thinking or related behaviors (Conti-Ramsden & Botting, 2008). These youth may have a greater level of perceived risk if their inability to express themselves is viewed as having limited empathy or remorse for their illegal acts or contributes to their nonparticipation in intervention programming (antisocial traits) when, in fact, they cannot fully express an understanding or have receptive language problems that prevent them from expressing themselves or participate in treatment programs.

Competency. In regard to competency, the impact that a juvenile's communication disorder has on his or her level of competency will likely be largely related to his or her type of communication disorder, as well as the severity of the communication impairment, and the level of impairment in verbal intelligence. In the case of a speech disorder that affects the youth's intelligibility and clarity when speaking, this disorder does not typically impair verbal intelligence as is the case for a language disorder. It is therefore reasonable to assume that a youth offender having a speech disorder would not significantly impact his or her factual or rational understanding of the court process. What would need to be considered, however, is the severity of the speech disorder and how it may affect the youth's ability to communicate with his or her attorney and assist in the defense.

In regard to language disorders, the level of severity of the expressive or receptive language component would be the primary consideration when determining the impact on competency. A youth with a disorder in receptive language may have difficulty fully understanding and comprehending what is occurring during the court process and trial and, therefore, while the youth may have factual knowledge of the procedures he or she may have a limited rational understanding. In the case of an expressive language disorder, a youth may have knowledge and understanding but have limited ability to express this knowledge and, therefore, demonstrate impairments in his or her ability to effectively communicate with the attorney and assist in the defense.

Remediation and restoration of competency will also likely depend on the type and severity of the impairment associated with the communication disorder. Speech disorders would be more remediable to restoration programs, particularly if the youth offender is able to receive an individualized one-to-one intervention program that can accommodate poor intelligibility of speech. Youth having language disorders, however, may be less responsive to remediation since, as with other disabilities discussed in this chapter, language disorders are a developmental disability and many of the impairments will be present across the person's lifespan. Intervention programs may improve a youth's expressive and receptive language skills, but the level of remediation achieved must be carefully evaluated to ensure that the restoration is successful.

References

Allen, G., & Courchesne, E. (2003). Differential effects of developmental cerebellar abnormality on cognitive and motor functions in the cerebellum: An fMRI study of autism. *The American Journal of Psychiatry, 160*(2), 262–273.

American Psychiatric Association. (1980). *Diagnostic and statistical manual of mental disorders* (3rd ed.). Washington, DC: Author.

American Psychiatric Association (2000). *Diagnostic and statistical manual for mental disorders* (4th ed. Text Revision). Washington, DC: Author.

American Psychiatric Association. (2013). *Diagnostic and statistical manual for mental disorders* (5th ed.). Washington, DC: Author.

Baltruschat, L., Hasselhorn, M., Tarbox, J., Dixon, D. R., Najdowski, A. C., Mullins, R. D., … Gould, E. R. (2011). Addressing working memory in children with autism through behavioral intervention. *Research in Autism Spectrum Disorders, 5*, 267–276.

Bandura, A. (1969). *Principles of behavior modification*. New York, NY: Holt.

Baron-Cohen, S. (1995). *Mindblindness. An essay on autism and theory of mind*. Cambridge, MA: MIT Press.

BBC (2012). Profile: Gary McKinnon. Retrieved from http://www.bbc.com/news/uk-19946902.

Benner, G. J., Nelson, R., & Epstein, M. H. (2002). Language skills of children with EBD: A literature review. *Journal of Emotional and Behavioral Disorders, 10*, 453–467. doi:10.1177/106342660201000105.

Bennetto, L., Pennington, B., & Rogers, S. J. (1996). Intact and impaired memory functions in autism. *Child Development, 67*(4), 1816–1835. doi:10.2307/1131734.

Billstedt, E., Gillberg, C., & Gillberg, C. (2005). Autism after adolescence: Population-based 13-to 22-year follow-up study of 120 individuals with autism diagnosed in childhood. *Journal of Autism and Developmental Disorders, 35*(3), 351–360. doi:10.1007/s10803-005-3302-5.

Bishop, D. V. M., & Hayiou-Thomas, M. E. (2008). Heritability of specific language impairment depends on diagnostic criteria. *Genes, Brain, and Behavior, 7*(3), 365–372. doi:10.1111/j.1601-183x.2007.00360.x.

Bluestone, C. D., & Klein, J. O. (2007). *Otitis media in infants and children* (4th ed.). Philadelphia, PA: WB Saunders.

Brambilla, P., Harden, A., di Nemi, S. U., Perez, J., Soares, J. C., & Barale, F. (2003). Brain anatomy and development in autism: Review of structural MRI studies. *Brain Research Bulletin, 61*(6), 557–569. doi:10.1016/j.brainresbull.2003.06.001.

Brame, R., Turner, M. G., Paternoster, R., & Bushway, S. D. (2012). Cumulative prevalence of arrest from ages 8 to 23 in a national sample. *Pediatrics, 129*(1), 21–27. doi:10.1542/peds.2010-3710.

Brookman-Frazee, L., Baker-Ericzen, M., Stahmer, A., Mandell, D., Haine, R. A., & Hough, R. L. (2009). Involvement of youth with autism spectrum disorders or intellectual disabilities in multiple public service systems. *Journal of Mental Health Research in Intellectual Disabilities, 2*(3), 201–219. doi:10.1080/19315860902741542.

Bryan, K., Freer, J., & Furlong, C. (2007). Language and communication difficulties in juvenile offenders. *International Journal of Language and Communication Disorders, 42*(5), 505–520. doi:10.1080/13682820601053977.

Bullock, L. M., & McArthur, P. (1994). Correctional special education: Disability prevalence estimates and teacher preparation programs. *Education and Treatment of Children, 17*, 347–355.

Burd, L., Fisher, W., & Kerbesbian, J. (1987). A prevalence study of pervasive developmental disorders in North Dakota. *Journal of the American Academy of Child and Adolescent Psychiatry, 26*, 700–703.

Casey, P., & Keilitz, I. (1990). Estimating the prevalence of learning disabled and mentally retarded juvenile offenders: A meta-analysis. In P. E. Leone (Ed.), *Understanding trouble and troubling youth* (pp. 82–101). Newbury Park, CA: Sage.

Center for Disease Control and Prevention. (2014). *Prevalence of autism spectrum disorder among children aged 8 years—Autism and Developmental Disabilities Monitoring Network, 11 sites, United States, 2010.* Atlanta, GA: Author.

Chakrabarti, S., & Fombonne, E. (2001). Pervasive developmental disorders in preschool children. *Journal of the American Medical Association, 285*(24), 3093–3099. doi:10.1001/jama.285.24.3093.

Charlop-Christy, M. H., Malmberg, D. B., Rocha, M. L., & Schreibman, L. (2008). Treating autistic spectrum disorder. In R. J. Morris & T. R. Kratochwill (Eds.), *The practice of child therapy* (4th ed., pp. 299–336). New York, NY: Lawrence Erlbaum.

Cheely, C. A., Carpenter, L. A., Letourneau, E. J., Nicholas, J. S., Charles, J., & King, L. B. (2012). The prevalence of youth with autism spectrum disorders in the criminal justice system. *Journal of Autism and Developmental Disorders, 42*(9), 1856–1862. doi:10.1007/s10803-011-1427-2.

Cohen, N. J., Barwick, M. A., Horodezky, N. B., & Vallance, D. D. (1998). Language, achievement, and cognitive processing psychiatrically disturbed children with previously identified and unsuspected language impairments. *Journal of Child Psychology and Psychiatry, 39,* 865–877.

Conti-Ramsden, G. M., & Botting, N. (2008). Emotional health in adolescents with and without a history of specific language impairment (SLI). *Journal of Child Psychology and Psychiatry, 49*(5), 516–525. doi:10.1111/j.1469-7610.2007.01858.x.

Cook, J. L., & Cook, G. (2008). *Child development principles and perspectives* (2nd ed.). New York, NY: Pearson.

Cooper, M., Thapar, A., & Jones, D. K. (2014). White matter microstructure predicts autistic traits in attention-deficit/hyperactivity disorder. *Journal of Autism and Developmental Disorders, 44,* 2742–2754. doi:10.1007/s10803-014-2131-9.

DeThorne, L. S., Hart, S. A., Petrill, S. A., Deater-Deckard, K., Thompson, L. A., Schatschneider, C., ... Davison, M. D. (2006). Children's history of speech-language difficulties: Genetic influences and associations with reading-related measures. *Journal of Speech, Language, and Hearing Research, 49*(6), 1280–1293. doi:10.1044/1092-4388(2006/092).

de Vries, M., Prins, P. J. M., Schmand, B. A., & Geurts, H. M. (2015). Working memory and cognitive flexibility training for children with an autism spectrum disorder: A randomized controlled trial. *Journal of Child Psychology & Psychiatry, 56,* 56–567. doi:10.1111/jcpp.12324.

Fergusson, D. M., & Horwood, L. (2002). Male and female offending trajectories. *Development and psychopathology, 14*(01), 159–177. doi:10.1017/s0954579402001098.

Fidler, D. J., Bailey, J. N., & Smalley, S. L. (2000). Macrocephaly in autism and other pervasive developmental disorders. *Developmental Medicine and Child Neurology, 42*(11), 737–740. doi:10.1111/j.1469-8749.2000.tb00035.x.

Frith, U., & Happe, F. (1994). Autism: Beyond "theory of mind". *Cognition, 50*(1), 115–132. doi:10.1016/0010-0277(94)90024-8.

Geurts, H. M., deVries, M., & van den Bergh, S. F. W. M. (2014). Executive functioning theory and autism. In S. Goldstein & J. A. Naglieri (Eds.), *Handbook of executive functioning* (pp. 121–141). New York, NY: Springer.

Grisso, T. (2013). *Forensic evaluation of juveniles* (2nd ed.). Sarasota, FL: Professional Resource Press.

Grisso, T., & Quinlan, J. (2005). Juvenile court clinical services: A national description. *Juvenile and Family Court Journal, 56*(4), 9–20. doi:10.1111/j.1755-6988.2005.tb00175.x.

Gopnik, M. (1990). Feature-blind grammar and dysphasia. *Nature, 344,* 715. doi:10.1038/344715a0.

Haar, S., Berman, S., Behrmann, M., & Dinstein, I. (2014). Anatomical abnormalities in autism?. *Cerebral Cortex, 35*(14) doi:10.1093/cercor/bhu242.

Harden, A. Y., Minshew, N. J., Mallikarjuhn, M., & Keshavan, M. S. (2001). Brain volume in autism. *Journal of Child Neurology, 16*(6), 421–424. doi:10.1177/088307380101600607.

Hart, B., & Risley, T. R. (1995). *Meaningful differences in the everyday experience of young American children.* Baltimore, MD: Paul H. Brookes.

Herbert, M. R. (2005). Large brains in autism: The challenge of pervasive abnormality. *The Neuroscientist, 11*(5), 417–440. doi:10.1177/1073858405278866.

References

Hirschi, T., & Hindelang, M. J. (1977). Intelligence and delinquency: A revisionist review. *American Sociological Review, 42*, 571–587. doi:10.2307/2094556.

Howlin, P. (2004). *Autism: Preparing for adulthood* (2nd ed.). London, England: Routledge.

Johnson, C. J., Beitchman, J. H., Young, A., Escobar, M., Atkinson, L., Wilson, B., … Wang, M. (1999). Fourteen-year follow-up of children with and without speech/language impairments: Speech/language stability and outcomes. *Journal of Speech, Language and Hearing, 42*(3), 744-760.doi:10.1044/jslhr.4203.744.

Johnson, M. H., Gliga, T., Jones, E., & Charman, T. (2015). Annual research review: Infant development, autism, and ADHD—early pathways to emerging disorders. *The Journal of Child Psychology & Psychiatry, 56*, 228–247.

Josepth, R. M., & Tanaka, J. (2003). Holistic and part-based faced recognition in children with autism. *Journal of Child Psychology and Psychiatry, 44*(4), 529–542. doi:10.1111/1469-7610.00142.

Just, M. A., Cherkassky, V. L., Keller, T. A., & Minshew, N. J. (2004). Cortical activation and synchronization during sentence comprehension in high-functioning autism: Evidence of underconnectivity. *Brain, 127*(8), 1811–1821. doi:10.1093/brain/awh199.

Kanner, L. (1943). Autistic disturbances of affective contact. *Nervous Child, 2*, 217–250.

Keilitz, I., & Dunivant, N. (1987). The learning disabled offender. In C. M. Nelson, R. B. Rutherford, & B. I. Wolford (Eds.), *Special education in the criminal justice system* (pp. 120–137). Columbus, OH: Merrill.

Kenworthy, L., Anthony, L. G., Naiman, D. Q., Cannon, L.,Wills, M. C., Luong-Tran, C., … & Bal, E. (2014).Randomized controlled effectiveness trial of executive function intervention for children on the autism spectrum. *Journal of Child Psychology and Psychiatry, 55*, 274–383.

King, C., & Murphy, G. H. (2014). A systematic review of people with autism spectrum disorder and the criminal justice system. *Journal of Autism and Developmental Disorder, 44*, 2717–2733. doi:10.1007/s10803-014-2046-5.

Klin, A., Jones, W., Schultz, R., Volkmar, F., & Cohen, D. (2002). Visual fixation patterns during viewing of naturalistic social situations as predictors of social competence in individuals with autism. *Archives of General Psychiatry, 59*(9), 809–816. doi:10.1001/archpsyc.59.9.809.

Koolhof, R., Loeber, R., Wei, E. H., Pardini, D., & D'Escury, A. C. (2007). Inhibition deficits of serious delinquent boys of low intelligence. *Criminal Behaviour and Mental Health, 17*(5), 274–292. doi:10.1002/cbm.661.

Kuder, S. J. (2012). *Teaching students with language and communication disabilities* (4th ed.). New York, NY: Pearson.

Larson, K. A. (1988). A research review and alternative hypothesis explaining the link between learning disabilities and delinquency. *Journal of Learning Disabilities, 21*(6), 257–263. doi:10.1177/002221948802100607.

Law, J., Garrett, Z., & Nye, C. (2004). The efficacy of treatment for children with developmental speech and language delay/disorder: A meta-analysis. *Journal of Speech, Language, and Hearing Research, 47*(4), 924–943.

Leonard, L. B. (1998). *Children with specific language impairment*. Cambridge, MA: MIT Press.

Leffert, J., Siperstein, G., & Widaman, K. (2010). Social perception in children with intellectual disabilities: The interpretation of benign and hostile intentions. *Journal of Intellectual Disability Research, 54*, 168–180. doi:10.1111/j.1365-2788.2009.01240.x.

Leyfer, O. T., Folstein, S. E., Bacalman, S., Davis, N. O., Dinh, E., Morgan, J., … Lainhart, J. E. (2006). Comorbid psychiatric disorders in children with autism: Interview development and rates of disorders. *Journal of Autism and Developmental Disorders, 36*(7), 849-861. doi:10.1007/s10803-006-0123-0.

Lord, C., & McGee, J. P. (2001). *Educating children with autism*. Washington, DC: National Academy Press.

Lotter, V. (1966). Epidemiology of autistic conditions in young children. *Social Psychiatry, 1*(3), 124–137. doi:10.1007/bf00584048.

Matson, J. L., Terlonge, C., & Minshawi, N. F. (2008). Children with intellectual disabilities. In R. J. Morris & T. R. Kratochwill (Eds.), *The practice of child therapy* (4th ed., pp. 337–362). New York, NY: Lawrence Erlbaum.

Mayes, S., & Calhoun, S. L. (2008). WISC-IV and WIAT-II profiles in children with high-functioning autism. *Journal of Autism and Developmental Disorders, 38*, 428–439.

Mayes, T. A. (2003). Persons with autism and criminal justice: Core concepts and leading cases. *Journal of Positive Behavior Interventions, 5*(2), 92–100. doi:10.1177/10983007030050020401.

McCready, B. (1926). Defects in the zone of language (word-deafness and word-blindness) and their influence in education and behavior. *American Journal of Psychiatry, 83*(2), 267–277.

McDermott, S., Durkin, M. S., Schupt, N., & Stein, Z. A. (2007). Epidemiology and etiology of mental retardation. In J. W. Jacobson, J. A. Mulikc, & J. Rojann (Eds.), *Handbook of intellectual and developmental disabilities* (pp. 3–40). New York, NY: Springer.

Mervis, C. B., & John, A. E. (2010). Intellectual disability syndromes. In K. O. Yeates, M. D. Ris, H. G. Taylor, & B. F. Pennington (Eds.), *Pediatric neuropsychology: Research, theory, and practice* (2nd ed., pp. 447–472). New York, NY: Springer.

O'Hearn, K., Asato, M., Ordaz, S., & Luna, B. (2008). Neurodevelopment and executive function in autism. *Development and psychopathology, 20*(04), 1103–1132. doi:10.1017/s0954579408000527.

Osher, D., Woodruff, D., & Sims, A. (2002). Schools make a difference: The relationship between education services for African American children and youth and their overrepresentation in the juvenile justice system. In D. Losen (Ed.), *Minority issues in special education* (pp. 93–116). Cambridge, MA: The Civil Rights Project, Harvard University and the Harvard Education.

Orton, S. T. (1937). *Reading, writing, and speech problems in children*. New York, NY: Norton.

Pennington, B. F., & Ozonoff, S. (1996). Executive functions and developmental psychopathology. *Journal of Child Psychology and Psychiatry, 37*(1), 51–87. doi:10.1111/j.1469-7610.1996.tb01380.x.

Peters, J. M., Taquet, M., Vega, C., Jeste, S. S., Fernandez, I. S., Tan, J., ... Warfield SK.et al. (2013). Brain functional networks in syndromic and non-syndromic autism: A graph theoretical study of EEG connectivity. *BMC Medicine, 11*, 54. doi:10.1186/1741-7015-11-54.

Quinn, M. M., Rutherford, R. B., Leone, P. E., Osher, D. M., & Poirier, J. M. (2005). Youth with disabilities in juvenile corrections: A national survey. *Exceptional Children, 71*(3), 339–345. doi:10.1177/001440290507100308.

Rapin, I. (1997). Autism. *New England Journal of Medicine, 337*, 97–104. doi:10.1056/nejm199707103370206.

Rescorla, L., Ross, G. S., & McClure, S. (2007). Language delay and behavioral/emotional problems in toddlers: Findings from two developmental clinics. *Journal of Speech, Language, and Hearing Research, 50*(4), 1063–1078. doi:10.1044/1092-4388(2007/074).

Rice, C. E., Baio, J., Van Naarden Braun, K., Doernberg, N., Meaney, F. J., & Kirby, R. S. (2007). A public health collaboration for the surveillance of autism spectrum disorders. *Pediatric and Perinatal Epidemiology, 21*(2), 179–190. doi:10.1111/j.1365-3016.2007.00801.x.

Rice, M. L., Oetting, J. B., Marquis, J., Bode, J., & Pae, S. (1994). Frequency of input effects on word comprehension of children with specific language impairment. *Journal of Speech, Language, and Hearing Research, 37*(1), 106–122. doi:10.1044/jshr.3701.106.

Rumsey, J. M. (1985). Conceptual problem-solving in highly verbal, nonretarded autistic men. *Journal of Autism and Developmental Disorders, 15*(1), 23–36. doi:10.1007/bf01837896.

Russell, J. (1997). *Autism as an executive disorder*. New York, NY: Oxford University Press.

Rutter, M. (1978). Language disorder and infantile autism. In M. Rutter & E. Schopler (Eds.), *Autism: A reappraisal of concepts and treatment* (pp. 85–104). New York, NY: Plenum Press.

Sanger, D. D., Moore-Brown, B., Magnuson, G., & Svoboda, N. (2001). Prevalence of language problems among adolescent delinquents: A closer look. *Communication Disorders Quarterly, 23*(1), 17–26. doi:10.1177/152574010102300104.

Schalock, R. L., Buntinx, W. H. E., Borthwick-Duffy, S., Bradley, V., Craig, E. M., Coulter, D. L., ... Yeager, M. H. (2010). *Intellectual disability: Definition, classification, and system of supports*. Washington, DC: American Association on Intellectual and Developmental Disabilities.

Schalock, R. L., Borthwick-Duffy, S. A., Buntinx, W. H. E., Coulter, D. L., & Craig, E. M. (2009). *Intellectual disability: Definition, classification, and systems of supports* (11th ed.). Washington, DC: American Association on Intellectual and Developmental Disabilities.

Shaywitz, S. E. (1998). Dyslexia. *New England Journal of Medicine, 338*(5), 307–312. doi:10.1056/nejm199801293380507.

References

Sigman, M., & McGovern, C. W. (2005). Improvement in cognitive and language skills from preschool to adolescence in autism. *Journal of Autism and Developmental Disorders, 35*(1), 15–23. doi:10.1007/s10803-004-1027-5.

Simonoff, E., Pickles, A., Charman, T., Chandler, S., Loucas, T., & Baird, G. (2008). Psychiatric disorders in children with autism spectrum disorders: Prevalence, comorbidity, and associated factors in a population-derived sample. *Journal of the American Academy of Child & Adolescent Psychiatry, 47*(8), 921–929. doi:10.1097/chi.0b013e318179964f.

Skinner, B. F. (1938). *The behavior of organisms*. New York, NY: Appleton-Century-Crofts.

Skinner, B. F. (1953). *Science and human behavior*. New York, NY: Macmillan.

Snowling, M. J., Bishop, D. V. M., Stothard, S. E., Chipchase, B., & Kaplan, C. (2006). Psychosocial outcomes at 15 years of children with a preschool history of speech-language impairment. *Journal of Child Psychology and Psychiatry, 47*(8), 759–765. doi:10.1111/j.1469-7610.2006.01631.x.

Snowling, M. J., & Hayious-Thomas, M. E. (2010). Specific language impairment. In K. O. Yeates, M. D. Ris, H. G. Taylor, & B. R. Pennington (Eds.), *Pediatric neuropsychology: Research, theory, and practice* (pp. 363–392). New York, NY: Springer.

Stahlberg, O., Anckarsater, H., & Nilsson, T. (2010). Mental health problems in youth committed to juvenile institutions: Prevalence and treatment needs. *European Child & Adolescent Psychiatry, 19*(12), 893–903. doi:10.1007/s00787-010-0137-1.

Tomblin, J. B., Records, N. L., Buckwalter, P., Zhang, X., Smith, E., & O'Brien, M. (1997). Prevalence of specific language impairment in kindergarten children. *Journal of Speech, Language and Hearing Research, 40*(6), 1245–1260. doi:10.1044/jslhr.4006.1245.

Ullman, M. T., & Pierpont, E. I. (2005). Speech language impairment is not specific to language: The procedural deficit hypothesis. *Cortex, 41*(3), 399–433. doi:10.1016/s0010-9452(08)70276-4.

Van der Lely, H. K. J. (1994). Canonical linking rules: Forward versus linking in normally developing and specifically language-impaired children. *Cognition, 51*(1), 29–72. doi:10.1016/0010-0277(94)90008-6.

Vermeiren, R., Jespers, I., & Moffitt, T. E. (2006). Mental health problems in juvenile justice populations. *Child and Adolescent Psychiatric Clinics of North America, 15*(2), 333–351. doi:10.1016/j.chc.2005.11.008.

Vernes, S. C., Newbury, D. F., Abrahams, B. S., Winchester, L., Nicod, J., Groszer, M., ... Fisher, S. E. (2008). A functional genetic link between distinct developmental language disorders. *New England Journal of Medicine, 359*(22), 2337-2345. doi:10.1056/nejmoa0802828.

Wainwright-Sharp, J. A., & Bryson, S. E. (1993). Visual orienting deficits in high-functioning people with autism. *Journal of Autism and Developmental Disorders, 23*, 1–13. doi:10.1007/bf01066415.

Webster, R. I., & Shevell, M. I. (2004). Topical Review: Neurobiology of specific language impairment. *Journal of Child Neurology, 19*(7), 471–481. doi:10.1177/08830738040190070101.

Whitmire, K. A. (2000). Adolescence as a developmental phase: A tutorial. *Topics in Language Disorders, 20*(2), 1–14. doi:10.1097/00011363-200020020-00003.

Wiig, E. H., Semel, E., & Secord, W. (2013). *Clinical evaluation of language fundamentals—Fifth edition (CELF-5)*. New York, NY: Pearson.

Winnepenninckx, B., Rooms, L., & Kooy, R. F. (2003). Mental retardation: A review of the genetic causes. *The British Journal of Developmental Disabilities, 49*(96), 29–44. doi:10.1179/096979503799104138.

World Health Organization (WHO). (1996). *Multiaxial classification of child and adolescent psychiatric disorders: The ICD-10 classification of mental and behavioral disorders in children and adolescents*. Cambridge, England: Cambridge University Press.

Chapter 8
Learning and Emotional Disabilities

The terms "specific learning disability" and "emotional disturbance" refer to disability diagnoses that are used within school settings and apply to those children and adolescents under 22 years of age who have received one or both of these diagnoses based on the IDEIA, 2004). As was discussed in Chap. 6, the IDEIA is a federal law mandating a free and appropriate education to all students, regardless of their disability, with the first iteration of this law being the EHA (or PL 94-142) that was passed by the US Congress in 1975. This act mandated that all states receiving federal support for the education of students must provide a free and appropriate public education (FAPE) to all eligible youth having a disability until their 22nd birthday. IDEIA further delineated the types of special education services to which all eligible students are entitled. Moreover, the EHA and IDEIA, as well as litigation involving incarcerated youth and other federal mandates, have further clarified that the guarantee of a FAPE applies to all eligible youth with a disability, independent of the educational setting such as a school within a juvenile detention center (Leone, Price, & Vitolo, 1986).

There are a variety of educational disability categories under IDEIA that can qualify a student for receiving special education services. While many DSM-5 diagnoses can qualify a youth for services under IDEIA, having a DSM-5 diagnosis does not automatically qualify a student for special education services, and not all DSM-5 diagnoses are encompassed under IDEIA. For example, while IDEIA]does have eligibility categories for intellectual disability and autism spectrum disorder, a youth with a DSM-5 diagnosis of major depressive disorder does not automatically fall under any IDEIA diagnostic category. Rather, the youth may be considered under the eligibility category of "other health impairment" or "emotional disability" if it is determined that the depression is preventing the student from effectively learning. This is also the case for the DSM-5 diagnosis of attention deficit hyperactivity disorder, with students having this diagnosis also falling under the IDEIA categories of other health impairment or emotional disability if their ability to learn and be educated is interfered with by their attention deficits and/or hyperactivity-related behaviors.

In a 2014 report to the US Congress, the US Department of Education identified specific learning disability (SLD) (also generally referred to as "learning disability") as the most common special education category, with 40.6 % of those in special education receiving services for a SLD. The next most common categories included speech or language impairments (18.2 % of those receiving special education services), other health impairments (13.2 %), autism (7.6 %), intellectual disabilities (7.3 %), and emotional disabilities (6.2 %). While the most common disability in the general student population is SLD, in the juvenile justice system emotional disturbance or emotional disability has been identified as the most prevalent education-related disability, though there is also a high prevalence of SLD (Quinn, Rutherford, Leone, Osher, & Poirier, 2005). This chapter will focus on these latter two disabilities, given their prevalence within the juvenile justice system. Many of the other disabilities that will qualify a student for special education services (e.g., ASD, intellectual disability, or speech-language impairment) were addressed in Chap. 7).

Specific Learning Disability

Since the implementation of PL 94-142, the number of children receiving services for a learning disability has increased exponentially, with the most common disability to be diagnosed among school-age children being SLD. It is a disorder in one or more of the basic psychological processes involved in understanding or in using language (spoken or written) that may manifest itself in difficulty with the ability to listen, think, speak, read, write, or perform math. Learning disabilities do not include learning problems that are primarily the result of visual, hearing, motor, intellectual, or emotional disabilities; rather, they occur with other specific processes related to learning and academic achievement, including reading, writing, and math APA, 2013; IDEA, 2004). According to a report from the US Department of Education (2014), approximately 3.4 % of all students in school receive special education services for a SLD, and of those students in special education, approximately 40 % are receiving services for SLD. Several categories of SLD are listed under IDEIA, with each involving deficits in reading, writing, math, and oral language skills. Since language deficits and related communication disorders have already been discussed in Chap. 6, this section will focus on SLD in the areas of reading, writing, and math.

Learning disabilities are more common in males than females (APA, 2013; US Department of Education, 2014). The reasons behind this are unclear, with some professionals suggesting that it may be largely environmental in that males are more readily identified as they tend to externalize behaviors, with others suggesting that there may be genetic links for SLD to the X chromosome (Sanger Institute, 2009). Although the causes connected to SLD are still being explored, neuroscience has supported differences in the brain and neurological functioning of individuals with SLD (Shaywitz, Mody, & Shaywitz, 2006).

Reading Disabilities

Reading disabilities are the most common type of SLD. In fact, it is estimated that as many as 80 % of all individuals diagnosed as having a SLD have a reading disability (US Department of Education, 2012). Consistent with other learning disabilities, reading disabilities are diagnosed more often in males than females (Flannery, Liederman, Daly, & Schultz, 2000).

A reading disability, otherwise known as *dyslexia*, is a SLD in which an individual fails to make significant progress in learning to read than what would be expected given his or her IQ level and in comparison to typical same-age/same-grade peers (APA, 2013). Reading disabilities, however, are *not related* to IQ; they do not result from a child or adolescent having a low level of intelligence. The unexpected inability to read has presented a conundrum to teachers and parents alike for more than a century, and educators have long reported on cases of children who appear typical in thinking and functioning but have a "word blindness" and unexplained inability to read (Kirk, 1976). The first written reports of this unexplained phenomenon were provided by Pringle Morgan, a physician, in 1896, when he wrote about his experience working with a 14-year-old boy who was unable to learn to read despite appearing to be of at least average intelligence and high functioning in other areas such as math (Critchley, 1970).

Children with dyslexia struggle to read words accurately and fluently, which can subsequently affect their ability to comprehend what they read (Shaywitz, Escobar, Shaywitz, Fletcher, & Makuch, 1992). Many people associate reversing letters (e.g., substituting "b" for "d") as a key indicator of dyslexia. While this can be one symptom of a reading disability, it is actually only a small characteristic in the pool of difficulties commonly observed in students having dyslexia. In addition, letter reversals and switching can occur in typically developing students or those with attention difficulties. Instead, the most notable deficit associated with dyslexia is a struggle at the most basic level to accurately hear the distinct units of words (e.g., Kirk, 1976; Smith, Pennington, Boada, & Shriberg, 2005). For example, while it may be very apparent to a typically developing child that the word "bed" has the distinct sounds of /b/ /e/ and /d/, students with dyslexia are often impaired in the ability to separate out sounds. This difficulty in *phonological awareness* then leads to difficulty in seeing the letter "b" and automatically associating it with the sound /b/. Further difficulties may be observed in a child with dyslexia struggling to associate sounds with the various letters or letter combinations (e.g., /th/ /sh/). These difficulties make learning and using phonics difficult, and subsequently, reading suffers as the child with dyslexia cannot easily and fluidly read words (Mather & Wendling, 2011a, 2011b).

In addition to phonological processing difficulties, students with dyslexia may take additional time to memorize words such as "when" or "while" and other words that cannot be sounded out. Students with dyslexia may also have difficulty in differentiating between similar-looking words such as "lint" and "hint." Because of these difficulties in the fundamental skills needed for reading, individuals with dyslexia take longer to learn to read, have difficulty reading smoothly, and have difficulty understanding what they are reading since their main focus is on figuring out each individual word of a sentence versus focusing on understanding the meaning of a sentence. In addition, these students often struggle to spell accurately, which can impair their ability to express themselves in writing. Difficulties with word problems in math can also occur, because of the reading comprehension required to complete math problems. As students with reading disabilities progress through school and the difficulty level of the school work increases, a variety of academic difficulties may also be observed outside of reading given that reading skills are critical in learning other curriculum topics as science and history. While a student's reading difficulties may first present initially as just a problem in his or her early reading ability in elementary school, the difficulty could become more pronounced and problematic as the complexity of the reading demands on the student increases in middle school or high school. This, in turn, could have a negative impact on the student's later learning and academic success unless special education services and appropriate accommodations are provided.

Both the DSM-5 (APA, 2013) and IDEIA recognize various types of reading disabilities. Specifically, they both acknowledge three main areas of deficits that can occur: (1) SLD with impairment in basic reading skills, (2) SLD with impairment in reading fluency, and (3) SLD with impairment in reading comprehension.

Etiology. While an under-stimulating environment in early childhood, poor parental intervention and support for school, and/or poor academic instruction can all be factors that contribute to reading delays, dyslexia is not due to environmental factors. Rather, dyslexia is a neurodevelopmental disorder, with research demonstrating that there are neurological and functional differences in the brains of individuals with dyslexia compared to their respective same-age typical peers. Using methods such as functional imaging (e.g., fMRIs or PET scans) that allow neuroscientists and others to view brain activity, researchers have identified that the brains of individuals with dyslexia process language and words differently than those without dyslexia. Specifically, the typically developing individual uses primarily the left hemisphere of the brain to read and understand printed words, whereas an individual with dyslexia uses both right and left hemispheres. In addition, individuals with dyslexia have been found to have less activation in certain areas of the brain, which leads to difficulties accurately processing the sounds in the words that they hear, using phonics to figure out a new word, and quickly identifying words that they see in print (Shaywitz & Shaywitz, 2004).

Diagnosis and Treatment. Reading disabilities are typically diagnosed in one of two ways: (1) through the student's school in which special education personnel conduct a psychoeducational evaluation to determine if the student meets the eligibility criteria for SLD with a reading disability, using the diagnostic criteria outlined by IDEIA, or (2) through a qualified private practitioner, such as a licensed psychologist, in which a psychoeducational evaluation is conducted to determine if the student meets diagnostic criteria for a SLD with a reading disability, using IDEA and/or DSM-5 criteria.

IDEA (2004) criteria for a reading disability include the following:

(a) The student does not achieve adequately for his or her given age or is not meeting state-approved grade-level standards when provided with appropriate learning experiences and instruction in the areas of *basic reading skills*, *reading fluency*, or *reading comprehension*.
(b) Insufficient progress can be determined in one of three ways: academic achievement that is significantly below intellectual ability; academic progress despite scientific, research-based intervention, or the student displays a pattern of strengths and weaknesses in performance and achievement relative to age, grade-level standards, or intelligence.
(c) The achievement difficulties are not due to a visual, hearing, or motor disability; intellectual disability; emotional disability; cultural factors; environmental factors; or limited language proficiency.

DSM-5 criteria for diagnosing a reading disability vary slightly but are overall consistent with IDEIA. These diagnostic criteria include:

(a) Difficulties learning and using academic skills despite intervention.
(b) Inaccurate or slow and effortful word reading.
(c) Difficulty understanding the meaning of what is read.
(d) The academic skills are substantially and quantifiably below those expected for the individual's age, cause impairment in functioning, and were present during school-age years.
(e) The learning difficulties are not due to intellectual disabilities, visual or auditory difficulties, other neurological or mental health disorders, socioeconomic disadvantage, limited language proficiency, or inadequate instruction (APA, 2013).

While individuals with a reading disability have difficulty mastering the basic skills needed for reading, this does not mean that they will be unable to learn to read adequately. Rather, since the brain of a person having dyslexia processes language and print words differently than his or her typical peers, he or she needs specialized reading instruction to accommodate the differences in learning. The majority of evidence-based programs designed for individuals with dyslexia are multisensory programs, meaning that they rely not only on verbal instruction but also visual cues and even tactile cues when teaching basic reading skills. In general, reading interventions focus heavily on helping students develop a stronger understanding of phonics and letter-sound combinations (Flanagan & Alfonso, 2010). In the school setting, interventions are typically provided in the least restrictive setting. Consequently, if a student is otherwise developing in a typical manner, he or she will likely be placed in a regular education classroom setting and receive additional reading instruction support services as necessary. This type of resource support can range from occurring only a few times per week at 30 min per session to daily depending on the needs of the student and how reading is impacting his or her performance in other academic areas. In addition to individualized reading instruction, accommodations will be provided to the student that may include the following: the teacher or aide reading a test or exam to the student to ensure reading comprehension does not prevent the student from demonstrating his or her knowledge in content area being examined, providing audio textbooks to the student, and/or allowing the student extended time to complete the test (Mather & Wendling, 2011a, 2011b).

Math Disabilities

Math is a difficult subject for many students in the public school system. The abstract, sequential thinking, problem-solving skills, and attention to detail required to be successful at math often make the content challenging to learn. In addition, math is a subject area that builds quickly on previous learning, so any failure to study or keep up with the required work on the part of a student being truant from school or suspended from school or having significant school absences, can significantly impact the student's success in math. For other students who do not have significant absences and who try to study, math is still difficult because they lack the underlying cognitive systems needed to learn even basic math skills (Barbaresi, Katusic, Colligan, Weaver, & Jacobson, 2005). Specifically, while students who have dyslexia have difficulty mastering the fundamental concepts of reading (e.g., phonological processing), students with math disabilities have difficulty learning and understanding the basic concepts needed for math.

For those who lack understanding of the basic concepts needed for math, difficulties are typically observed in three main areas: *number sense, overlearning and memorizing basic math facts*, and/or *following rules and procedures of various math problems*. In regard to number sense, even a young child who is developing in a typical manner can quickly see that "●●●" is a larger quantity than "●●" and later that "●●● = *3*." As they age, children also begin to understand that while both numbers "7" and "8" are larger numbers than "1" and "2," the difference between them is the same as the difference between the numbers "1" and "2." An individual with a math disability, however, lacks this number sense. For example, they may need to individually count the symbols in "●●●" to determine the quantity, *nn* and do not have an internal number line that helps them understand that the increment between "7" and "8" is *not* actually any larger than that between "1" and "2." Similarly, research has found that students with math disabilities struggle to memorize basic math facts, such as simple addition problems or multiplication tables (e.g., Geary, Hamson, & Hoard, 2000; Jordan, Hanich, & Kaplan, 2003). Because of these deficits in number sense and memorizing basic math facts, when completing even basic addition and subtraction, these students must rely on inefficient strategies such as counting on fingers or making tic marks to help them understand the meaning of the numbers before them. This can slow down their math performance and make it extremely difficult to understand more complex math since as more complex math is presented to students, it is assumed that the students have overlearned these latter basic math skills. In addition to these difficulties in basic skills, children with math disabilities are more likely to make procedural errors (e.g., misaligning double-digit numbers during subtraction or borrowing incorrectly), which contribute to more difficulties with early math skills (Geary, Hoard, Byrd-Craven, Nugent, & Numtee, 2007).

Etiology. While there is considerable research examining the etiology and neurological underpinnings of reading and reading disabilities, considerably less is known about math disabilities. Studies have found that children with math disabilities often have cognitive deficits in the areas of IQ, working memory, and processing speed. For example, research has suggested that those persons with math disabilities typically have low average IQs (Mazzocco, 2007). In addition to low average IQ, deficits in working memory have been found in students with math disabilities (e.g., Geary et al., 2007; Swanson & Sachse-Lee, 2001). Working memory is essentially "memory in action," as it is the ability to hold something in short-term memory and then perform an action with it such as hearing directions and then completing a task based on the instructions. Working memory relies on attention and focus, and it is an important component in academic achievement. For math, working memory is important in completing multiple-step problems (e.g., division, double-digit addition, or subtraction). Studies have found that students with math disabilities perform well below average on working memory tasks (e.g., Geary et al., 2007; Swanson & Sachse-Lee, 2001). Processing speed deficits have also been observed in children with math disabilities (e.g., Murphy, Mazzocco, Hanich, & Early, 2007; Swanson & Sachse-Lee, 2001). Processing speed is essentially one's ability to process information quickly and efficiently. In regard to math, these students are more likely to process and complete basic tasks much more slowly, making learning new procedures and completing math tasks more difficult.

Similar to other types of learning disabilities, a genetic component to math disabilities has been recognized, with family members being several times more likely to be diagnosed with a math disability (Shavlev et al., 2001). Math disabilities have also been found to co-occur with other disabilities. For example, studies have found that nearly 60 % of students with math disabilities also have reading disabilities (Barbaresi et al., 2005). In addition, children with attention deficit hyperactivity disorder have been shown to have difficulty more often with math, presumably because of the negative impact that working memory and attention deficits have on math performance.

Diagnosis and Treatment. As in the case of SLD, math disabilities are typically diagnosed in one of two ways: (1) through the student's school in which special education personnel conduct a psychoeducational evaluation to determine if the student meets the eligibility criteria for SLD with a math disability, using the diagnostic criteria outlined by IDEIA (2004) or (2) through a qualified private practitioner, such as a licensed psychologist, in which a psychoeducational evaluation is conducted to determine if the student meets diagnostic criteria for a SLD for math, using IDEIA and/or DSM-5 criteria.

The IDEIA (2004) criteria for a math disability include the following:

(a) The student does not achieve adequately for their given age or is not meeting state-approved grade-level standards when provided with appropriate learning experiences and instruction in the areas of *mathematics calculation* or *mathematics problem solving*.
(b) Insufficient progress can be determined in one of three ways: achievement that is below general intelligence; insufficient academic progress despite scientific, research-based intervention, or the child displays a pattern of strengths and weaknesses in performance and achievement relative to age, grade-level standards, or intelligence.
(c) The achievement difficulties are not due to a visual, hearing, or motor disability; intellectual disability; emotional disability; cultural factors; environmental factors; or limited language proficiency.

The DSM-5 criteria for diagnosing a math disability vary slightly from reading disability but are overall consistent with IDEIA. These diagnostic criteria include:

(a) Difficulties learning and using academic skills despite intervention.
(b) Difficulties mastering number sense, number factors, or calculation or difficulties with mathematical reasoning.
(c) The academic skills are substantially and quantifiably below those expected for the individual's age, cause impairment, and were present during school-age years.
(d) The learning difficulties are not due to intellectual disabilities, visual or auditory difficulties, other neurological or mental health disorders, socioeconomic disadvantage, limited language proficiency, or inadequate instruction (APA, 2013).

Evidence-based math interventions are much less common than evidence-based interventions for reading disabilities (see, e.g., Morris & Thompson, 2008). The National Mathematics Advisory Panel has provided some guidelines and advised that teacher-guided, explicit instruction that occurs over a long period of time is the most effective type of math intervention (Gersten et al., 2008). In the school setting, students will typically receive individualized instruction, with the amount of instruction increasing as needed to meet the needs of the student (Wendling & Mather, 2008). Generally, if math is the only area of weakness, then the student will remain in the general regular education classroom and attend resource support services when it is time for math instruction. Accommodations may also be provided, such as allowing the student to use a calculator on tests and extra time to complete tests.

Writing Disabilities

Writing is a complex process that is difficult for many individuals, largely because it involves a variety of skills, processes, and mechanisms. The creative aspect of writing relies heavily on language skills (vocabulary, expressive language, comprehension), while the actual act of writing relies heavily on motor and visual skills.

In order to write well, a student needs to be able to generate ideas, organize his or her thoughts coherently and in a logical manner, and then have the spelling skills and motor ability to transfer the ideas onto paper in a neat and legible fashion. Not surprisingly, a deficit in one of these areas can have an appreciable impact on one's ability to write (Berninger & Richards, 2002).

While significant impairments in one's ability to write legibly does not alone qualify an individual for having a SLD diagnosis, the inability to accurately form letters, write neatly, and use correct spacing typically relates to other writing problems. The example below is of a student with *dysgraphia*, which is a writing disability associated with poor transcription (see Fig. 8.1). Students having dysgraphia may have the language capacity needed to express ideas but also have cognitive and/or motor difficulties that otherwise result in handwriting that is extremely difficult to read and, therefore, impairs their ability to write.

In other cases, a student with a writing disability may be able to form letters accurately but have a language impairment that negatively impacts his or her ability to write thoughts on paper in a coherent manner (see Fig. 8.2). Students with this type of difficulty may also have problems expressing themselves orally, through writing, or in both domains.

Finally, a third subgroup of individuals with writing disabilities includes those with difficulties due primarily to their limited ability to spell accurately (see Fig. 8.3). They may have the fine motor and language skills needed to write, but because of a reading disability, their ability to effectively spell negatively impacts their writing at a level that presents as largely incoherent.

Fig. 8.1 Writing sample of a 14-year-old boy with dysgraphia. "I do not like to write"

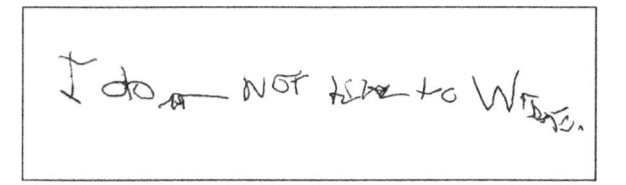

Fig. 8.2 Writing sample of a 10-year-old girl with attention deficit hyperactivity disorder and a SLD in written expression. "The boy is skating"

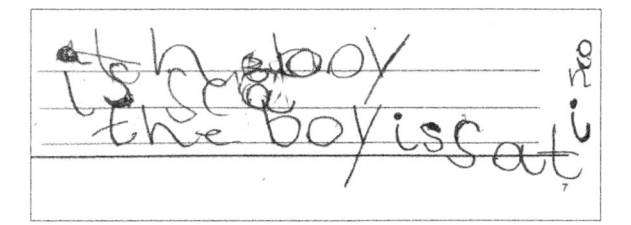

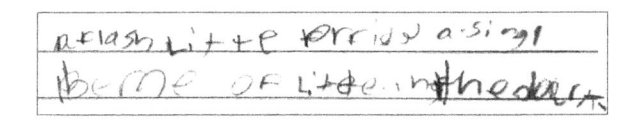

Fig. 8.3 Writing sample from a 13-year-old boy who was diagnosed with attention deficit hyperactivity disorder and a reading disability. "A flashlight provides a single beam of light in the dark"

Writing disabilities are estimated to occur in approximately 5 % of the public school student population (National Center for Education Statistics, 2009), with more males than females experiencing these difficulties (Katusic, Colligan, Weaver, & Barbaresi, 2009; Wiznitzer & Scheffel, 2009). While a writing disability can occur in isolation, this is actually relatively uncommon. Rather, studies have found that nearly three-quarters of students with a writing disability also have learning problems or a SLD in other areas (Flanagan & Alfonso, 2010). For example, Katusic et al. (2009) found that 75 % of students with a writing disability also had reading difficulties. Other studies have found a high incidence of writing disability in youth with attention deficit hyperactivity disorder, with the speculation for this being the similarity in the cognitive difficulties in children having each type of disability or disorder (e.g., DeBono et al., 2012; Rodriguez et al., 2009).

Etiology. Given the multiple systems involved in writing, it is not surprising that there are multiple factors known to be associated with writing disabilities, including genetic, neurological, neuropsychological, and medical conditions. In regard to genetic and neurological factors, family studies have suggested a genetic link to the presence and severity of writing disabilities (e.g., Berninger, Nielsen, Abbott, Wijsman, & Raskind, 2008; Gubbay & de Klerk, 1995). Other studies have suggested that there may be functional differences in the brains of those having a writing disability. For example, researchers at the University of Washington completed a study that utilized fMRIs for children with and without dysgraphia, asking them to write letters. Results found differences in neural connections between the groups, with the results indicating that those with dysgraphia essentially required more neuronal activity to accomplish the same task as those who did not have dysgraphia (Richards et al., 2015).

Several neuropsychological deficits have also been observed in students with writing disabilities. Most notably, studies have found executive functioning deficits to be highly related to writing difficulties (Feifer & De Fina, 2002). As has been discussed previously, executive functioning skills are those higher-level skills that regulate one's behavior. These skills include attention, impulse control, planning, organization, and flexible thinking. Executive functioning deficits are typically observed in individuals having attention deficit hyperactivity disorder, so it is also not surprising that there is a high comorbidity between this mental disorder and writing disabilities. In addition to executive functioning deficits, language impairments are highly associated with writing disabilities, given the critical role of language in written expression (Flanagan & Alfonso, 2010).

Diagnosis and Treatment. As in the case of other learning disabilities, a writing disability is typically diagnosed in one of two ways: (1) through the student's school in which special education personnel conduct a psychoeducational evaluation to determine if the student meets the eligibility criteria for a writing disability, using the diagnostic criteria outlined by IDEIA (2004) or (2) through a qualified private practitioner, such as a licensed psychologist, in which a psychoeducational evaluation is conducted to determine if the student meets diagnostic criteria for a writing disability, using IDEIA or DSM-5 criteria.

IDEIA (2004) criteria for a writing disability include the following:

(a) The student does not achieve adequately for their given age or is not meeting state-approved grade-level standards when provided with appropriate learning experiences and instruction in the areas of *written expression*.
(b) Poor achievement in writing is demonstrated by writing achievement that is significantly below general intelligence, insufficient academic progress in writing despite the use of research-based interventions, or a pattern of performance that shows weak writing and related cognitive abilities, yet strengths in other academic areas and cognitive abilities.
(c) The achievement difficulties are not due to a visual, hearing, or motor disability; intellectual disability; emotional disability; cultural factors; environmental factors; or limited language proficiency.

The DSM-5 criteria for diagnosing a writing disability vary slightly, particularly with the inclusion of spelling difficulties being independently classified, whereas IDEIA does not allow poor spelling alone to qualify a student with a writing disability. DSM-5 diagnostic criteria include the following:

(a) Difficulties learning and using academic skills despite intervention.
(b) Difficulties with spelling or difficulties with written expression.
(c) The academic skills are substantially and quantifiably below those expected for the individual's age, cause impairment, and were present during school-age years.
(d) The learning difficulties are not due to intellectual disabilities, visual or auditory difficulties, other neurological or mental health disorders, socioeconomic disadvantage, limited language proficiency, or inadequate instruction (APA, 2013).

As can be seen, while definitions of SLD involving a writing disability vary slightly between IDEIA and DSM-5, ultimately a diagnosis is based on the clinical evidence that a child or adolescent is unable to effectively express himself or herself in writing at a level that would be expected given his or her age and ability level.

Since there are a variety of factors that contribute to a writing disability (e.g., fine motor deficits, language impairments, dyslexia, executive functioning deficits), treatments for this form of SLD vary considerably. Ultimately, it is important to understand the primary cause of the writing disability in order to identify the most effective intervention. For example, for those children having dysgraphia (who also have the most trouble with the motoric aspects of writing), occupational therapy to improve fine motor skills may be a primary intervention (Berninger, 2007). In addition, these youth may require more individualized instruction in forming letters and accurately spacing words, as well as computer/typing instruction and, possibly, accommodations that use dictation software. On the other hand, youth whose primary source of difficulty is executive functioning deficits and related difficulties in expressing themselves in written words, they will need interventions geared toward helping them learn organization and idea building strategies (Flanagan & Alfonso, 2010).

Much less is known about writing disabilities than reading disabilities, but there are still many evidence-based strategies shown to improve the writing skills of those with writing disabilities (see, for example, Berninger et al., 2008). In general, students with writing disabilities will require accommodations that allow them to use a keyboard and receive extra time when writing, and they will need individualized instruction that explicitly teaches them skills and strategies to organize their writing, effectively construct and combine sentences, and edit their final work (e.g., Cutler & Graham, 2008; Graham & Perin, 2007).

Impact of Specific Learning Disability on Functioning

Impairments in academic functioning are inherent in the diagnosis of any form of SLD, as academic achievement difficulties must be present in order for a student to qualify for this diagnosis. However, it should also be noted that the impact that a SLD diagnosis has on a youth's school success is more far reaching than just difficulties with reading, writing, and/or math. These youth have significantly more suspensions and expulsions in school, and they are also at an increased risk of dropping out of school compared to their typically developing and same-age peers (US Department of Education, 2014). In addition, students with SLD are more likely to experience school failure, have poor grade point averages, be retained a grade level, and are less likely to attend secondary education (National Center for Learning Disabilities, 2013).

As described above in the etiology section of the various learning disabilities, SLD is associated with a variety of cognitive impairments. These vary depending on the type of SLD, but deficits have been observed in working memory, attention, processing speed, and language skills (Flanagan & Alfonso, 2010). These cognitive deficits are likely directly related to the actual learning difficulty, but they also have secondary implications. For example, research has found that many students with learning disabilities also struggle socially (Bender & Wall, 1994), with some studies reporting that as many as 75 % of students with learning disabilities also have social difficulties (Kavale & Forness, 1996). There have been a variety of explanations for this, with a common position being that children with learning disabilities have cognitive processing deficits that lead to difficulties processing social cues and understanding social context (Bauminger, Edelsztein, & Morash, 2005). Interpreting social situations is a critical part in participating in social exchanges with others. The receiver needs to understand the social cues and social contexts of what the speaker is communicating to fully understand the speaker's message. On the other hand, the speaker needs to convey his or her message using his or her knowledge of social communication so that the receiver can interpret what is being conveyed. Having cognitive processing difficulties can have a negative effect on one's ability to participate in a social exchange, making social relationships more difficult to form.

In this regard, Bauminger et al. (2005) found that children with learning disabilities had greater deficits in nonverbal communication skills and, subsequently, had more trouble understanding complex emotions in social situations. These researchers provided social vignettes to students with and without learning disabilities and found that those with learning disabilities had more trouble encoding social cues in each story, understanding social contexts within a story, understanding social goals of those participating in each social exchange, thinking of social responses for the characters in each story, and understanding the relationship between social goals and social solutions. In addition, results found that the students with learning disabilities struggled to understand complex and mixed emotions, with them struggling to identify emotions like anger, loneliness, pride, guilt, and embarrassment. These researchers concluded that students with learning disabilities may not understand the phases of social information processing, which leads to difficulty piecing together what they learned from previous social exchanges and applying it to novel social experiences, influencing their ability to communicate with social goals in mind.

Tur-Kaspa and Bryan (1994) also argued that children with learning disabilities have difficulty with social information processing due to a deficit in perceptual capabilities that negatively impact their ability to encode social situations, while Margalit and Tur-Kaspa (1998) concluded that children with learning disabilities are impulsive with their social responses due to a deficit in self-regulation (and executive functioning) skills. Slower information processing speed has also been implicated in negative emotional states and delays in emotional understanding in social contexts (e.g., Bauminger et al., 2005; Bryan, Sullivan-Burstein, & Mathur, 1998). In addition, students with learning disabilities have reported higher levels of social isolation and distress (Hogan, McLellan, & Bauman, 2000) and may be at a greater risk of being bullied by their peers (e.g., Flanagan & Alfonso, 2010; Martlew & Hodson, 1991).

In addition to causing learning difficulties and thinking deficits, learning disabilities have been associated with emotional difficulties. For example, Gallegos, Langley, and Villegas (2012) found that those students with learning disabilities reported higher levels of depression and anxiety than did their typical peers who did not have a SLD. The causal relationship between these is relatively unclear, as there are two general arguments for this relationship, one argument being that learning difficulties lead to social problems and self-esteem problems or other emotional difficulties and the other that the social and emotional difficulties are due to information processing deficits that contribute to a SLD (Bauminger et al., 2005). Regardless, it is clear that learning disabilities impact a child or adolescent in more ways than in just how they perform academically in the classroom.

Emotional Disabilities

IDEIA uses the category of "emotional disturbance" to describe children whose emotional disabilities are serious enough to impair their academic performance for a long period of time. Criteria used to determine if a student qualifies for an emotional disturbance under IDEIA include (a) an inability to learn that cannot be explained by intellectual, sensory, or health factors; (b) an inability to build or maintain satisfactory interpersonal relationships with peers and teachers, (c) inappropriate types of behavior or feelings under normal circumstances, (d) a general pervasive mood of unhappiness or depression, and/or (e) a tendency to develop physical symptoms or fears associated with personal or school problems (IDEIA, 2004). In order to be considered for special education services, IDEIA mandates that a student must demonstrate at least one of these characteristics for a long period of time and to a degree that his or her educational performance is significantly impaired.

While some students may qualify under IDEIA for having an emotional disturbance (or emotional disability) while they are in early elementary school, the majority are diagnosed in later elementary or middle school (US Department of Education, 2014). Children with an emotional disability typically have a long history of difficulty transitioning between activities or environments, as well as manifest disruptive behaviors in the classroom, low frustration tolerance, "emotional outbursts, and/or early difficulties building friendships and interacting appropriately with peers. It is these latter behaviors that often disrupt the classroom environment that are also viewed as contributing factors to a youth being identified as having an emotional disability, since they typically have significant more difficulty functioning in the typical learning environment than their same-age typically developing peers.

Although the terms "emotional disability" and "emotional disturbance"" are often used synonymously within educational settings, they are not necessarily synonymous with the DSM-5 term "mental disorder" or the terms "mental health disability" and "mental health disorder." The reason for this is that a youth who receives special education services for an emotional disability within the school setting is *not required* under IDEIA to meet the diagnostic criteria for a DSM-5 mental disorder (or mental health disability or disorder). Rather, the primary factor considered for an IDEIA diagnosis of emotional disturbance is whether the youth's emotional difficulties negatively impact his or her school performance. Conversely, while having a diagnosis of a mental health disorder can help a youth qualify for an IDEIA diagnosis of an emotional disturbance, the presence of such a diagnosis does not automatically qualify the student for special education services under the category of an emotional disturbance.

The fact that emotional disability and mental health disability are not synonymous is due partially to the fact that some mental disorders are excluded from the IDEIA criteria for emotional disturbance. For example, a DSM-5 diagnosis of "conduct disorder" or "oppositional defiant disorder" can lead to obvious school and classroom difficulties; however, these latter disruptive behavior disorders are typically considered within schools to be related to "social maladjustment" which is an *exclusionary criterion*" for receiving special education services under the IDEIA category of emotional disturbance. Therefore, while disruptive behaviors are often characteristics found in youth having a DSM-5 diagnosis of conduct disorder, those who qualify for an IDEIA diagnosis of emotional disturbance must display social or emotional difficulties other than social maladjustment that interfere with their learning at school.

There is a fair degree of controversy regarding whether disorders such as conduct disorder are, in fact, "only" indicative of social maladjustment, or whether social maladjustment and emotional disability are actually two terms for similar behavioral difficulties (e.g., Merrell & Walker, 2004; Smith, Katsiyannis, Losinski, & Ryan, 2015). Nevertheless, according to IDEIA, those students who are considered to have "social maladjustment" would not qualify as having an emotional disturbance or emotional disability. This exclusion of social maladjustment has led some researchers to suggest that emotional disability in children and adolescents may be underdiagnosed in the youth offender population, since the disruptive and antisocial behaviors of these youth may be attributed to social maladjustment when, in fact, these youth are manifesting emotional difficulties (e.g., Weber, 2009).

Despite being one of the more prevalent disabilities within the juvenile justice system, emotional disturbance is diagnosed in less than 1 % of the general regular education population (US Department of Education, 2014). Of those students receiving special education services, approximately 6.2 % are receiving services for an emotional disturbance (US Department of Education, 2014). Significantly more males than females are identified as having an emotional disturbance, and these students are also more likely to be of minority status, from low socioeconomic backgrounds, and from single-parent households (e.g., Achilles, McLaughlin, & Croninger, 2007; US Department of Education, 2014). In contrast, in their national survey of juvenile delinquents receiving special education services, Quinn et al. (2005) found that of those delinquents receiving special education services, as many as 50 % of them were receiving services under the category of emotional disability.

Impact on Functioning

As discussed below, emotional disabilities can cause a significant negative impact on a student's daily functioning; therefore, it is not surprising that these students have the poorest prognosis for long-term success in school (US Department of Education, 2014).

Cognitive Impairments. Studies have found that students with an emotional disability or disturbance often have language difficulties (e.g., Benner, Nelson, & Epstein, 2002; Nelson, Benner, & Cheney, 2005; Nelson, Benner, Neill, & Stage, 2006; Wagner, Kutash, Duchnowski, Epstein, & Sumi, 2005), with deficits observed in all areas of language skills including expressive, receptive, and pragmatic language. However, the research findings concerning the nature of cognitive deficits in these youth are quite varied. This variability is not necessarily due to the fact that no cognitive difficulties exist in these youth but, rather, due to the heterogeneity of the symptoms and characteristics of the students in school who comprise this diagnostic category. For example, if a student is classified under IDEIA as having an emotional disability and is also diagnosed under DSM-5 as having attention deficit hyperactivity disorder or bipolar disorder, then this student would have the potential for having cognitive deficits in executive functioning (e.g., Coghill, Hayward, Rhodes, Grimmer, & Matthews, 2014; Martinussen, Hayden, Hogg-Johnson, & Tannock, 2005). Furthermore, the level of severity of a person's emotional disability may have an effect on his or her cognitive deficits. For example, although there is no evidence to suggest that students having an emotional disability will also have lower levels of IQ, there is some evidence to suggest that those students with more severe emotional disabilities do present with lower IQs than those students with less severe emotional disabilities (Mattison, 2011).

Academic Difficulties. As is consistent with all educational disabilities covered under IDEIA, in order to be diagnosed with an emotional disability, a history of poor academic performance must be demonstrated (IDEIA, 2004). Emotional disabilities also often co-occur with the presence of a SLD (US Department of Education, 2014), so it is not surprising that research has demonstrated that students with such emotional difficulties are at an increased risk of academic failure. In this regard, researchers have reported that the academic difficulties displayed by students with emotional disabilities are significantly greater than those having other types of disabilities (e.g., Trout, Nordness, Pierce, & Epstein, 2003; Wagner & Cameto, 2004).

This level of risk of academic difficulties is increased further for those students whose emotional disability is significant enough to require placement in a special education classroom versus being educated in the regular education classroom and receiving resource support services. A study by Lane, Barton-Arwood, Nelson, and Wehby (2008), for example, examined the academic achievement levels of students with an emotional disability who were being educated in a self-contained special education classroom and found that these students scored well below average (i.e., <25th percentile) in all academic achievement areas. Other research has found that students with emotional disabilities perform 1–2 years below grade level, with notable academic deficits in math, basic reading skills, reading comprehension, and writing (e.g., Anderson, Kutash, & Duchnowski, 2001; Lane, Carter, Pierson, & Glaeser, 2006; Reid, Gonzalez, Nordness, Trout, & Epstein, 2004; Trout et al., 2003). Interestingly, studies have also found that even when the academic performance levels of students having an emotional disability are consistent with those students having another IDEIA classification, their respective teachers still rated the academic achievement of students with emotional disabilities lower than that of their peers (Lane et al., 2006). As a result of the academic difficulties experienced by students having an emotional disability, they are also more likely to be retained than their peers, despite research showing such retention to be relatively ineffective (Anderson et al., 2001).

The poor academic achievement demonstrated by students having an emotional disability is likely due, in part, to the impact that their emotional difficulties have on their ability to learn. For example, the presence of a low frustration tolerance in many of these students and difficulties with attention and concentration plus poor interpersonal skills make learning difficult for any student, and these are identifying traits of students with emotional difficulties (IDEIA, 2004). In addition to intrinsic factors that may negatively impact learning, students having emotional disability are more likely to be removed from the classroom for behavioral problems, be suspended, and have higher rates of truancy and poor attendance, all of which will limit the instructional time available to them and hinder their learning (Whitcomb & Merrell, 2012).

Consistent with their high rates of academic failure, students with an emotional disability are at the highest risk of school dropout among youth having an IDEIA diagnosis, even though the dropout percentages have fallen over the years from 55.9 % in 2003 to less than 39 % in 2012 (US Department of Education, 2014). In addition, research has found that less than 20 % of those who graduate high school go on to higher education (Wagner et al., 2005).

Social and Mental Health Difficulties. Social relationship difficulties are an identifying characteristic of students having an emotional disability, to a degree that such difficulties often lead to them being referred for a special education evaluation and later diagnosed as having an emotional disability (e.g., Kauffman, 2001; Walker, Ramsey, & Gresham, 2004). For example, the National Longitudinal Transition Study (2006) found that teachers and parents rated nearly half of those students with an emotional disability as being well below average in regard to social skills.

Consistent with the IDEIA diagnostic criteria for an emotional disturbance, many of these youth struggle to build and maintain satisfactory relationships with either adults or peers, and research has consistently found that these students are more likely to be socially isolated, have fewer friendships, and have more negative interactions with others (e.g., Lane et al., 2006; Wagner et al., 2005). These difficulties may be related to poor social competence and limited social skills, which can interfere with their ability to understand social situations and accurately interact and communicate with their peers or adults. In addition, the social difficulties that they experience may be related to poor emotional regulation and the behavior difficulties that they frequently display in school. Such behaviors are likely to result in negative reactions from parents, teachers, school personnel, and peers, which can make both adult and peer relationships more difficult to develop (e.g., Rose & Espelage, 2012).

Behavioral Implications. As is evident in the IDEIA classification of emotional disturbance, students who qualify for special education services typically lack prosocial behaviors and the ability to interact positively in their environment. These deficits contribute to the academic and social difficulties and behavior difficulties commonly observed. Although behavior difficulties are not the only symptoms that can indicate the possible presence of an emotional disability, students demonstrating behavior difficulties are more likely to be flagged and identified by school personnel, since these *externalizing behaviors* often negatively impact the learning environment for all students (Wagner & Cameto, 2004). This is in contrast to those students with *internalizing behaviors* who are experiencing anxiety and/or depression and who may not be identified as quickly or as early as those with externalizing behaviors. However, both sets of students have the potential for being classified under IDEIA as having an emotional disturbance and are likely to have more difficulty, in comparison to their typically developing same-age peers, to participate in school work within peer groups, follow classroom rules, and not be disruptive in the classroom (Kauffman & Landrum, 2009).

In general, students with emotional disabilities also have a low frustration tolerance, are highly sensitive to changes in their environments, are impulsive, and have poor emotional regulation. These traits can lead to behavior difficulties such as tantrums, aggressive outbursts, or other impulsive, emotionally volatile behavior toward others or themselves (Kauffman & Landrum, 2009). Self-injurious behaviors can also occur in some students with a more severe emotional disability, with a student potentially engaging in such behaviors as scratching, cutting, or head banging when frustrated (Whitcomb & Merrell, 2012).

Given the types of externalizing and internalizing behaviors that could be observed in students classified as having an emotional disability, these students are more likely to be suspended or expelled compared to their typical regular education same-age peers or even in comparison to students classified as having another type of disability under IDEIA (US Department of Education, 2014). In addition, these students are more likely to have interaction with the juvenile justice system given their inclination toward engaging in externalizing behaviors when upset.

School-Based Interventions for Emotional Disabilities

Since students who meet the criteria for an emotional disability represent a heterogeneous population, this can lead to many challenges in providing effective interventions and, subsequently, is a contributing factor to the poor intervention outcomes for these youth (Kern, 2015). As mentioned earlier, these students often present with significant learning or academic difficulties and have poor behavioral regulation, social difficulties, and difficulty interacting positively within their school environment. Given the behavior patterns often demonstrated by many of these students, interventions for this population are frequently multifaceted. For example, it is not uncommon for parents or other care providers to consult with psychiatrists or other medical personnel outside of the school setting to determine if their respective children should be placed on a medication regimen to help manage their behaviors and/or emotions. It is also not uncommon for the same student to be seen within a therapeutic program by a mental health professional outside of the school setting. Not all students will be placed on a regimen of medication or be seen by a mental health professional outside of the school setting.

Interventions within the school setting in which students have an emotional disability include a broad range of programs such as behavioral support, social skills training, or alternative classroom or alternative school placements. Behavioral support may include positive reward systems and behavior plans, which have been shown to be effective in increasing desirable behaviors in the school environment (Bradshaw, Mitchell, & Leaf, 2010). Social skills training may include individual and small group work that focuses on building social competence and appropriate social skills. Interestingly, despite the social difficulties present among this population of students, research has been mixed in regard to the effectiveness of social skills training in improving these skills in children with emotional disabilities (e.g., Cook et al., 2008; Greshman, 2014; Maag, 2006).

Alternative placements are often used for students with more severe emotional disabilities, and these may include a self-contained classroom that is designed only for those students with emotional disabilities, or it could include a placement in an alternative school setting that is designed to meet the needs of students with severe emotional disabilities (US Department of Education, 2014). IDEIA (2004) requires that services be provided to students with disabilities in the least restrictive environment possible. While the types and intensity of services provided vary considerably depending on the needs of a student, the levels of support could broadly be categorized into the following categories, ranging from least restrictive to most restrictive:

(a) *General education classroom with behavioral support.* Students with the lowest level of need will typically remain in a general education classroom but be provided resource support to meet the student's behavioral and emotional needs. For example, the student with emotional disability may have an individualized behavior plan, receive a predetermined amount of counseling services at school each week, and/or have classroom accommodations that attempt to help the student deal with issues presented because of the emotional disability. If these interventions are not successful, then the intensity of services can be increased and additional instructional, behavioral, and counseling support can be provided.

(b) *Self-contained classroom.* If it is determined that a student with an emotional disability cannot be successful in the general education classroom despite increased resource support, he or she may be considered for placement in a self-contained classroom. These special education classrooms are typically very small (7–10 students), have a low student-to-teacher ratio (typically one classroom teacher and two or more teacher aides), have a teacher certified to teach students with emotional disabilities, and are designed to accommodate the special emotional and behavioral needs of students with severe emotional disabilities. It is not uncommon for these classrooms to include students across grade levels (e.g., 3rd to 5th grade).

(c) *Specialized day school for students with severe emotional disabilities.* If a student is unsuccessful in a self-contained classroom, a more restrictive setting may be a school that accommodates only those children with severe emotional disabilities. These are highly specialized schools with special education teachers and teacher aides trained to work with these high-needs students. For a student to qualify for this restricted type of setting, he or she would typically need to have demonstrated that he or she has a significant risk to themselves or others and is unable to learn in the general education school despite additional support.

(d) *Residential treatment center.* The most intensive level of support is a residential treatment center, which would provide intensive emotional, behavioral, and educational support. This type of setting would typically only be used after all other options have been exhausted or the student presents a very high risk to himself or herself or others (e.g., highly aggressive, suicidal ideation or attempt (IDEA, 2004).

As noted above, even with the appropriate educational interventions and accommodations provided, students with emotional disabilities are at a considerable risk for a low level of long-term success (Kent, 2015). In addition, given the poor emotional regulation and disruptive behaviors common in this population, it is not surprising that students with emotional disabilities are overrepresented in the juvenile delinquency population.

Learning and Emotional Disabilities and Juvenile Delinquency

It is estimated that 10–13 % of general regular education students receive special education services for educational disabilities, while studies have found that between 30 and 75 % of youth in the juvenile justice system qualify for having at least one disability and, therefore, eligible to receive special education services (e.g., Morris & Morris, 2006; National Center for Education Statistics, 2009; Quinn et al., 2005; US Department of Education, 2014). As discussed earlier in the book, the wide range in percentage values may be due to a variety of factors, such as the definition of disability and/or type of classification system used in a particular study, the specific assessment instruments and/or evaluation procedure used by the diagnosticians, and the methodology used by researchers in collecting data. However, independent of these limitations, the research literature has repeatedly shown that there is an overrepresentation of juvenile offenders who have a disability in both short-term detention and long-term correctional facilities, particularly youth identified as having an emotional disability (e.g., Morris & Morris, 2006).

In this regard, according to Quinn et al. (2005), the majority of youth in juvenile correctional facilities served under IDEIA were those with a classification of emotional disturbance (47.7 %), followed by SLD (38.6 %) and intellectual disability (9.7 %). A study by Cruise, Evans, and Pickens (2011) examined data of over 3799 juvenile delinquents and found that nearly 40 % of the sample qualified for special education services, with the most common educational disabilities being learning disability and emotional disability. These researchers also found that male juvenile delinquents were found to be 1.33 times more likely to have a special education classification, with SLD and other health impaired being the two most prevalent IDEIA categories; however, females were found to be 1.37 times more likely to have an emotional disability. In addition, it was found that age of first offense was related to special education status, with those delinquents whose first arrest occurred at an earlier age being more likely to have been receiving special education services. There are several hypotheses regarding the reasons that students with learning and emotional difficulties are overrepresented in the juvenile justice system, including the school failure hypothesis, susceptibility theory, and differential treatment hypothesis (see Chap. 4 for an explanation of these various theories).

This high percentage of youth in juvenile correctional facilities who are classified as having a disability under IDEIA (2004) presents a unique set of challenges for juvenile justice personnel. For example, these youth may present with many information processing, cognitive, and language impairments that negatively impact their ability to fully participate in court-related programming. Research findings have shown that there is a relationship between cognitive functioning and the presence of a learning disability in youth. Specifically, even though the IQ level of these youth may be average, deficits have been found to be common in areas such as language and executive functioning (Flanagan & Alfonso, 2010).

Youth with learning and emotional disabilities are also at a greater risk for social, emotional, and behavioral difficulties, which may also increase the likelihood of them being arrested and becoming involved in the juvenile justice system. In addition, in our opinion, these youth may have difficulty fully understanding the social expectations of court hearings, have difficulty acting appropriately during a court hearing and while they are in detention or another secure setting, and have difficulty fully understanding the nuances and nonverbal cues needed to socially navigate through the juvenile court process. The executive functioning deficits common in individuals with learning and/or emotional disabilities may also be related to poor emotional regulation and behavioral regulation, as executive functioning skills are responsible for self-regulation skills such as impulse control and flexible thinking (Kolb & Winshaw, 2008). While having a learning or emotional disability does not explain all situations in which a youth offender may become emotionally dysregulated or act impulsively, we believe that it is important for court personnel to take into consideration the impact that these types of disabilities may have on juvenile offenders during various phases of the juvenile court process in order to avoid misinterpreting a youth's actions as defiance or antisocial behavior versus being representative of his or her disability.

Finally, as has been discussed earlier, youth having a learning or emotional disability have unique educational needs that, in our opinion, need to be considered when adjudicating a case and deciding, if necessary, on placement and other required interventions. For example, if truancy has been an ongoing issue for a youth, it may be beneficial to review his or her education history and determine whether there is a pattern of academic failures present, particularly in reading, which merits a referral for a psychoeducational evaluation in order to determine if, in fact, the youth has a SLD. The reason for this is that students with learning disabilities are at a greater risk of truancy and dropout compared to their same-age peers (US Department of Education, 2014). If the youth is found to have a SLD, this information could be helpful to court personnel regarding ordering the youth to have frequent and regular tutoring by a qualified learning disability specialist. Although online schooling or placement at a self-paced alternative school is often considered for youth having a SLD, Flanagan and Alfonso (2010) suggest that these programs are not typically designed for a youth who has a SLD, since it is often assumed in these programs that the youth has mastered basic reading skills and that the student is motivated, attentive, and organized—all skills which may be weak in students having a SLD, particularly youth offenders with a SLD.

In terms of placement, it may be especially problematic when youth offenders having a learning and/or emotional disability are placed in a secure setting for extended periods of time, since the level of special education services that are available may not be equal to those found in the public school setting. In this regard, Morris and Thompson (2008) indicated that even though short-term and long-term correctional facilities are required to provide special education services as mandated under IDEIA, these settings face a variety of challenges in providing comprehensive services. For example, correctional settings may have more difficulty accurately identifying delinquents with disabilities given the limited history of educating the youth and inconsistent or unavailable school records; they often do not have the resources to provide individualized education programs and related services, and the secure, confined setting may make it more difficult to comply with procedural safeguards and disciplinary procedures when working with juvenile offenders who have educational disabilities.

Even acknowledging the fact that the juvenile justice system is designed largely to protect the public, it remains our opinion that educational concerns should be taken into account in the disposition of a case. This is particularly important given that research has demonstrated the impact an educational disability can have on a youth's functioning, as well as the fact that research has also found that academic remediation can reduce recidivism (Archwamety & Katsiyannis, 2000).

Impact on Risk and Risk Assessment

Research has repeatedly found that youth with learning or emotional disabilities are more likely to re-offend than are their typical peers (e.g., Barrett, Katsiyannis, & Zhang, 2009; Zhang, Hsu, Katsiyannis, Barrett, & Ju, 2011). For example, a study by Zhang, Barrett, Katsiyannis, and Yoon (2011) examined a large sample of youth with and without educational disabilities. They had over 100,000 juvenile delinquents in their sample, with nearly half receiving special education services. The results of this study indicated that juvenile delinquents with disabilities were more likely male, Black, referred at an earlier age, had a family history of criminality, and came from lower socioeconomic families. Delinquents with learning and emotional disabilities were also referred to the juvenile justice system twice as often, had more adjudications and probations, and were three times as likely to commit a third offense than were their nondisabled peers. Results also found that these youth offenders were typically detained for longer periods of time.

In a study examining risk factors of recidivism for male and female youth offenders, Thompson and Morris (2013) examined a sample of 3287 delinquents. A variety of variables were examined, including special education status. Results of this study found that 33.7 % of male delinquents were receiving special education services and 17.5 % of female delinquents were enrolled in special education. While learning disabilities were not related to total number of offenses, the diagnosis of an emotional disability was a significant predictor of recidivism for both male and female delinquents. Additionally, analyses found that while youth offenders with emotional disabilities did not differ from other offenders in regard to offense severity, delinquents with emotional disabilities committed significantly more offenses and more offenses against persons than did those without emotional disabilities. Therefore, while the causal nature of the exact relationship is likely moderated by several other variables, it does appear that juvenile delinquents having a disability (specifically, an emotional disability) are more likely to re-offend.

When determining a youth offender's overall level of risk, his or her disability should be considered both in regard to the impact it may have on the probability of re-offending and in regard to the youth appearing to be more antisocial or defiant than he or she typically is based on the presence of difficulties in executive functioning that are directly related to his or her disability. For example, when determining the juvenile's *risk of dangerousness*, there is some evidence to suggest that juveniles with disabilities may engage in more severe offenses than their nondisabled peers (Zhang, Barrett et al., 2011), but there are no data to indicate whether these more severe offenses are premeditated cruel and aggressive acts or impulsive responses to situations. Youth having an emotional disability are more inclined toward irritability, emotional reactivity, emotional outbursts, and impulsive aggression, so this would be important to consider when determining risk of dangerousness versus only looking at history of offense severity. In addition, when considering whether a youth offender lacks remorse or empathy, it is suggested that a determination be made whether the youth presents as if he or she has no empathy or remorse because of his or her impaired social skills or communication difficulties.

Similarly, in regard to *sophistication and maturity*, the level of impulsivity of the offense(s) should be carefully considered in light of the executive functioning deficits that commonly occur in youth with learning or emotional disabilities. Sophisticated adult criminal and youth offender acts require a high level of thinking and decision-making. The presence of a SLD does not imply that a youth offender cannot engage in higher-level thinking, but it suggests that problems may exist in this youth in the area of sophistication and maturity; therefore, we believe that youth having a SLD should be evaluated to further determine if their lack of sophistication and maturity is directly related to the presence of a SLD.

In regard to *treatment amenability*, when examining responsiveness to treatment, we feel that one of the most important considerations should be whether the treatment programs have been, or will be, compatible with the youth's disability. For example, given that language deficits are common in learning and emotional disabilities, juvenile delinquents having these disabilities may have more difficulty being successful in group "talk therapy" programs or other procedures that rely heavily on expressive or receptive language skills. In addition, research has found that academic remediation programs have been helpful in reducing offending (Archwamety & Katsiyannis, 2000). Therefore, if a juvenile offender with a learning or emotional disability has not been successful in treatment programming, it would be beneficial to consider the type of intervention program that was being provided and whether it was appropriate given the youth's disability. As mentioned earlier, the failure to fulfill a requirement such as writing a letter of apology may not be indicative of defiance and poor treatment amenability if the youth offender has a SLD that negatively impacts his or her ability to write.

Competency

As has been described in previous chapters, competency is determined by evaluating two different capacities: (1) the degree of reasonable understanding that a youth offender has in regard to the juvenile court process and (2) the youth's ability to sufficiently participate in the court trial and collaborate with his or her attorney. Competence to stand trial assumes that the youth has both a factual *and* rational understanding of the juvenile justice system and court process. Given the impact that an educational disability can have on functioning, it is our position that it would be important to evaluate a juvenile's competency when he or she has a history of receiving special education services. For example, language difficulties are common in youth having a SLD, so it would be important to have an objective assessment conducted of a youth offender's expressive and receptive language skills to determine his or her ability to comprehend what he or she hears and be able to effectively communicate with his or her attorney.

If a youth offender who has a learning or emotional disability is not found to be competent, then the type of program and instructional method proposed to restore competency becomes very important. Specifically, programs that rely heavily on reading or language skills may be more difficult for a youth offender having an SLD than those that provide visual cues and information in a variety of contexts. In addition, it would be important to ensure that a youth with a reading disability is not provided critical information in written format.

References

Achilles, G. M., McLaughlin, M. J., & Croninger, R. G. (2007). Sociocultural correlates of disciplinary exclusion among students with emotional, behavioral, and learning disabilities in the SEELS national dataset. *Journal of Emotional and Behavioral Disorders, 15*(1), 33–45. doi:10.1177/10634266070150010401.

American Psychiatric Association. (2013). *Diagnostic and statistical manual for mental disorders (DSM-5®)*. Washington, DC: Author.

Anderson, J. A., Kutash, K., & Duchnowski, A. J. (2001). A comparison of the academic progress of students with EBD and students with LD. *Journal of Emotional and Behavioral Disorders, 9*(2), 106–115. doi:10.1177/106342660100900205.

Archwamety, T., & Katsiyannis, A. (2000). Academic remediation, parole violations, and recidivism rates among delinquent youth. *Remedial and Special Education, 21*(3), 161–170. doi:10.1177/074193250002100306.

Barbaresi, W. J., Katusic, S. K., Colligan, R. C., Weaver, A. L., & Jacobson, S. J. (2005). Math learning disorder: Incidence in a population-based cohort, 1976-82, Rochester, Minn. *Ambulatory Pediatrics, 5*(5), 281–289. doi:10.1367/a04-209r.1.

Barrett, D. E., Katsiyannis, A., & Zhang, D. (2009). Predictors of offense severity, adjudication, incarceration and repeat referrals for juvenile offenders: A multicohort replication study. *Remedial and Special Education, 31*, 261–275. doi:10.1177/0741932509355990.

Bauminger, N., Edelsztein, H. S., & Morash, J. (2005). Social information processing and emotional understanding in children with LD. *Journal of Learning Disabilities, 38*(1), 45–61. doi:10.1177/00222194050380010401.

References

Bender, W. N., & Wall, M. (1994). Social-emotional development of students with learning disabilities. *Learning Disabilities Quarterly, 17*(4), 323–341. doi:10.2307/1511128.

Benner, G. J., Nelson, J. R., & Epstein, M. H. (2002). Language skills of children with EBD: A literature review. *Journal of Emotional and Behavioral Disorders, 10*(1), 43–56. doi:10.1177/106342660201000105.

Berninger, V. (2007). Written language during early and middle childhood. In R. J. Morris & N. Mather (Eds.), *Evidence-based interventions for students with learning and behavioral challenges*. New York, NY: Routledge Press.

Berninger, V. W., Nielsen, K. H., Abbott, R. D., Wijsman, E., & Raskind, W. (2008). Gender differences in severity of writing and reading disabilities. *Journal of School Psychology, 46*(2), 151–172.

Berninger, V. W., & Richards, T. L. (2002). *Brain literacy for educators and psychologists*. San Diego, CA: Academic Press.

Bradshaw, C. P., Mitchell, M., & Leaf, P. J. (2010). Examining the effects of schoolwide positive behavioral interventions and support on student outcomes: Results from a randomized controlled effectiveness trial in elementary schools. *Journal of Positive Behavior Interventions, 12*(3), 133–148. doi:10.1177/1098300709334798.

Bryan, T., Sullivan-Burstein, K., & Mathur, S. (1998). The influence of affect on social-information processing. *Journal of Learning Disabilities, 31*(5), 418–426. doi:10.1177/002221949803100501.

Coghill, D. R., Hayward, D., Rhodes, S. M., Grimmer, C., & Matthews, K. (2014). A longitudinal examination of neuropsychological and clinical functioning in boys with attention deficit hyperactivity disorder (ADHD): Improvements in executive functioning do not explain clinical improvement. *Psychological Medicine, 44*(5), 1087–1099. doi:10.1017/s0033291713001761.

Cook, C. R., Gresham, F. M., Kern, L., Barreras, R. B., Thornton, S., & Crews, S. D. (2008). Social skills training for secondary students with emotional and/or behavioral disorders: A review and analysis of the meta-analytic literature. *Journal of Emotional and Behavioral Disorders, 16*, 131–144. doi:10.1177/1063426608314541.

Critchley, M. (1970). *The dyslexic child* (2nd ed.). Springfield, IL: Charles C. Thomas.

Cruise, K. R., Evans, L. J., & Pickens, I. B. (2011). Integrating mental health and special education needs into comprehensive service planning for juvenile offenders in long-term custody settings. *Learning and Individual Differences, 21*(1), 30–40. doi:10.1016/j.lindif.2010.11.004.

Cutler, L., & Graham, S. (2008). Primary grade writing instruction: A national survey. *Journal of Educational Psychology, 100*(4), 907–919. doi:10.1037/a0012656.

DeBono, T., Hosseini, A., Cairo, C., Ghelani, K., Tannock, R., & Toplak, M. E. (2012). Written expression performance in adolescents with attention-deficit/hyperactivity disorder (ADHD). *Reading and Writing, 25*(6), 1403–1426.

Education for All Handicapped Children Act of 1975, Pub. L. No. 94-142.

Feifer, S. G., & De Fina, P. A. (2002). *The neuropsychology of written language disorders: Diagnosis and intervention*. Middletown, MD: School Neuropsych Press.

Flanagan, D. P., & Alfonso, V. C. (2010). *Essentials of specific learning disability identification*. Hoboken, NJ: Wiley.

Flannery, K. A., Liederman, J., Daly, L., & Schultz, J. (2000). Male prevalence for reading disability is found in a large sample of black and white children free from ascertainment bias. *Journal of the International Neuropsychology Society, 6*(4), 433–442. doi:10.1017/s1355617700644016.

Gallegos, J., Langley, A., & Villegas, D. (2012). Anxiety, depression, and coping skills among Mexican school children: A comparison of students with and without learning disabilities. *Learning Disability Quarterly, 35*(1), 54–61.

Geary, D. C., Hamson, C. O., & Hoard, M. K. (2000). Numerical and arithmetical cognition: A longitudinal study of process and concept deficits in children with learning disability. *Journal of Experimental Child Psychology, 77*(3), 236–263. doi:10.1006/jecp.2000.2561.

Geary, D. C., Hoard, M. K., Byrd-Craven, J., Nugent, L., & Numtee, C. (2007). Cognitive mechanisms underlying achievement deficits in children with mathematical learning disability. *Child Development, 78*(4), 1343–1359. doi:10.1111/j.1467-8624.2007.01069.x.

Gersten, R., Ferrini-Mundy, J., Benbow, C., Clements, D. H., Loveless, T., Williams, V., & Arispe. I. (2008). Report of the task group on instructional practices. In National Mathematics Advisory Panel, *Reports of the task groups and subcommittees* (pp. 606-624). Washington, DC: United States Department of Education.

Graham, S., & Perin, D. (2007). *Writing next: Effective strategies to improve writing of adolescents in middle and high schools*. A Report to Carnegie Corporation of New York. Washington, DC: Alliance for Excellent Education.

Greshman, F. (2014). Evidence-based social skills interventions for students at risk for EBD. *Remedial and Special Education, 36*, 100–104. doi:10.1177/0741932514556183.

Gubbay, S. S., & de Klerk, N. H. (1995). A study and review of developmental dysgraphia in relation to acquired dysgraphia. *Brain and Development, 17*(1), 1–8. doi:10.1016/0387-7604(94)00110-j.

Hogan, A., McLellan, L., & Bauman, A. (2000). Health promotion needs of young people with disabilities: A population study. *Disability and Rehabilitation, 22*(8), 352–357. doi:10.1080/096382800296593.

Individuals with Disabilities Education Improvement Act of 2004, Pub. L. No. 108-446.

Jordan, N. C., Hanich, L. B., & Kaplan, D. (2003). Arithmetic fact master in young children: A longitudinal investigation. *Journal of Experimental Child Psychology, 85*(2), 103–119. doi:10.1016/s0022-0965(03)00032-8.

Katusic, S. K., Colligan, R. C., Weaver, A. L., & Barbaresi, W. J. (2009). The forgotten learning disability: Epidemiology of written-language disorder in a population-based birth cohort (1976-1982), Rochester, Minnesota. *Pediatrics, 123*(5), 1306–1313. doi:10.1542/peds.2008-2098.

Kauffman, J. M. (2001). *Characteristics of emotional and behavioral disorders for children and youth* (7th ed.). Columbus, OH: Merrill.

Kauffman, J. M., & Landrum, T. J. (2009). *Characteristics of emotional and behavioral disorders of children and youth* (9th ed.). Upper Saddle River, NJ: Prentice Hall.

Kavale, K. A., & Forness, S. R. (1996). Social skill deficits and learning disabilities: A meta-analysis. *Journal of Learning Disabilities, 29*(3), 226–237. doi:10.1177/002221949602900301.

Kern, L. (2015). Addressing the needs of students with social, emotional, and behavioral problems: Reflections and visions. *Remedial and Special Education, 36*(1), 24–27. doi:10.1177/0741932514554104.

Kirk, S. A. (1976). Personal perspectives. In J. M. Kauffman & D. P. Hallahan (Eds.), *Teaching children with learning disabilities* (pp. 238–269). Columbus, OH: Merrill.

Kolb, B., & Winshaw, I. Q. (2008). *Fundamentals of human neuropsychology* (6th ed.). New York, NY: Macmillan.

Lane, K. L., Barton-Arwood, S. M., Nelson, J. R., & Wehby, J. (2008). Academic performance of students with emotional and behavioral disorders served in a self-contained setting. *Journal of Behavioral Education, 17*(1), 43–62. doi:10.1007/s10864-007-9050-1.

Lane, K. L., Carter, E. W., Pierson, M. R., & Glaeser, B. C. (2006). Academic, social, and behavioral characteristics of high school students with emotional disturbances or learning disabilities. *Journal of Emotional and Behavioral Disorders, 14*(2), 108–117. doi:10.1177/10634266060140020101.

Leone, P. E., Price, T., & Vitolo, R. K. (1986). Appropriate education for all incarcerated youth: Meeting the spirit of PL. 94–142 in youth detention facilities. *Remedial and Special Education, 7*(4), 9–14. doi:10.1177/074193258600700404.

Maag, J. W. (2006). Social skills training for students with emotional and behavioral disorders: A review of reviews. *Behavioral Disorders, 32*, 4–17.

Margalit, M., & Tur-Kaspa, H. (1998). LD: A multi-dimensional neurodevelopment model. *Psychology, 7*, 64–76.

References

Martlew, M., & Hodson, J. (1991). Children with mild learning difficulties in an integrated and in a special school: Comparisons of behaviour, teasing, and teachers' attitudes. *British Journal of Educational Psychology, 61*(3), 355–372. doi:10.1111/j.2044-8279.1991.tb00992.x.

Martinussen, R., Hayden, J., Hogg-Johnson, S., & Tannock, R. (2005). A meta-analysis of working memory impairments in children with attention-deficit/hyperactivity disorder. *Journal of the American Academy of Child and Adolescent Psychiatry, 44*(4), 377–384. doi:10.1097/01.chi.0000153228.72591.73.

Mather, N., & Wendling, B.J. (2011). *Essentials of dyslexia assessment and intervention*. Hoboken, NJ: John Wiley & Sons, Inc.

Mather, N., & Wendling, B.J. (2011). How SLD manifests in writing. In D.L. Flanagan and V.C. Alfonso (Eds.), *Essentials of specific learning disability identification*. (pg.65-88). Hoboken, NJ: John Wiley & Sons, Inc.

Mattison, R. E. (2011). Comparison of students classified ED in self-contained classrooms and a self-contained school. *Education and Treatment of Children, 34I*(1), 15–33. doi:10.1353/etc.2011.0003.

Mazzocco, M. M. M. (2007). Defining and differentiating mathematical learning disabilities and difficulties. In D. B. Berch & M. M. M. Mazzocco (Eds.), *Why is math so hard for some children? The nature and origins of mathematical learning difficulties and disabilities* (pp. 29–48). Baltimore, MD: Brookes.

Merrell, K. W., & Walker, H. M. (2004). Deconstructing a definition: Social maladjustment vs. emotional disturbance and moving the EBD field forward. *Psychology in the Schools, 41*(8), 899–910.

Morris, K. A., & Morris, R. J. (2006). Disability and juvenile delinquency: Issues and trends. *Disability and Society, 21*(6), 613–627. doi:10.1080/09687590600918339.

Morris, R. J., & Thompson, K. C. (2008). Juvenile delinquency and special education laws: Policy implementation issues and directions for future research. *Journal of Correctional Education, 59*(2), 173–190.

Murphy, M. M., Mazzocco, M. M. M., Hanich, L. B., & Early, M. C. (2007). Cognitive characteristics of children with mathematics learning disability (MLD) vary as a function of the cutoff criterion used to define MLD. *Journal of Learning Disabilities, 40*(5), 458–478. doi:10.1177/00222194070400050901.

National Center for Education Statistics. (2009). *Digest of education statistics, 2008 (NCES 2009–020), Chapter 2*. Washington, DC: US Department of Education.

National Center for Learning Disabilities. (2013). *The state of learning disabilities* (3rd ed.). New York, NY: Author.

National Longitudinal Transition Study-2. (2006). *The social adjustment of elementary and middle school students with disabilities*. Washington, DC: US Department of Education, Institute for Educational Sciences.

Nelson, J. R., Benner, G. J., & Cheney, D. (2005). An investigation of language skills of students with emotional disturbance served in public school settings. *The Journal of Special Education, 39*(2), 97–105. doi:10.1177/00224669050390020501.

Nelson, J. R., Benner, G. J., Neill, S., & Stage, S. A. (2006). Interrelationships among language skills, externalizing behavior, and academic fluency and their impact on the academic skills of students with ED. *Journal of Emotional and Behavioral Disorders, 14*(4), 209–216. doi:10.1177/10634266060140040401.

Quinn, M. M., Rutherford, R. B., Leone, P. E., Osher, D. M., & Poirier, J. M. (2005). Youth with disabilities in juvenile corrections. A national survey. *Exceptional Children, 71*(3), 339–345. doi:10.1177/001440290507100308.

Reid, R., Gonzalez, J., Nordness, P. D., Trout, A., & Epstein, M. H. (2004). A meta-analysis of the academic status of students with emotional/behavioral disturbance. *The Journal of Special Education, 38*(3), 130–143. doi:10.1177/00224669040380030101.

Richards, T. L., Grabowski, T. J., Boord, P., Yagle, K., Askren, M., Mestre, Z., ... Berninger, V. (2015). Contrasting brain patterns of writing-related DTI parameters, fMRI connectivity, and DTI-fMRI connectivity correlations in children with and without dysgraphia or dyslexia. *NeuroImage: Clinical, 8*, 408-421. doi:10.1016/j.nicl.2015.03.018

Rodriguez, C., Alvarez, D., Gonzalez-Castro, P., Garcia, J. N., Alvarez, L., Nunez-Perez, J.C., ... Bernado, A. (2009). ADHD and writing learning disabilities: Comorbidity in basis of attention and working memory. *European Journal of Education and Psychology, 2(3)* 181–198.

Rose, C. A., & Espelage, D. L. (2012). Risk and protective factors associated with the bullying involvement of students with emotional and behavioral disorders. *Behavior Disorders, 37*(3), 133–148.

Sanger Institute (2009). *The genetic X-factor: Nine new X chromosome genes associated with learning disabilities.* Retrieved from http://www.sanger.ac.uk/about/press/2009/090419.html

Shavlev, R. S., Manor, O., Kerem, B., Ayali, M., Badichi, N., Friedlander, Y., & Gross-Tsur, V. (2001). Developmental dyscalculia is a familial learning disability. *Journal of Learning Disabilities, 34*(1), 59-65. doi:10.1177/002221940103400105.

Shaywitz, S. E., Escobar, M. D., Shaywitz, B. A., Fletcher, J. M., & Makuch, R. (1992). Evidence that dyslexia may represent the lower tail of a normal distribution of reading ability. *New England Journal of Medicine, 326*(3), 145–150. doi:10.1056/nejm199201163260301.

Shaywitz, S. E., Mody, M., & Shaywitz, B. A. (2006). Neural mechanisms in dyslexia. *Current Directions in Psychological Science, 15*(6), 278–281.

Shaywitz, S. E., & Shaywitz, B. A. (2004). Reading disability and the brain. *Educational Leadership, 61*(6), 6–11.

Smith, C. R., Katsiyannis, A., Losinski, M., & Ryan, J. B. (2015). Eligibility for students with emotional or behavioral disorders: The social maladjustment dilemma continues. *Journal of Disability Policy Studies, 25*(4), 252–259.

Smith, S. D., Pennington, B. F., Boada, R., & Shriberg, L. D. (2005). Linkage of speech sound disorder to reading disability loci. *Journal of Child Psychology and Psychiatry, 45*(10), 1057–1066.

Swanson, H. L., & Sachse-Lee, C. (2001). Mathematical problem solving and working memory in children with learning disabilities: Both executive and phonological processes are important. *Journal of Experimental Child Psychology, 79*(3), 294–321. doi:10.1006/jecp.2000.2587.

Thompson, K. C., & Morris, R. J. (2013). Predicting recidivism among juvenile delinquents: Comparison of risk factors for male and female offenders. *Office of Juvenile Justice and Delinquency Prevention, 36.*

Trout, A. L., Nordness, P. D., Pierce, C. D., & Epstein, M. H. (2003). Research on the academic status of children with emotional and behavioral disorders: A review of the literature from 1961 to 2000. *Journal of Emotional and Behavioral Disorders, 11*(4), 198–210. doi:10.1177/10634266030110040201.

Tur-Kaspa, H., & Bryan, T. H. (1994). Social information-processing skills of students with learning disabilities. *Learning Disabilities Research & Practice, 9*, 12–23.

US Department of Education. (2012). *Twenty-fourth annual report to Congress on the implementation of the Individuals with Disabilities Education Act.* Washington, DC: Author.

US Department of Education. (2014). *Thirty-sixth annual report to Congress on the implementation of the Individuals with Disabilities Education Act.* Washington, DC: Author.

Wagner, M., & Cameto, R. (2004). The characteristics, experiences, and outcomes of youth with emotional disturbances. A report from the national longitudinal transition study-2. *National Center on Secondary Education and Transition, 3*(2).

Wagner, M., Kutash, K., Duchnowski, A. J., Epstein, M. H., & Sumi, W. C. (2005). The children and youth we serve: A national picture of the characteristics of students with emotional disturbances receiving special education. *The Journal of Emotional and Behavioral Disorders, 13*(2), 79–96. doi:10.1177/10634266050130020201.

Walker, H. M., Ramsey, E., & Gresham, F. M. (2004). *Antisocial behavior in school: Evidence-based practices* (2nd ed.). Belmont, CA: Wadsworth/Thomson Learning.

References

Weber, M. C. (2009). The IDEA eligibility mess. *Buffalo Law Review, 57*, 83–160.

Wendling, B. J., & Mather, N. (2008). *Essentials of evidence-based academic interventions.* Hoboken, NJ: Wiley.

Whitcomb, S., & Merrell, K. W. (2012). *Behavioral, social, and emotional assessments of children and adolescents* (4th ed.). New York, NY: Routledge.

Wiznitzer, M., & Scheffel, D. L. (2009). Learning disabilities. In R. B. David, J. B. Bodensteiner, D. E. Mandelbaum, & B. Olson (Eds.), *Clinical pediatric neurology* (pp. 479–492). New York, NY: Demos Medical.

Zhang, D., Barrett, D. E., Katsiyannis, A., & Yoon, M. (2011). Juvenile offenders with and without disabilities: Risks and patterns of recidivism. *Learning and Individual Differences, 21*(1), 12–18. doi:10.1016/j.lindif.2010.09.006.

Zhang, D., Hsu, H. Y., Katsiyannis, A., Barrett, D. E., & Ju, S. (2011). Adolescents with disabilities in the juvenile justice system: Patterns of recidivism. *Exceptional Children, 77*(3), 283–298. doi:10.1016/j.lindif.2010.09.006.

Part III
Mental Health Disabilities

Chapter 9
Mental Health Disorders

In 1999, the first ever US Surgeon General's report on mental health was published (U.S. Department of Health and Human Services, 1999). This empirically based report identified mental health disorders as an "urgent health concern" and indicated that they were the second leading cause of disability in the United States. At the time that this report was released, approximately 21 % of children between 9 and 17 years of age were receiving services for some type of mental health difficulty that impaired their daily functioning. Consistent with this, other research studies have found that up to 50 % of adolescents may meet the criteria for a mental health disorder at some point during childhood or adolescence (Merikangas et al., 2010). In fact, more than half of the lifetime cases of mental health disorders begin by the age of 14, with only 20 % of children and adolescents with mental health disorders being identified and receiving mental health services (US Public Health Service, 2000).

The above findings present a concern for society, since untreated mental health disorders often lead to more serious mental health problems and increases in suicide risk (e.g., Kessler, Chiu, Demler, & Walters, 2005; Shaffer & Craft, 1999). In addition, adolescents with mental health difficulties are at risk for a variety of additional problems such as school or social difficulties. For example, a longitudinal study that followed children throughout elementary school found that those with mental health disorders, particularly comorbid disorders, had greater levels of social, academic, and physical impairment than those without mental health disorders (Essex et al., 2009). As noted in the previous chapter, there is also a relationship between juvenile delinquency and emotional disability, with a high number of juvenile delinquents qualifying for at least one mental health disorder diagnosis (Shufelt & Cocozza, 2006). Over the past few decades, numerous studies have examined mental health in delinquents and identified both the high need for services for these youth and the diverse array of mental health disorders that exist in these youth (e.g., Teplin, Abram, McClelland, Dulcan, & Mericle, 2002; Welch-Brewer, Stoddard-Dare, & Mallett, 2011).

What Is a Mental Health Disorder?

The DSM-5 (APA, 2013), as well as the previous editions of the *Diagnostic and Statistical Manual of Mental Disorders* of the American Psychiatric Association, is the most commonly recognized manual for psychiatrists, psychologists, and other mental health professionals to assist them in the diagnosis of mental health disorders. It has become the standard reference handbook for mental health professionals. The manual has been revised several times since the publication of the first edition in 1952, with the most recent revision being released in 2013. The DSM-5 includes nearly 300 recognized mental health disorders that are broadly classified into a number of different categories including, but not limited to, neurodevelopmental disorders, psychotic disorders, bipolar disorders, depressive disorders, anxiety disorders, trauma-related disorders, sleep disorders, sexual disorders, disruptive disorders, substance-related disorders, and personality disorders.

Commonly Used Terms

The DSM-5 defines a mental health disorder as the following:

> A mental disorder is a syndrome characterized by clinically significant disturbance in an individual's cognition, emotion regulation, or behavior that reflects a dysfunction in the psychological, biological, or developmental processes underlying a mental functioning. Mental disorders are usually associated with significant distress or disability in social, occupational, or other important activities. An expectable or culturally approved response to a common stressor or loss, such as the death of a loved one, is not a mental disorder. Socially deviant behavior (e.g., political, religious, or sexual) and conflicts that are primarily between the individual and society are not mental disorders unless the deviance or conflict results from a dysfunction in the individual, as described above (APA, 2013, p. 20).

There are many commonly used descriptors and definitions associated with mental health disorders. Informal classifications often include terms such as *serious mental illness* or *personality disorders*. The term "serious mental illness" includes mental health disorders that involve psychosis and/or other symptoms severe enough to require a high level of care such as intensive inpatient treatment or hospitalization. *Schizophrenia* and *bipolar disorder* are the most common types of disorders that are included under the term serious mental illness. Bipolar disorder is addressed in Chap. 10 of this book; however, because of the very low incidence of schizophrenia both in the general adolescent population and the juvenile delinquency population, neither this nor other psychoses are discussed in this book. Personality disorders include those mental health disorders that are characterized by an ongoing, enduring pattern of behavior that is markedly different from cultural norms and expectations (APA, 2013). This ingrained and often maladaptive pattern of behavior typically begins manifesting itself in adolescence or early adulthood, causes marked impairment or distress in the individual's functioning, and is stable over time, contrary to other mental health disorders which typically are evident for a shorter period of time. There are several personality disorders, including *antisocial personality disorder*, *borderline personality disorder*, and *narcissistic personality disorder*. Personality disorders are not diagnosable until adulthood, so they will not be discussed in this book.

Other terms that are frequently used when discussing mental health disorders are the following:

1. *Diagnostic criteria.* This term indicates the specific symptoms that must be present in order for an individual to qualify for a mental health disorder under the DSM-5. For example, while sadness is common in those who are depressed, being sad does not qualify one for the diagnosis of depression. Rather, sadness is just one of several diagnostic criteria that must be present for the person to qualify for the diagnosis of depression. For example, in addition to sadness an adolescent must also present with at least four other symptoms, such as weight change, difficulty sleeping, fatigue, difficulty concentrating, or recurrent thoughts of death (APA, 2013).
2. *Comorbidity.* The term comorbidity is used to indicate that an individual meets the criteria for more than one mental health disorder. For example, a youth may be diagnosed with both an anxiety disorder and depression. In this regard, a national study that was published in 2010 surveyed over 10,000 adolescents between 13 and 18 years of age and found that of those qualifying for a mental health disorder, 40 % also qualified for more than one mental health disorder (Merikangas et al., 2010).
3. *Severity.* The severity of a mental health disorder is typically determined by the total number of symptoms with which an individual presents, with fewer symptoms indicating a milder level. In addition, severity is often determined by the negative impact that the symptoms have on one's functioning. If the symptoms make it difficult for an individual to attend school or work, the mental health disorder may be perceived as more severe than if the symptoms affect the individual's functioning in a milder way, such as negative mood or difficulty sleeping (APA, 2013). The severity level of a disorder is important to understand as it has direct implications on the youth's ability to function as well as on treatment recommendations.
4. *Significant impact on functioning.* This relates to the impact that the mental health disorder has on one's ability to function and be successful in his or her environment. A mental health disorder could affect one's social functioning, including interpersonal skills, ability to form and maintain relationships, and general socialization. A disorder could impact occupational functioning, or work performance, or it could impair school functioning, such as a youth's ability to attend school and be successful in coursework. A disorder could also impact daily living (e.g., personal hygiene and ability to care for oneself) or physical well-being. In general, severe mental health disorders will have more of a significant impact on a youth's functioning.
5. *Rule out.* This is often abbreviated in the form of R/O and may precede a diagnosis (e.g., "R/O bipolar disorder"). This essentially implies that there are some symptoms of a disorder present, but the individual does not meet criteria at this time for a diagnosis. Therefore, when a youth has several R/O diagnoses, it implies that while there are several symptoms or behaviors consistent with various mental health disorders, no actual diagnosis is being given.

6. *Unspecified.* This term applies to a diagnosis when an individual presents with many significant symptoms but does not fully meet the criteria for a diagnosis. This may occur because of the complex presentation of many disorders or in situations where a practitioner has limited time or ability to gather information about the individual's symptom history (e.g., hospital emergency room) (APA, 2013). For example, if all symptoms of generalized anxiety disorder are present except the duration has been five months instead of six months, the practitioner may provide a diagnosis of "unspecified anxiety disorder." In previous editions of the APA (2000), e.g., APA, this was annotated as *not otherwise specified* (NOS).

Mental Health Disorders in the Juvenile Justice System

As previously reported, research has indicated that approximately 20 % of youth in the general population have a mental health disorder (U.S. Department of Health and Human Services, 1999). In contrast, a study by Wasserman, McReynolds, Ko, Katz, and Carpenter (2005) found that up to 50 % of juvenile offenders reported a mental health concern, with other studies estimating the prevalence of mental health disorders in this population to be as high as 75 % (e.g., Skowyra & Cocozza, 2007; Teplin et al., 2002; Wasserman, McReynolds, Schwalbe, Keating, & Jones, 2010). These mental health disorders range from the less obvious disorders such as anxiety, depression, and post-traumatic stress disorder to the more overt disorders such as conduct disorder, oppositional defiant disorder, and attention deficit hyperactivity disorder. Research has found that the most common mental health disorders among youth offenders are depressive disorders (13–40 % of those with a mental health disorder), anxiety disorders (as high as 25 %), attention deficit hyperactivity disorder (as high as 50 %), disruptive behavior disorders (30–80 %), and substance use disorders (30–70 %) (e.g., Kinscherff, 2012; Shufelt & Cocozza, 2006).

Comorbid mental health disorders among youth offenders are also common. For instance, Shufelt and Cocozza (2006) reported that 21 % of the youth offenders that they studied had one mental health disorder, 17 % had two, 19 % had three, and 43 % had four or more mental disorders. These researchers also found that youth offenders with at least one mental health disorder were also found to have a higher comorbidity with substance use disorders (60.8 %). Mallet (2014) provided a review of the prevalence of mental health disorders in the general population versus those who were incarcerated. Their review of studies found that 33–80 % of incarcerated youth met the criteria for mental health disorders versus 9–18 % of youth in the general population. With regard to maltreatment history, Mallet (2014) found that 26 to 60 % of delinquent youth had a history of child maltreatment versus approximately 1 % in the general population. With regard to the presence of substance abuse disorders, estimates of 30–70 % of delinquents meet the criteria for this disorder versus 4–5 % of youth in the general population (e.g., Chassin, 2008, Grisso, 2008, Washburn et al., 2008).

Differences in the prevalence rates of mental health disorders in juvenile offenders may be due to a variety of factors, including diagnostic criteria used or reporting method used (e.g., psychological or psychiatric evaluation versus use of a brief screening procedure, review of case records, or youth's self-report). For example, some studies identify the prevalence of mental health disorders based on youth's self-reported symptoms, while others use a self-report a rating scale provided to the youth or identify symptoms via a diagnostic interview (e.g., Teplin et al., 2002). This can result, in many cases, in the overreporting of mental health problems or even inaccurate mental health diagnoses. Other studies may review the mental health records of referred youth and include in the reported prevalence data the primary diagnosis listed in each case record (e.g., Mallet et al., 2009). While this method provides researchers with a more verifiable mental health disorder diagnosis in comparison to using self-report data, it excludes those youth who have not been referred for mental health services or those whose mental health records were not available at the time that a particular study was conducted.

In addition to research methodology, variations in prevalence rates may be due to the fact that some studies have found differences in mental health symptoms for male versus female youth offenders. For example, Shufelt and Cocozza (2006) reported a higher prevalence of most types of mental health disorders among females (81 %) than males (66.8 %). In particular, anxiety disorders and mood disorders were more prevalent for females (56 % and 29.2 %, respectively) in comparison to males (26.4 % and 14.3 %, respectively). However, both males and females had generally equivalent rates for substance use disorders and disruptive behavior disorders. Another study conducted by Cauffman, Piquero, Broidy, Espelage, and Mazerolle (2004) found that female juvenile delinquents with more serious offenses were more likely to have internalizing symptoms, such as high levels of trauma, than did male juvenile delinquents. Moreover, in an earlier study conducted by Calhoun (2001) on sex-related differences in social-emotional functioning among 88 juvenile offenders, it was found that female juvenile offenders were more likely than male offenders to report poorer relationships with their parents, low self-esteem, and an external locus of control (Calhoun, 2001). A study by Welch-Brewer et al. (2011) also found a sex-related relationship between mental health difficulties and juvenile delinquency. These researchers examined data from 341 juvenile delinquents. Among other findings, their results indicated that nearly 74 % of females met criteria for a mental health disorder, while 55 % of males qualified for a mental health diagnosis.

In addition to differences in sex, research has suggested that mental health problems among juvenile delinquents may differ by race or ethnicity. For example, Teplin et al. (2002) found that over 80 % of White, 70 % of Hispanic, and 65 % of Black juvenile offenders had mental health diagnoses. Moreover, internalizing disorders were found to be 19 times more prevalent among White juvenile offenders and that these latter youth were also found to be seven times more likely to have a comorbid internalizing and externalizing disorder. Similarly, in a study conducted by Welch-Brewer et al. (2011), approximately 24 % of Black juveniles met criteria for a substance abuse disorder and 72 % met criteria for a mental health disorder. Although a smaller proportion of Black females met criteria for a substance abuse disorder and a smaller proportion of Black males met criteria for a mental health disorder, a higher proportion of Black males met criteria for a substance abuse disorder.

Although the data are consistent in that there is an overrepresentation of mental health disorders among youth within the juvenile justice system, what is not as clear is *why* so many juvenile delinquents have mental health problems. There are a variety of plausible explanations, including both theories of causation and findings from correlational studies. For example, in Grisso's summary of adolescent offenders having mental health disorders, he divided these explanations into three categories: *clinical*, *socio-legal*, and *intersystemic*. From a clinical perspective, he argues that the same symptoms of a mental health disorder that increase the likelihood of aggression also increase the likelihood that these youth will be detained for longer periods of time. Symptoms often include impulsivity, anger, and irritability, which can contribute to these youth being less manageable and lead to less favorable interactions with the courts. With regard to the socio-legal perspective, Grisso indicates that the more punitive nature of laws over the past few decades has resulted in more of a blanket approach to punishment rather than to an individualized approach that allows the court more discretion to help youth with mental health disorders to receive diversion and community services. Grisso's intersystemic perspective suggests that the reduction in the availability of community mental health services has left many youth without appropriate treatment and as a result the juvenile justice system is now filling the gap. This is evidenced by federal statistics that demonstrated that over 12,000 youth have been detained at some point in the juvenile justice system merely to obtain mental health services (e.g., U.S. General Accounting Office, 2003).

Like most other disabilities, mental health disorders typically do not act independently with regard to their association with juvenile delinquency. Rather, most juvenile delinquents with mental health disorders also have a variety of other risk factors such as academic difficulties, familial instability, and low socioeconomic status. Subsequently, while there is a significant amount of research examining the relationship between mental health disorders and juvenile delinquency, few have focused on specific mental health problems as being considered contributing factors to delinquent acts. In fact, while research has found that some behavioral and emotional difficulties may predate delinquency (e.g., Barrett, Katsiyannis, Zhang, & Zhang, 2013; McReynolds, Schwalbe, & Wasserman, 2010), there is some evidence to suggest that mental health disorders such as depression are actually secondary to juvenile delinquency in that the mental health problems occurred (or became exacerbated) *after* the youth became involved with the juvenile justice system.

In this regard, Defoe, Farrington, and Loeber (2013) concluded in their study that depression was secondary to juvenile delinquency. This study utilized data from over 1000 male delinquents between ages 7 and 19 years of age and included a variety of factors shown to be related to juvenile delinquency, including hyperactivity, impulsivity, attention deficits, low academic achievement, depressive symptoms, and socioeconomic status. Advanced statistical modeling was used to determine any potential causal relationship among these factors, with the results indicating that hyperactivity and low socioeconomic status were independent causal factors of low academic achievement. In addition, poor academic achievement was found to be a causal factor for juvenile delinquency, and then, subsequently, juvenile delinquency was a causal factor for depression. In other words, from our point of view, Defoe et al. (2013) are suggesting the following (see Fig. 9.1).

Hyperactivity Low SES → Poor Achievement → Delinquency → Depression

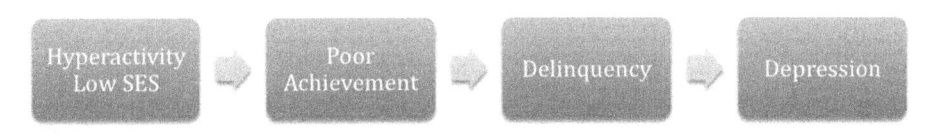

Fig. 9.1 Causal model for mental health in delinquents (Defoe et al., 2013)

Regardless of the causal relationship, there is sufficient research available to indicate that there is a high prevalence of mental health disorders among juvenile offenders, with the most common disorders involving internalizing and externalizing disorders.

Substance use disorders. Another important consideration when examining the presence of mental health problems among juvenile offenders is substance abuse. While not all juvenile delinquents qualify for a substance abuse diagnosis, substance abuse is a common occurrence among the juvenile offender population, with the most common illegal drug used prior to a youth's offense being marijuana (Mulvey, Schubert, & Chassin, 2010). However, the causal relationship between substance use and juvenile offending is unclear at this time, as risk factors for substance use are very similar to risk factors of delinquency (Iacono, Malone, & McGue, 2008). Nevertheless, research has repeatedly substantiated that youth offenders engaging in substance use—or those with identified substance use disorders—are at an increased risk of reoffending and engaging in more serious offending (e.g., Collin et al., 2011; Johnston, O'Malley, Bachman, & Schulenberg, 2012).

Many courts have attempted to accommodate for the difficulties related to substance use by establishing drug courts that can more appropriately respond to the needs of juvenile offenders who abuse drugs and alcohol. However, this can also be difficult because of the various factors that may link substance abuse with offending. For example, Mulvey et al. (2010) point out that substance abuse can have both direct and indirect contributions to juvenile delinquency. With regard to direct impacts, a youth may be caught in the possession of drugs or drug-related paraphernalia, he or she may be caught using illegal drugs, or he or she may be charged with selling or distributing drugs. Indirectly, those youth who use substances are more likely to associate with juvenile offending peers, may engage in property crimes as a way to gather income to purchase drugs, or they may make poor decisions and engage in delinquent activity while under the influence of drugs or alcohol (Mulvey et al., 2010).

As is acknowledged throughout the following chapters, increased substance use is also associated with many mental health disorders both in the general population and juvenile offender population (APA, 2013). The relationship between substance use, disability, and juvenile offending is one that is incredibly complex. While significant research is available that examines etiology, risk factors, and impact on functioning of individuals in the general population, the research regarding the juvenile offender population is less clear. This is likely due to the complex presentation of juvenile offenders, the high rates of substance use in this population, and the high comorbidity with other disorders (e.g., Mallet, 2014; Shufelt & Cocozza, 2006; Teplin et al., 2002). Fortunately, most juvenile justice systems have begun acknowledging the prevalence of substance use among juvenile offenders, incorporating substance abuse screenings, substance abuse-focused courts, and substance abuse treatment as regular components of programming (Chassin, 2008). Given the complexity of substance use in this population, as well as the fact that there is limited evidence-based research in this area, substance use disorders are not specifically covered in the following chapters. Rather, issues related to substance use with each disability are discussed as appropriate.

References

American Psychiatric Association. (2000). *Diagnostic and statistical manual for mental disorders* (4th ed. Text Revision). Washington, DC: Author.

American Psychiatric Association. (2013). *Diagnostic and statistical manual for mental disorders* (5th ed.). Washington, DC: Author.

Barrett, D. E., Katsiyannis, A., Zhang, D., & Zhang, D. (2013). Delinquency and recidivism: A multicohort, matched-control study of the role of early adverse experiences, mental health problems, and disabilities. *Journal of Emotional and Behavioral Disorders, 22*, 3–15. doi:10.1177/1063426612470514.

Calhoun, G. B. (2001). Differences between male and female juvenile offenders as measured by the BASC. *Journal of Offender Rehabilitation, 33*(2), 87–96. doi:10.1300/j076v33n02_06.

Cauffman, E., Piquero, A. R., Broidy, L., Espelage, D. L., & Mazerolle, P. (2004). Heterogeneity in the association between social-emotional adjustment profiles and deviant behavior among male and female serious juvenile offenders. *International Journal of Offender Therapy and Comparative Criminology, 48*(2), 235–252. doi:10.1177/0306624x03261255.

Chassin, L. (2008). Juvenile justice and substance use. *The Future of Children, 18*(2), 165–183. doi:10.1353/foc.0.0017.

Collins, D., Abadi, M. H., Johnson, K., Shamblen, S., & Thompson, K. (2011). Non-medical use of prescription drugs among youth in an Appalachian population: Prevalence, predictors, and implications for prevention. *Journal of Education, 41*, 309–326.

Defoe, I. N., Farrington, D. P., & Loeber, R. (2013). Disentangling the relationship between delinquency and hyperactivity, low achievement, depression, and low socioeconomic status: Analysis of repeated longitudinal data. *Journal of Criminal Justice, 41*(2), 100–107. doi:10.1016/j.jcrimjus.2012.12.002.

Essex, M. J., Kraemer, H. C, Slattery, M. J., Burk, L. R., Boyce, W. T., Woodward, H. R., & Kupfer, D. J. (2009). Screening for childhood mental health problems: Outcomes and early identification. *Journal of Child Psychology and Psychiatry, 50*(5), 562–570. doi:10.1111/j.1469-7610.2008.02015.x

Grisso, T. (2008). Adolescent offenders with mental disorders. *The Future of Children, 18*(2), 143–164. doi:10.1353/foc.0.0016.

Iacono, W., Malone, S., & McGue, M. (2008). Behavioral disinhibition and the development of early-onset addiction: Common and specific influences. *Annual Review of Clinical Psychology, 4*, 325–348.

Johnston, L. D., O'Malley, P. M., Bachman, J. G., & Schulenberg, J. E. (2012). *Monitoring the future national results on adolescent drug use: Overview of key findings, 2011*. Bethesda, MD: National Institute on Drug Abuse.

Kessler, R. C., Chiu, W. T., Demler, O., & Walters, E. E. (2005). Prevalence, severity, and comorbidity of twelve-month DSM-IV disorders in the National Comorbidity Survey Replication (NCS-R). *Archives of General Psychiatry, 62*(6), 617–627. doi:10.1001/archpsyc.62.6.617.

Kinscherff, R. (2012). *A primer for mental health practitioners working with youth involved in the juvenile justice system.* Washington, DC: Technical Assistance Partnership for Child and Family Mental Health.

Mallet, C. A. (2014). Youthful offending and delinquency: The comorbid impact of maltreatment, mental health problems, and learning disabilities. *Child and Adolescent Social Work Journal, 31*(4), 369–392. doi:10.1007/s10560-013-0323-3.

Mallett, C. A., Stoddard-Dare, P. A., & Seck, M. M. (2009). Predicting juvenile delinquency: The nexus of childhood maltreatment, depression, and bipolar disorder. *Criminal Behavior and Mental Health, 19*(4), 235–246. doi:10.1002/cbm.737.

McReynolds, L. S., Schwalbe, C. S., & Wasserman, G. A. (2010). The contribution of psychiatric disorder to juvenile recidivism. *Criminal Justice and Behavior, 37*(2), 204–216. doi:10.1177/0093854809354961.

Merikangas, K. R., He, J. P., Burstein, M., Swanson, S. A., Avenevoli, S., Cui, L., ... Swendsen, J. (2010). Lifetime prevalence of mental disorders in US adolescents: results from the National Comorbidity Survey Replication–Adolescent Supplement (NCS-A). *Journal of the American Academy of Child & Adolescent Psychiatry, 49*(10), 980-989. doi:10.1016/j.jaac.2010.05.017

Mulvey, E. P., Schubert, C. A., & Chassin, L. (2010). *Substance use and delinquent behavior among serious adolescent offenders.* Washington, DC: Office of Juvenile Justice and Delinquency Prevention.

Shaffer, D., & Craft, L. (1999). Methods of adolescent suicide prevention. *Journal of Clinical Psychiatry, 60*, 70–74.

Shufelt, J. L., & Cocozza, J. J. (2006). *Youth with mental health disorders in the juvenile justice system: Results from a multi-state prevalence study.* Delmar, NY: National Center for Mental Health and Juvenile Justice.

Skowyra, K. R., & Cocozza, J. J. (2007). *Blueprint for change: A comprehensive model for the identification and treatment of youth with mental health needs in contact with the juvenile justice system.* Delmar, NY: Policy Research.

Teplin, L. A., Abram, K. M., McClelland, G. M., Dulcan, M. K., & Mericle, A. A. (2002). Psychiatric disorders in youth in juvenile detention. *Archives of General Psychiatry, 59*(12), 1133–1143. doi:10.1001/archpsyc.59.12.1133.

U.S. Department of Health and Human Services. (1999). *Mental health: A report of the Surgeon General.* Rockville, MD: Author.

U.S. General Accounting Office. (2003). *Child Welfare and Juvenile Justice—Federal agencies should play a stronger role in helping states reduce the number of children placed solely to obtain mental health services.* Washington, DC: Author.

U.S. Public Health Service Report. (2000). *Report of the Surgeon General's Conference on Children's Mental Health: A national Action Agenda.* Washington, DC: Department of Health and Human Services.

Washburn, J. J., Teplin, L. A., Voss, L. S., Simon, C. D., Abram, K. M., & McClelland, G. M. (2008). Psychiatric disorders among detained youth: a comparison of youth processed in juvenile court and adult criminal court. *Psychiatric Services, 59*(9), 965–973. doi:10.1176/appi.ps.59.9.965.

Wasserman, G. A., McReynolds, L. S., Ko, S. J., Katz, L. M., & Carpenter, J. R. (2005). Gender differences in psychiatric disorders at juvenile probation intake. *American Journal of Public Health, 95*(1), 131. doi:10.2105/ajph.2003.024737.

Wasserman, G. A., McReynolds, L. S., Schwalbe, C. S., Keating, J. M., & Jones, S. A. (2010). Psychiatric disorder, comorbidity, and suicidal behavior in juvenile justice youth. *Criminal Justice and Behavior, 37*(12), 1361–1376. doi:10.1177/0093854810382751.

Welch-Brewer, C. L., Stoddard-Dare, P., & Mallett, C. A. (2011). Race, substance abuse, and mental health disorders as predictors of Juvenile court outcomes: do they vary by gender? *Child and Adolescent Social Work Journal, 28*(3), 229–241. doi:10.1007/s10560-011-0229-x.

Chapter 10
Mood Disorders

While disruptive behavior disorders (i.e., attention deficit hyperactivity disorder, oppositional defiant disorder, and conduct disorder) are the most common diagnoses among the juvenile offender population, research has also found a high prevalence of internalizing disorders in these youth. Internalizing disorders include those mental health disorders that are characterized by symptoms internal to the individual (e.g., negative thoughts, beliefs, and/or feelings). There are several internalizing disorders included in the DSM-5, such as major depressive disorder, generalized anxiety disorder, bipolar disorder, and post-traumatic stress disorder. This chapter discusses the most common internalizing *mood disorders* found in the juvenile offender population. The term "mood disorder" is a generic term commonly used to describe mental health disorders that have significant negative impact on one's daily mood, with these disorders including *depressive disorders*, *mood dysregulation disorder*, and *bipolar disorder*.

Depressive Disorders

Depressive disorders are broadly characterized by the presence of a sad, empty, and/or irritable mood. Symptoms include cognitive (thought), affective (emotional), and physical (behavioral and physiological) changes that negatively impact an individual's ability to function on a regular basis. There are several mental health disorders that are included in the general category of depressive disorders, such as *major depressive disorder*, *persistent depressive disorder*, *premenstrual dysphoric disorder*, *substance-/medication-induced depressive disorder*, and *depressive disorder due to another medical condition*. These latter disorders are similar in that they are characterized by a sad, empty, or irritable mood; however, they have different causes for the depressive symptoms, as well as different DSM-5 diagnostic criteria. The most commonly observed depressive disorders in the juvenile offender population include major depressive disorder and persistent depressive disorder.

In order to be diagnosed with a major depressive disorder, the DSM-5 (APA, 2013) requires that at least five symptoms related to negative mood be present over a two-week period. Possible diagnostic symptoms that may occur when a person is depressed include:

- Depressed mood nearly every day, which often presents in children as irritability rather than sadness.
- Decreased interest or pleasure in daily activities.
- Weight gain or loss, changes in appetite.
- Sleep difficulties, such as insomnia or sleeping more than normal.
- Physical agitation and restlessness *or* retardation and slowed movements.
- Loss of energy.
- Ongoing feelings of guilt or worthlessness.
- Difficulty concentrating, indecisiveness.
- Suicidal ideation and recurring thoughts of death (APA, 2013).

The DSM-5 also indicates that in order for a person to be considered as having a depressive disorder (rather than just being "sad" or "down"), these symptoms must cause significant impairment in one's functioning. In adults, this may often be observed in the workplace, with a depressed employee showing up late to work, not completing work in a timely manner, or struggling to focus on work. In children and adolescents, impairment may be observed in poor schoolwork, not finishing homework, reduced participation in extracurricular activities, or failing to do other required activities such as chores or follow household rules. Like many other disorders, depression is typically described in terms of severity, which is based on the number of diagnostic criteria one meets for the disorder and the level of impairment the symptoms have on an individual's daily functioning (APA, 2013).

Persistent depressive disorder, which is also known as *dysthymia*, is diagnosed when one has experienced chronic major depressive disorder. It is similar to major depressive disorder except that the symptoms are chronic, lasting more than a year for children and adolescents and more than 2 years for adults (APA, 2013). According to the DSM-5, because of the chronic depression that these individuals experience, they are also at a greater risk for anxiety disorders and substance use disorders.

According to the National Institute of Mental Health (2014), approximately 11 % of adolescents meet criteria for a depressive disorder by 18 years of age, with approximately 5 % of youth qualifying for moderate to severe depression at any given time. Research has also found higher rates of depression in juvenile offenders in comparison to the general population. For example, a meta-analysis conducted by Fazel, Doll, and Langstrom (2008) found approximately 10.6 % of delinquent males to be diagnosed with depression and 29.2 % of female delinquents diagnosed with depression. In fact, after conduct disorder, oppositional defiant disorder, and attention deficit hyperactivity disorder, depressive disorders have been found to be one of the most prevalent mental health disorders among juvenile offenders, with studies estimating that between 13 % and 40 % of juvenile offenders qualify as having a diagnosis of depressive disorder (Kinscherff, 2012).

Interestingly, a study conducted by Stoddard-Dare, Mallett, and Boitel (2011) found a prevalence of depression as high as conduct disorder in their random sample of 341 adjudicated delinquents, with 12.9 % having a diagnosis of depression and 11.4 % having a diagnosis of conduct disorder.

Etiology and Treatment

No single cause of depression has been identified in the research literature; rather, research has suggested that there are a variety of factors that may contribute to depression. For example, neurological differences in the brain functioning of people experiencing depression have been identified, including differences in hormone levels and disruption in neurotransmitters, both of which are important in the regulation of mood and behavior (Kolb & Whishaw, 2008). Related to this, there has been a genetic component found in depression, with adolescents with a family history of depression being more inclined to experience depression (APA, 2013). In addition to biological and neurological factors, environmental influences have been found to increase the likelihood that depression will be diagnosed in certain people, with such influences including early exposure to trauma early trauma and related stressors and appreciable family disruption (Saveanu & Nemeroff, 2012).

In terms of theoretical perspectives, some theories have hypothesized that the core of depression is a pessimistic and negative thought pattern. Specifically, the *cognitive theory of depression* posits that individuals who think negatively are more prone toward depression as they frequently and continually perceive or think about events, persons, and situations around them in a negative manner, which leads to a negatively biased view of the world (Beck, 1967).

A variety of treatments are available to treat depression in children and adolescents, including various modalities of psychotherapy and pharmacological interventions. One of the most empirically supported forms of therapeutic treatment for depression in children and youth is CBT (e.g., Compton et al., 2004; Curry, 2001). CBT is based on the assumption that depression is largely influenced by negative thoughts and related behaviors, with the goal of CBT to improve depression by changing the negative thoughts and restructuring the way an individual thinks about and responds to a situation or event. CBT is considered a short-term therapy and typically lasts under 20 sessions (Weersing & Brent, 2013). A licensed mental health provider trained in conducting CBT should provide the therapy. In addition to CBT, *interpersonal therapy* (IPT) has been found to be effective in treating depression in children and youth (Mufson et al., 2004). This therapy focuses on difficulties resulting from interpersonal relationships, encouraging adolescents to focus on one of four areas that are primary sources of difficulty: grief, role disputes, role transitions, and interpersonal or social skill deficits. The goal of IPT is to help a youth develop more effective coping strategies to deal with these difficulties, including better communication, affect expression, and social skills (e.g., Jacobson & Mufson, 2012; Kaslow et al., 2008).

Medication has also been found to be an effective form of treatment for youth having depression, and antidepressant medications are often prescribed for these youth (Delate, Gelenberg, Simmons, & Motheral, 2004). Specifically, at the time of this publication the Food and Drug Administration (FDA) has approved the use of certain selective serotonin reuptake inhibitors (SSRIs) for treating depression in youth, including fluoxetine (Prozac) and escitalopram (Lexapro) (FDA, 2015). Individuals taking antidepressant medications must receive ongoing medical care—typically by a child psychiatrist—in order to closely monitor dosage levels and usage frequency to ensure adequate outcome results. In addition, it is important to monitor for possible side effects, since a major warning that accompanies the use of antidepressants is related to the sudden stopping of the medication, as this can lead to withdrawal symptoms or relapse in major depressive symptoms (Kaslow et al., 2008).

Both CBT and medication have been proven to be effective interventions for the treatment of depression in adolescents (e.g., Kaslow et al., 2008). The Treatment for Adolescents with Depression Study (TADS) is one of the most comprehensive experimental studies conducted to determine the effectiveness of various treatments for depression. This study examined the effectiveness of therapy, medication, and combination treatment (CBT+medication) in a sample of 439 youth across the United States and found that combination treatment is the most effective way to treat depression in adolescents. Specifically, researchers found that after the first 12 weeks of treatment, 71 % of the youth who were receiving a combination treatment saw improvement in their symptoms, while 61 % taking medication only saw symptom improvement, and 44 % with therapy alone had improved symptoms (March et al., 2004). Across time, combination treatment remained the most effective form of treatment. Specifically, at 36 weeks, 86 % receiving combination treatment saw improvement, and nearly 80 % of those receiving medication or therapy reported improved symptoms (March et al., 2007).

In addition to therapeutic and psychotropic interventions within the home and community settings, the school setting can also be a place that provides support for youth having depression. Schools are often the first place to observe or identify problems given the amount of time a youth spends in the school setting, as many schools have early prevention and identification programs (Reinemann, Stark, Molnar, & Simpson, 2006). While it is not a setting to provide intensive therapeutic support, school counseling services may be available for those experiencing symptoms of depression at school. For those students whose depression is chronic and severe enough to significantly interfere with learning, special education services may be considered under the IDEIA category of emotional disability (IDEA, 2004). If special education services are not warranted under IDEIA, then accommodations may be provided under a Section 504 plan of the *Rehabilitation Act* (1973). Accommodations for depression may include modifications such as schedule changes, assignment substitutions, extra time for test taking, and alternative requirements or deadlines.

Implications on Functioning

The symptoms related to depression can cause significant impairments in a youth's daily life. Research has found that depression in children and adolescents is related to behavioral difficulties, social difficulties, academic difficulties, and even cognitive impairments (e.g., Cash, 2008; Fite, Rubens, Preddy, Raine, & Pardini, 2014; Kaslow et al., 2008; Lundy, Silva, Kaemingk, Goodwin, & Quan, 2010).

Cognitive and Academic Implications. Mood disturbance is typically associated with depressive disorders. Although cognitive impairments are not listed in the diagnostic criteria for depression, deficits in thinking skills have long been associated with depression and can cause significant difficulties in daily functioning (e.g., Kaslow et al., 2008). The majority of available research on this topic relates to the significant memory and attentional difficulties observed in depressed adults (e.g., Andrews et al., 2007; Shelton & Kirwan, 2013); however, there are research findings that indicate that thinking difficulties are also observed in depressed youth. For example, a study by Lundy et al. (2010) examined the relationship between symptoms of depression and cognitive functioning in 335 children. These researchers found that children with depression performed worse on several cognitive domain measures, including general intelligence, language, visual-spatial skills, attention, processing speed, memory, executive functioning skills, and academic performance.

Given that mood and depression can affect attention and concentration, memory, and motivation, it is not surprising that youth having depression typically begin having more academic difficulties. Depression can manifest itself in the school setting by the depressed student having difficulty paying attention in class, withdrawing from school activities, having increased truancy, or having a sudden drop in grades and grade point average (Cash, 2008; Eisenberg, Golberstein, & Hunt, 2009; Hysenbegasi, Hass, & Rowland, 2005). Students with emotional issues such as depression are also at a higher risk of dropping out of school (US Department of Education, 2014). The causal connection between depression and academic difficulties is unknown, but it may be related to the cognitive difficulties that occur, as learning is more difficult when one has impairments in attention and memory. Sleep difficulties and lethargy are also common with depression (APA, 2013), which can make it more difficult for a student to wake early in the morning and have energy to focus and learn throughout the day. Finally, the anhedonia and poor motivation associated with depression can lead to decreased motivation for school and studying.

Behavioral and Social Implications. Depression in children and adolescents typically manifests itself differently than in adults. While depression in adults is primarily characterized by sad and lethargic mood, in children and adolescents it is typically observed by increased irritability, anger, and defiance. The DSM-5 diagnostic criteria for depression are similar for youth and adults; however, the DSM-5 provides that "irritable mood" can substitute for "sad mood" when diagnosing children and adolescents with depression (APA, 2013). As noted by the American Academy of Child and Adolescent Psychiatry ([AACAP], 2013), this chronically irritable mood can contribute to a low frustration tolerance and the child or adolescent subsequently becoming defiant, angry, or hostile more quickly. These youth may be more inclined to be defiant or argumentative with parents or teachers, and they may be more inclined to anger outbursts or tantrums because of this sadness and irritability. This is not to imply that these youth are more likely to initiate violence or aggression but rather that they may be more inclined to *react* aggressively once provoked.

Fite et al. (2014) examined aggressiveness in children with depression and confirmed that children with depression were more inclined toward acting aggressively. However, these researchers also found that while children were at a greater risk of displaying reactive aggression (i.e., reacting negatively to a situation) in comparison to their typical nondepressed peers, there was no difference in proactive aggression (i.e., initiating an aggressive event). In addition, a study by Ebesutani, Kim, and Young (2014) that examined the role of negative mood and violence exposure with child and adolescent aggression found that negative mood was a major contributing factor of and predictive factor for aggressive behavior. The relationship between aggression and depression in youth is appreciable enough that studies have suggested that this relationship is similar to that of aggression that is typically observed in youth having externalizing disorders. For example, Cabiya-Morales et al. (2007) examined 176 children with attention deficit hyperactivity disorder and found that depressed mood for both male and female children was a significant predictor of aggressive behavior. As discussed below, research has also found that depressive disorders are associated with juvenile delinquency in regard to the increased presence of physical aggression and acts of stealing (Loeber & Keenan, 1994; Takeda, 2000).

In addition to behavioral disruptions, social difficulties are common among depressed youth. The aggression and irritability that are often present can disrupt relationships with parents and other family members, with parents reporting higher levels of distress at home with teenagers experiencing depression (AACAP, 2013). A depressed adolescent may more likely to become quickly angry, act defiantly, argue more, and engage in more rule-breaking behaviors in the household or with friends, which can also negatively impact peer and familial relationships (Kaslow et al., 2008). In addition to these behavioral difficulties disrupting interpersonal relationships, the tendency for individuals with depression to withdraw from social groups and other activities can have obvious implications on social relationships. Youth with depression are also less likely to be involved in school sports or other extracurricular activities, reducing socialization time (APA, 2013).

Mood Dysregulation Disorder

Mood dysregulation disorder is a new classification included in the DSM-5 under the category of depressive disorders. It was added to the DSM-5 as a way to address the possible misdiagnosis of chronically irritable and explosive youth who were previously diagnosed as having bipolar disorder (APA, 2013). Specifically, since the early 2000s, there has been an increase by almost 500 % in the diagnosis of bipolar disorder in children and adolescents (Stringaris, 2013). The suggested explanation for this increase on the part of many clinicians and researchers is due to the observation that many practitioners have applied the diagnosis of bipolar disorder to a children or adolescents because they manifest severe irritability (Margulies, Weintraub, Basile, Grover, & Carlson, 2012). However, in fact, such irritability may not be related to mania/hypomania in bipolar disorder but, instead, to a distinct type of behavioral dysregulation, irritability, and anger now labeled mood dysregulation disorder (e.g., Althoff, Verhulst, Rettew, Hudziak, & Van der Ende, 2010; Copeland, Angold, Costello, & Egger, 2012; Jucksch et al., 2011; Margulies et al., 2012). The DSM-5 provides a number of diagnostic criteria that must be met in order for a child or adolescent to qualify for this diagnosis:

(a) Frequent temper outbursts that include verbal rages or aggressive outbursts toward people or property, with these outbursts being significantly out of proportion with the situation. For example, this could be a 12-year-old male who has an aggressive tantrum and outburst after being told he cannot wear his old torn sneakers to school.
(b) These outbursts must be inconsistent with developmental level. In this regard, while tantrum behaviors may be expected for a 2-year-old female, they are not expected to be present for a 12-year-old female.
(c) The outbursts occur frequently, on average of three times or more per week.
(d) The child or adolescent presents with a daily mood that is described as chronically irritable or angry.
(e) The outbursts happen in at least two of three settings. This implies that if the outbursts occur *only* at home or *only* at school, then the child would not meet criteria for the disorder. Rather, the outbursts would need to occur at home and school or both at home and with friends (APA, 2013).

Mood dysregulation disorder can only be diagnosed in children and adolescents from the ages of 6–18 years, and the behaviors must not be better explained by depression, a developmental disability such as ASD, oppositional defiant disorder, or other disability. This diagnosis is relatively new, and consequently few studies exist which examine the prevalence of mood dysregulation disorder in children and adolescents. In the DSM-5, it is estimated that the prevalence of this diagnosis is between 2 and 5 % of children and adolescents in the general population, with rates likely higher for males (APA, 2013). Copeland et al. (2012) examined data from a variety of community studies with 3258 youth from 2 to 17 years of age and found prevalence rates for this disorder ranging from 0.8 to 3.3 %, with it being much less prevalent in adolescents than in early childhood. Interestingly, these researchers also found that mood dysregulation disorder is a highly comorbid disorder, with it occurring with another disorder 62–92 % of the time. The primary comorbid disorder being depression and oppositional defiant disorder.

No statistics are currently available regarding the prevalence of mood dysregulation disorder in the youth offender population, though the study by Copeland et al. (2012) did find that 8.8 % of those who met criteria for mood dysregulation disorder also had involvement with the juvenile justice system. Given the high prevalence of oppositional defiant disorder and depressive disorders in youth offenders, it is reasonable to expect that this disorder might occur at a higher rate than in the general child and adolescent population.

Diagnosis and Treatment

Similar to other mental health disorders, mood dysregulation disorder is typically diagnosed through a comprehensive clinical interview with a youth and the youth's parents. Information should also obtained from other individuals who interact closely with the youth, such as weekend caregivers or teachers, in order to ensure that the behaviors are occurring in settings outside of the home. No standardized rating scales are available at this point to specifically assess symptoms related to mood dysregulation disorder; rather, the diagnosis relies solely on the clinician's clinical judgment based on the youth's background history and subjective reports of his or her behaviors. The DSM-5 also points out that practitioners need to be able to differentiate symptoms of mood dysregulation disorder from those of bipolar disorder and externalizing disorders (APA, 2013). This is important since the aggressive behaviors observed in mood dysregulation disorder could be misinterpreted as resulting from the antisocial or aggressive tendencies found in conduct disorder and oppositional defiant disorder or from the poor impulse control demonstrated by youth having attention deficit hyperactivity disorder (Leibenluft, 2011; Margulies et al., 2012).

Since the diagnostic category of mood dysregulation disorder is relatively new, little empirical research is available that discusses evidence-based treatment approaches. However, based on the presentation of symptoms, it is our belief that the most likely interventions that will be studied initially will include individual therapy such as CBT and IPT to address the irritability and anger control issues that youth manifest who have this disorder (see, e.g., Kaslow et al., 2008), parent training to teach parents strategies that can be implemented whenever their child or adolescent engages in violent outbursts and related aggressive behaviors (see, e.g., Barkley, 2013; Kazdin & De Los Reyes, 2008), and medication that focuses on stabilizing the youth's mood swings (see, e.g., Johnson & Fruehling, 2008).

Implications on Functioning

In addition to the lack of evidence-based therapy research available for treating youth having mood dysregulation disorder, there is limited research available that examines specific impairments that are present in these children and adolescents. Our speculation, however, is that youth with this disorder will have appreciable difficulties in their respective relationships with family members and peers and in their learning and related academic achievement levels at school. Consistent with this view, a study by Copeland et al. (2012) examined estimated prevalence rates of mood dysregulation disorder from other community studies and found that over half of the children meeting the criteria for mood dysregulation disorder had impairment in parental relations and nearly a quarter had poor sibling relations. High rates of school suspension and teacher difficulties were also found. Studies have also found that adolescents with a history of emotional lability and mood dysregulation are at an increased risk of other internalizing problems such as anxiety and depression (Leibenluft, 2011). In addition, in comparison to those youth not having this diagnosis, Copeland, Shanahan, Egger, Angold, and Costello (2014) found that youth having this diagnosis are more likely to have increased contact with the legal system, have poor educational success, and enter into low socioeconomic status in adulthood. These researchers also reported that in analyzing the data of over 1400 youth, it was found that those with severe mood dysregulation had significantly more felony charges, more accounts of police contact, and more episodes of fighting.

Bipolar Disorder

Bipolar disorder is included under the category of mood disorders, since the defining feature of this mental health disorder is the presence of distinct periods of mood imbalance. Bipolar disorder is *not* characterized by frequent moodiness or rapid mood swings throughout the day; rather, it is diagnosed after the presence of clear hypomanic or manic episodes have been observed, with these episodes each typically lasting a minimum of four days. There are two types of bipolar disorder, *Bipolar I disorder* and *Bipolar II disorder*. To qualify for Bipolar I, a *manic episode* must have been present, with the criteria being the following for a manic episode:

(a) A distinct period of at least a week in which abnormally elevated, expansive, or irritable mood is present, as well as high energy levels. The mood during a manic episode may be described as one feeling as though he or she is invincible or feeling "on top of the world." Excessive irritability during this period is common (APA, 2013).
(b) Changes in mood and behavior, such as inflated self-esteem or grandiosity, decreased need for sleep, pressured speech, talkative and tangential during speech, distractibility, increase in activity, or excessive involvement in high-risk activities (APA, 2013). In delinquents, mania may be observed in the forms of risky drug use or other high-risk, impulsive behaviors such as shoplifting, cutting off an ankle monitor, running away, or stealing a car.

Similar to other disorders, these changes in mood and behaviors must cause significant impairment in a person's functioning. To meet the criteria for a manic episode, the individual's level of impairment must be to a degree that it requires hospitalization *or* there is some level of psychosis present. A depressive episode is *not* required for a diagnosis of Bipolar I disorder, though depression often precedes or follows a manic episode. Bipolar I disorder is typically rated as *mild, moderate, or severe*, depending on the type and severity of symptoms present (APA, 2013).

Bipolar II is similar to Bipolar I disorder in regard to the presence of an elevated mood; however, this mood disturbance and change in activity level *do not impair functioning* sufficiently to require hospitalization or result in the presence of psychosis (APA, 2013). The elevated period in Bipolar II disorder is referred to as *hypomania*, and to qualify for a diagnosis, the hypomania would need to last for at least four days. In contrast to Bipolar I disorder, Bipolar II *does* require the presence of a depressive disorder in order to qualify for a diagnosis. Specifically, an individual would need to experience at least one hypomanic episode plus one or more major depressive episodes to qualify for this diagnosis (APA, 2013).

While the DSM-5 suggests that bipolar disorder is prevalent in less than 1 % of the population in the United States (APA, 2013), no prevalence data are listed that are specific for children and adolescents. Although there may be several reasons for this omission, one possible explanation is that the symptoms of bipolar disorder typically present themselves in late adolescence and, therefore, the symptoms may not be fully recognized by parents or teachers until early adulthood. Children or adolescents demonstrating high levels of irritability or mania-like symptoms do not typically have bipolar disorder (e.g., Horwitz et al., 2010; Margulies et al., 2012; Stringaris, 2013). With regard to juvenile delinquency, studies have estimated that 3–7 % of youth offenders have been diagnosed with bipolar disorder (e.g., Mallett, Stoddard-Dare, & Seck, 2009; Teplin, Abram, McClelland, Dulcan, & Mericle, 2002); however, there is no clear indication that these diagnoses are accurate given the difficulties associated with diagnosing bipolar disorder in children and adolescents.

The specific cause(s) of bipolar disorder is unknown, but a variety of factors have been identified as being associated with the cause of bipolar disorder. Bipolar disorder is largely considered to be a neurobiological disorder in that its causes are primarily associated with dysfunction in the brain, though environmental factors are thought to exacerbate symptoms and affect treatment success (Hart, Brock, & Jeltova, 2014). Research has identified a genetic link to bipolar disorder, with there being a higher likelihood of developing bipolar disorder if it is present in first-degree relatives (e.g., Althoff, Faraone, Rettew, Morley, & Hudziak, 2005; Kato, 2008). Contrary to many other mental health disorders, however, there do not appear to be any major gender differences in the prevalence or clinical presentation of symptoms of bipolar disorder, though there is some evidence to support differences in subtypes and age of onset (e.g., Biederman et al., 2004; Staton, Volness, & Beatty, 2008).

A common theoretical model that has been used to explain bipolar disorder is the *diathesis-stress model*, which asserts that while an individual has a biological predisposition for the disorder, various environmental stressors can exacerbate symptoms (Zuckerman, 1999). Consistent with this, a variety of environmental factors have been found to contribute to or exacerbate symptoms of bipolar disorder. In this regard, research has found that stimulant medication that is used for a child being treated for attention deficit hyperactivity disorder can increase mania, as can family conflict or other psychosocial stressors (e.g., Birmaher, Arbelaez, & Brent, 2002; Leahy, 2007; Reichart & Nolen, 2004; Youngstrom, Birmaher, & Findling, 2008; Zuckerman, 1999). This is evidenced, in part, by the fact that there is a high incidence of trauma history in individuals with bipolar disorder, with some studies estimating that as many as 50 % of adults with bipolar disorder experienced childhood trauma (Assion et al., 2009).

Diagnosis and Treatment

A psychiatrist, psychologist, or other mental health professional typically provides the diagnosis of bipolar disorder. Given the difficulty in accurately diagnosing this disorder in children and adolescents, a detailed background history that includes information from multiple sources should be obtained. This is particularly important considering that many parents are likely to overreport childhood behaviors and irritability as manic-like (Horwitz et al., 2010). Youngstrom, Findling, Youngstrom, and Calabrese (2005) provided a comprehensive guideline regarding recommendations for professionals involved in the diagnosis of pediatric bipolar disorder. These researchers suggested that the most important considerations/practices for ensuring an accurate diagnosis involve consideration of the base rates and likelihood of the disorder occurring in the setting in which the evaluation is conducted. For example, a male middle school youth who is in a psychiatric hospital because of serious mental health symptoms is more likely to have a diagnosis of bipolar disorder than is a same-age youth sitting in a pediatrician's office who was referred by his mother because of disruptive behaviors at home.

When diagnosing bipolar disorder, a comprehensive evaluation should also include an examination of the youth's family history of bipolar disorder, as well as using standardized assessment instruments. A variety of standardized screening instruments and diagnostic tools exist to assist in making a valid diagnosis of bipolar diagnoses in youth; however, these instruments are not often used since they require specific training in order to administer (e.g., Renou, Hergueta, Flament, Mouren-Simeoni, & Lecrubier, 2004). Nevertheless, given the appreciable negative impact that bipolar disorder can have on an individual's functioning, some professionals have recommended that there be a screening assessment for bipolar disorder when individuals are referred for severe depressive symptoms, suicidal ideation, or after delinquent offenses (Culver, Arnow, & Ketter, 2007).

Although there is no cure for bipolar disorder, treatment approaches typically include a combination of psychotherapy and medication. Medication is the most common type of treatment, with a variety of medications available to help regulate the mood and emotional difficulties that are present in a person having bipolar disorder (AACAP, 2014). Presently, there are no well-established therapy methods available, but research does support family-oriented psychoeducational approaches to help educate the family regarding the causes and symptoms of bipolar disorder, as well as to help them build skills to more effectively handle a child or adolescent having bipolar disorder (e.g., Fristad & MacPherson, 2014; Miklowitz et al., 2008).

While the number of evidence-based studies is limited, it has been suggested that CBT may be efficacious in helping regulate symptoms of bipolar disorder by focusing on the person's negative thought patterns during depressive episodes and implementing behavior management strategies (Fristad & MacPherson, 2014). Given the complexity of bipolar disorder, a multisystemic approach involving psychotherapy, parent education, and medication treatment requires consistency and frequent monitoring and should be provided by trained (and licensed) clinicians, especially since treatment adherence on the part of clients is often low in persons with severe mood disorders such as bipolar disorder (Gearing & Mian, 2005).

Implications on Functioning

Bipolar disorder is associated with serious complications and difficulties in the lives of those it affects. While the majority of research focuses on the impact of bipolar disorder on adults, available research with youth suggests that children and adolescents having this disorder also experience serious difficulties. The level of negative impact will vary depending on the age of onset and severity of the disorder (McClure-Tone, 2010).

Similar to depressive disorders, cognitive impairments have been associated with bipolar disorder. Specifically, while there is no indication that the overall IQ of youth having bipolar disorder is lower than their typically developing peers, significant deficits have been most notable in the area of verbal memory and executive functioning skills, including working memory and attention (Nieto & Castellanos, 2011). Considerable processing speed deficits have also been observed in individuals with bipolar disorder, with this likely to be partially related to the cognitive slowing effects of many medications that are prescribed for bipolar disorder (e.g., Horn, Roessner, & Holtmann, 2011; Mattis, Papolos, Luck, Cockerham, & Thode, 2011).

The behaviors associated with bipolar disorder (e.g., irritability or mood instability) can contribute to difficulties for youth in the classroom environment, since they are more likely to have difficulties concentrating, dealing with frustrating academic content, managing their behaviors in a structured environment, and adapting to changing demands of the classroom (Lofthouse & Fristad, 2008). In addition, the cognitive deficits associated with the disorder, as well as medications used to treat the disorder, can make learning more difficult; therefore, it should not be unexpected that these youth will often experience more academic difficulties than their typically functioning and same-age peers. Academic difficulties may also be due, in part, to the sleep difficulties common among children and adolescents with bipolar disorder as these youth tend to have difficulty falling asleep, staying asleep, and waking up in the morning in a timely manner (Roybal et al., 2011). In addition, there is some limited research suggesting that learning disabilities are more common in students with bipolar disorder than found in their typically developing peers (Biederman, Faraone, Chu, & Wozniak, 1999; Wozniak et al., 1995).

Social-Emotional and Behavioral Implications. In regard to social implications, as mentioned earlier, bipolar disorder can significantly affect both peer and familial relationships. Research has found that while a close, supportive family environment can serve as a protective factor for youth having bipolar disorder (Miklowitz & Johnson, 2009), many parents are more likely to use corporal punishment, have a more distant relationship with their child or adolescent, spend less time with him or her, and have a more volatile relationship with the youth and increased family conflict (e.g., Keenan-Miller & Miklowitz, 2011; Geller et al., 2000; Sullivan & Miklowitz, 2010).

Social relationships have also been found to be problematic in children and adolescents having bipolar disorder, which can negatively impact their quality of life (e.g., Freeman et al., 2009). For example, Geller et al. (2000) found that children with bipolar disorder were more likely to report difficulties with bullying, have few friendships, and generally present with poor social skills compared to youth without bipolar disorder. These difficulties with peer relationships are likely related to the irritability and mood dysregulation common in these youth, but may also be related to poor social perception and awareness. In this regard research has found that youth with bipolar disorder are more likely to have difficulty interpreting the emotions of others and are inclined to misinterpret these latter emotions as negative or threatening (e.g., Deveney, Brotman, Decker, Pine, & Leibenluft, 2012; Guyer et al., 2007; Rich et al., 2006).

Bipolar disorder is often comorbid with at least one other mental health disorder, with a common pattern being that the other disorder(s) *preceded* the diagnosis of bipolar disorder (Henin et al., 2007). Some researchers have argued that the high comorbidity between bipolar disorder and other mental health disorders such as attention deficit hyperactivity disorder may be overreported given the similarities in some symptoms (e.g., a review by Kowatch, Youngstrom, Danielyan, and Findling [2005] found that nearly 62 % of those with bipolar disorder would also meet the criteria for attention deficit hyperactivity disorder), but nevertheless a high rate of other disorders has been found. Substance use disorders are of particular concern in youth and adults with bipolar disorder, since these individuals are at a very high risk of engaging in substance use (Wilens et al., 2008). This has led some professionals to recommend that screening for substance use should begin in children as young as 10 years of age (Goldstein & Bukstein, 2010). The high prevalence of substance use in those with bipolar disorder has been attributed to biological (Kerner, Lambert, & Muthén, 2011) and social-emotional factors related to the disorder (Lorberg, Wilens, Martelon, Wong, & Parcell, 2010), with substance use being shown to decrease when the symptoms of bipolar disorder are treated with medication (Joshi & Wilens, 2009).

Comorbid externalizing disorders appear to be more common in males having bipolar disorder, while comorbid internalizing disorders appear to be more common in females (e.g., Masi et al., 2006; McIntyre et al., 2006). With regard to externalizing behaviors, given that bipolar disorder is often associated with irritability and anger outbursts, it is not surprising to learn that in addition to attention deficit hyperactivity disorder, there is a high comorbidity with conduct disorder and oppositional defiant disorder (Joshi & Wilens, 2009). These youth are more likely to act out more than their typical peers and be more likely to engage in problem behaviors such as arguing, fighting, and stealing (Kovacs, Kovacs, & Pollack, 1995). However, some of the externalizing behaviors such as aggression have also been reported to be more disorganized and impulsive in comparison to others (Joshi & Wilens, 2009).

In general, those persons having comorbid diagnoses with bipolar disorder tend to have more problematic symptoms and impairment in functioning (e.g., Arnold et al., 2011; Diler, Uguz, Seydaoglu, Erol, & Avci, 2007). It should also be noted that when bipolar disorder is comorbid with other mental health disorders, this is considered a risk factor for suicidal ideation, given that between 25 and 50 % of youth with bipolar disorder have attempted suicide (e.g., Goldstein et al., 2005; Goldstein, Olubadewo, Redding, & Lexcen, 2005; Moor, Crowe, Luty, Carter, & Joyce, 2012).

Mood Disorders in the Juvenile Justice System

Although mood disorders, especially depression, are more common among the youth offender population than in the general population of children and adolescents, research findings vary with respect to the association between type of offense(s) committed and mood disorders. For example, a study by Stoddard-Dare et al. (2011) examined detained delinquents and found that those with bipolar disorder were more likely to be detained for a crime against persons. Obeidallah and Earls (1999) examined the association between depression and delinquency in a sample of 754 delinquents and found that those with depression were more likely to commit property crimes than did those youth without depressive symptoms. Other studies, however, have reported conflicting findings, with some reporting that mood disorders are more related to property crimes, while others reported more of an association with offenses against persons (e.g., McReynolds, Schwalbe, & Wasserman, 2010; Takeda, 2000).

Like most studies involving juvenile offenders, the variability in results may be due to the fact that juvenile offenders are a complex and heterogeneous population, with many studies not controlling for the sex, race, socioeconomic status, and the presence versus absence of a learning disability, a trauma history, or an intellectual, emotional, cognitive, or language disability in the youth being studied. Variability in findings may also be related to the type of mood disorders in the sample studied. For example, mood dysregulation disorder is characterized by aggressive outbursts, so it would be expected that youth with this disorder are more likely to be arrested for a more violent crime like assault against person or destruction of property versus shoplifting.

While there is a strong relationship between mental health disorders and juvenile delinquency, there is limited evidence that these disorders specifically *cause* delinquency. For example, Kofler et al. (2011) examined a sample of over 3600 adolescents between 12 and 17 years of age, gathering data at three separate time points over a 12-month period. They found depressive symptoms to be a predictive factor for delinquency, with those youth having depression being at a greater risk to engage in later delinquent behavior. The risk was especially high for females with depression. A study by Defoe and colleagues (2013), however, concluded that depression was secondary to delinquency. This study examined data from over 1000 delinquents and found that depressive symptoms were typically exacerbated by delinquency rather than depression contributing to or being independent of delinquency. Given these examples of variability in findings, it seems most reasonable to assume that the presence of mental health disorders in youth offenders further complicates the risk factors and difficulties associated with these youth committing illegal acts.

As is the case with juvenile offenders having developmental and/or educational disabilities, the presence of a mood disorder can present additional challenges to the juvenile justice system beginning with the moment of arrest. While youth with mood disorders do not necessarily present with the same cognitive impairments evident in youth having developmental or learning disabilities, the instability in mood can negatively impact a youth's behavior and interactions with the arresting police officers and subsequent processing through the juvenile justice system.

There are also a variety of factors that can be considered when determining whether to arrest, detain, and/or adjudicate a youth, and the behaviors and symptoms commonly observed in youth with mood disorders may result in more negative results in each of these areas. Particularly for mood disorders such as mood dysregulation disorder or bipolar disorder, which are largely characterized by impulsive outbursts and unpredictable behavior, youth with mood disorders may be more at risk for increased difficulties during the initial police contact. For example, if a police officer decides to transport a youth to a detention facility after being arrested, it would be reasonable to assume that the youth having a mood disorder may be more inclined toward suicidal ideation, violent outbursts, or aggressive threats and would need to be closely monitored.

Emotional instability is a defining feature of mood disorders, and the related symptoms could be exacerbated by high-stress situations such as being arrested or placed in a detention facility. Any explosive or otherwise disruptive behaviors that occur during this time period have the potential for leading to additional charges filed against the youth; therefore, it is our belief that documenting whether there is a history of mood disorder in a particular youth should be considered during an initial hearing when evaluating any additional behaviors or offenses that occurred during arrest.

Similarly, the chronic irritability and low frustration tolerance often observed in youth with mood disorders should be considered by court personnel as a possible indication of a mental health disorder versus antisocial behavior. While having the diagnosis of a mood disorder should in no way excuse a juvenile offender of the need to act in prosocial ways when working with court staff, it is important to consider that these behaviors do occur in these youth and that they should be taken into consideration when determining appropriate intervention, placement, or related sanctions. In this regard, it is our view that the interventions chosen for these youth be appropriate—and wherever possible, evidence based—for the mental health disorder diagnosis. For example, while a group anger management program may outwardly appear to be an appropriate intervention, there is no empirical evidence that this procedure would be effective for a youth offender whose anger outbursts are related to mania and the presence of a bipolar disorder.

Impact on Offending and Risk Assessment

The research literature is not consistent in regard to the contribution that mental health disorders may have on the committing of illegal acts by youth, especially whether they are primary causal factors or secondary to other risk factors. Moreover, some studies have not found an association between the presence of mental health problems in youth offenders and recidivism (e.g., Colins et al., 2011). However, the majority of available findings on this topic do suggest that mental health problems may be related to re-offending youth offenders, with those youth having mood disorders or other mental health problems being found to have significantly more offenses (e.g., Colins et al., 2011; Schubert, Mulvey, & Glasheen, 2011; Stouthamer-Loeber, Loeber, Wei, Farrington, & Wikström, 2002).

McReynolds et al. (2010) examined a sample of 915 youth and found that half of those included in the study had one mental health disorder, with about 25 % of them being diagnosed with a substance use disorder, 20 % being diagnosed with an anxiety disorder, and 20 % being diagnosed as having a disruptive behavior disorder. Overall, disruptive behavior and substance use disorders were found to double a juvenile's risk for recidivism. Although internalizing disorders (e.g., depression or anxiety) alone were not found to be associated with recidivism, when they were comorbid with an externalizing disorder, it increased a juvenile offender's risk of recidivism, with this effect being found for both male and female youth offenders. In addition, females were four times as likely to recidivate if they had a comorbid mood disorder and substance use disorder in comparison with females without any comorbid disorder.

Another study by Hoeve, McReynolds, and Wasserman (2013) examined a sample of 340 delinquents in Alabama and also found that when internalizing disorders were comorbid with disruptive behaviors, there was a sixfold increase in recidivism compared to those juvenile offenders without mental health disorders. The results of these and other studies suggest that when determining whether the presence of a mood disorder is going to affect risk for re-offending, a primary consideration should be whether a comorbid disruptive behavior disorder is also present.

In addition to mental health disorders being related to recidivism, some studies have found that these disorders may be related to the types of offenses being committed. For example, Zara and Farrington (2013) utilized a prospective longitudinal dataset to determine if there were differences in early onset (prior to age 21) versus late onset (age 21 or later) offending on a number of specific risk factors. Participants in this study included 411 males, of which 31 % were early onset offenders, and each was assessed on four risk scales that measured antisocial behavior, family risk, socioeconomic factors, and internalizing problems. The results indicated that mental health issues, especially internalizing problems, predicted late onset offending, whereas antisocial behavior (e.g., serious conduct problems) predicted early onset offending. In addition, the researchers found that participants with serious conduct problems by 7 years of age were up to 19 times as likely to have a higher rate of offending by their mid-20s. In addition, as mentioned earlier, Stoddard-Dare et al. (2011) examined a random sample of 342 adjudicated youth and found that those youth with bipolar disorder were at a greater risk of being incarcerated for a crime against persons than were youth having attention deficit hyperactivity disorder or conduct disorder. In fact, the results of this study found that those youth having bipolar disorder were more than eight times higher than those without to be detained for a personal crime.

In regard to specific categories of risk assessment, determining the *risk of dangerousness* can be complicated in youth having mood disorders, since there is evidence to suggest that these youth are likely to commit an offense against persons and are inclined toward disruptive or violent outbursts and related aggressive behaviors (e.g., Joshi & Wilens, 2009; Stoddard-Dare et al., 2011). However, there is no evidence to suggest that such behaviors are directly related to poor empathy or antisocial or psychopathic features on the part of these youth. As indicated earlier, the outbursts in youth with mood disorders are more likely to be impulsive and reactive rather than premeditated, and as described by Joshi and Wilens (2009), these aggressive outbursts in mood disorders are typically more impulsive and disorganized in nature. In addition, these behaviors are likely to decrease when appropriate therapy and medication protocols are being implemented. It is our view that there is an increased risk of dangerousness on the part of youth having mood disorders, but this risk is more likely due to the symptoms of their mental health disorder rather than due to antisocial tendencies.

With respect to level of *sophistication and maturity*, there is no indication that having a mood disorder will lead to significant cognitive impairment or the inability to act in a sophisticated, mature manner. It is our view, however, that a final determination of a youth's level of sophistication and maturity can only be made once his or her level of impulsivity has been evaluated in regard to his or her performance of the illegal act(s). This evaluation should result in a determination of whether the act(s) was directly related to the youth's mood disorder. Executive functioning deficits have been observed in individuals with mood disorders, but otherwise there is little indication that IQ is affected (Nieto & Castellanos, 2011). Therefore, there is no empirical evidence that a mood disorder would directly impact sophistication or maturity of offending.

In terms of *treatment amenability*, there are two primary factors that need to be considered in regard to youth having mood disorders. First, a determination needs to be made whether a youth presents with comorbid disruptive behavior disorders. The presence of these comorbid disorders is associated with a weak prognosis regarding treatment amenability for bipolar disorder and is likely to contribute to an exacerbation of socially unacceptable behaviors and symptoms of the youth's mood disorder (Arnold et al., 2011). A second consideration involves whether the youth is being treated for his or her mood disorder with evidence-based methods and by a licensed mental health professional since, in our opinion, a youth receiving this form of consistent treatment with regular follow-up monitoring is more likely to experience success in reducing the frequency and intensity of the symptoms associated with the mood disorder and, therefore, reducing his or her risk of re-offending.

Competency

The presence in adults of a severe disability such as intellectual disability or psychosis is often given important consideration in court proceedings when determining whether a mental disorder may impact a person's competency (Duvall & Morris, 2006; Nicholson & Kugler, 1991). However, there are no specific cognitive impairments generally agreed upon by professionals who work within the juvenile justice system regarding which mental health disorders can negatively impact competency, especially since children and adolescents are already developmentally, emotionally, and cognitively immature compared to typical adults. There are no specific cognitive impairments related to mood disorders that would be expected to impair a juvenile's understanding of the court process. In addition, there are no inherent social impairments or other symptoms related to mood disorders that would *ipso facto* mean that they would significantly interfere with the youth offender's ability to participate and collaborate during his or her trial.

Nevertheless, it is our position that a youth's factual and rational understanding and ability to cooperate could be negatively impacted depending on the type of and severity of his or her mood disorder. It is therefore our position that juvenile offenders having mood disorders should be evaluated on a case-by-case basis by a licensed mental health professional to determine if a youth's behaviors, thoughts, and feelings, as well as any comorbid mental disorders that may be present, are sufficiently severe that they would likely interfere with the youth's ability to participate fully in his or her defense and trial.

For example, in the case of depression, those with severe depression are more inclined toward severe thinking deficits, attention deficits, and grossly impaired daily functioning (APA, 2013). This, in turn, may make it extremely difficult for the youth to participate in the trial. In regard to a youth offender having bipolar disorder, the type, severity, and current symptoms also need to be evaluated to determine if he or she is able to fully participate in the trial. For example, if the youth is currently in a hypomanic episode, he or she may likely display erratic and impulsive thinking and have difficulty with rational decision-making. If the youth is currently exhibiting mania, he or she may likely be unable to fully collaborate with his or her attorney during the entire court process. By providing the court with case-by-case evaluations of youth offenders having mood disorders, it is our opinion that the court will be in a better position to determine competency in these youth.

Remediation for youth having a mood disorder is likely to rest largely on the type and consistency of intervention. The research literature suggests that the symptoms associated with bipolar disorder are unlikely to be stabilized without a consistent medication regimen (e.g., Gearing & Mian, 2005; AACAP, 2014), while severe depression may necessitate both medication and therapy to improve functioning (e.g., Brent et al., 2008; Weersing & Brent, 2013). Following the appropriate evidence-based treatment, it is expected that restoration would be achieved within a reasonable amount of time, assuming that there are no additional delimiting factors.

References

Althoff, R. R., Verhulst, F. C., Rettew, D. C., Hudziak, J. J., & Van der Ende, J. (2010). Adult outcomes of childhood dysregulation: A 14-year follow up study. *Journal of the American Academy of Child and Adolescent Psychiatry, 49*(11), 1105–1124. doi:10.1097/00004583-201011000-00004.

Althoff, R. R., Faraone, S. V., Rettew, D. C., Morley, C. P., & Hudziak, J. J. (2005). Family, twin, adoption, and molecular genetic studies of juvenile bipolar disorder. *Bipolar Disorders, 7*, 598–609. doi:10.1111/j.1399-5618.2005.00268.x.

American Academy for Child and Adolescent Psychiatry. (2013). *Facts for families: The depressed child*. Washington, DC: Author.

American Academy for Child and Adolescent Psychiatry. (2014). *Bipolar disorder: Parents' medication guide for bipolar disorder in children and adolescents*. Washington, DC: Author.

American Psychiatric Association. (2013). *Diagnostic and statistical manual for mental disorders* (5th ed.). Washington, DC: Author.

Andrews, P. W., Aggen, S. H., Miller, G. F., Radi, C., Dencoff, J. E., & Neale, M. C. (2007). The functional design of depression's influence on attention: A preliminary test of alternative control-process mechanisms. *Evolutionary Psychology, 5*(3), 584–604.

Arnold, L. E., Demeter, C., Mount, K., Frazier, T. W., Youngstrom, E. A., Fristad, M., et al. (2011). Pediatric bipolar spectrum disorder and ADHD: Comparison and comorbidity in the LAMS clinical sample. *Bipolar Disorders, 13*, 509–521. doi:10.1111/j.1399-5618.2011.00948.x.

Assion, H.-J., Brune, N., Schmidt, N., Aubel, T., Edel, M.-A., Basilowski, M., et al. (2009). Trauma exposure and post-traumatic stress disorder in bipolar disorder. *Social Psychiatry and Psychiatric Epidemiology, 44*, 1041–1049. doi:10.1007/s00127-009-0029-1.

Barkley, R. (2013). *Defiant children: A clinician's manual for assessment and parent training* (3rd ed.). New York: Guilford Press.

Beck, A. T. (1967). *Depression: Clinical, experimental, and theoretical aspects*. Philadelphia, PA: University of Pennsylvania Press.

Biederman, J., Faraone, S. V., Chu, M. P., & Wozniak, J. (1999). Further evidence of a bidirectional overlap between juvenile mania and conduct disorder in children. *Journal of the American Academy of Child and Adolescent Psychiatry, 38*, 468–476.

Biederman, J., Kwon, A., Wozniak, J., Mick, E., Markowitz, S., Fazio, V., et al. (2004). Absence of gender differences in pediatric bipolar disorder: Findings from a large sample of referred youth. *Journal of Affective Disorders, 83*, 207–214. doi:10.1016/j.jad.2004.08.005.

Birmaher, B., Arbelaez, C., & Brent, D. (2002). Course and outcome of child and adolescent major depressive disorder. *Child and Adolescent Psychiatric Clinics of North America, 11*, 619–638. doi:10.1016/S1056-4993(02)00011-1.

Brent, D., Emslie, G., Clarke, G., et al. (2008). Switching to another SSRI or to venlafaxine with or without cognitive behavioral therapy for adolescents with SSRI-resistant depression: The TORDIA randomized controlled trial. *Journal of the American Medical Association, 299*, 901–913.

Cash, R. E. (2008). *Depression in adolescence: What can schools do*. Bethesda, MD: National Association of School Psychologists.

Cabiya-Morales, J. J., Padilla, L., Sayers-Montalvo, S., Pedrosa, O., Perez-Pedrogo, C., & Manzano-Mojica, J. (2007). Relationship between aggressive behavior, depressed mood, and other disruptive behavior in Puerto Rican children diagnosed with attention deficit and disruptive behavior disorders. *Puerto Rico Health Sciences Journal, 26*(1), 43–49.

Colins, O., Vermeiren, R., Vahl, P., Markus, M., Broekaert, E., & Doreleijers, T. (2011). Psychiatric disorder in detained male adolescents as risk factor for serious recidivism. *Canadian Journal of Psychiatry, 56*(1), 44–50. doi:10.1016/j.eurpsy.2011.01.001.

Compton, S. N., March, J. S., Brent, D. A., Albano, A. M., Weersing, V. R., & Curry, J. F. (2004). Cognitive-behavioral psychotherapy for anxiety and depressive disorders in children and adolescents: An evidence-based medicine review. *Journal of the American Academy of Child and Adolescent Psychiatry, 43*(8), 930–959. doi:10.1097/01.chi.0000127589.57468.bf.

Copeland, W. E., Angold, A., Costello, E. J., & Egger, H. (2012). Prevalence, comorbidity, and correlates of DSM-5 proposed disruptive mood dysregulation disorder. *The American Journal of Psychiatry, 170*(2), 173–179.

Copeland, W. E., Shanahan, L., Egger, H., Angold, A., & Costello, E. J. (2014). Adult diagnostic and functional outcomes of DSM-5 disruptive mood dysregulation disorder. *The American Journal of Psychiatry, 171*(6), 668–674. doi:10.1176/appi.ajp.2014.13091213.

Culver, J. L., Arnow, B. A., & Ketter, T. A. (2007). Bipolar disorder: Improving diagnosis and optimizing integrated care. *Journal of Clinical Psychology, 63*, 73–92. doi:10.1002/jclp.20333.

Curry, J. F. (2001). Specific psychotherapies for childhood and adolescent depression. *Biological Psychiatry, 49*(12), 1091–1100. doi:10.1016/s0006-3223(01)01130-1.

David-Ferdon, C., & Kaslow, N. J. (2008). Evidence-based psychosocial treatments for child and adolescent depression. *Journal of Clinical Child & Adolescent Psychology, 37*, 62–104.

Deveney, C. M., Brotman, M. A., Decker, A. M., Pine, D. S., & Leibenluft, E. (2012). Affective prosody labeling in youth with bipolar disorder or severe mood dysregulation. *Journal of Child Psychology and Psychiatry, 53*, 262–270. doi:10.1111/j.1469-7610.2011.02482.x.

Diler, R. S., Uguz, S., Seydaoglu, G., Erol, N., & Avci, A. (2007). Differentiating bipolar disorder in Turkish prepubertal children with attention-deficit hyperactivity disorder. *Bipolar Disorders, 9*, 243–251. doi:10.1111/j.1399-5618.2007.00347.x.

Defoe, I. N., Farrington, D. P., & Loeber, R. (2013). Disentangling the relationship between delinquency and hyperactivity, low achievement, depression, and low socioeconomic status: Analysis of repeated longitudinal data. *Journal of Criminal Justice, 41*(2), 100–107. doi:10.1016/j.jcrimjus.2012.12.002.

Delate, T., Gelenberg, A. J., Simmons, V. A., & Motheral, B. R. (2004). Trends in the use of antidepressants in a national sample of commercially insured pediatric patients, 1998–2002. *Psychiatric Services, 55*, 387–391.

Duvall, J., & Morris, R. J. (2006). Assessing mental retardation in death penalty cases: Critical issues for psychology and psychological practice. *Professional Psychology: Research and Practice, 37*, 658–665.

Ebesutani, C., Kim, E., & Young, J. (2014). The role of violence exposure and negative affect in understanding child and adolescent aggression. *Child Psychiatry and Human Development, 45*(6), 736–745. doi:10.1007/s10578-014-0442-x.

Eisenberg, D., Golberstein, E., & Hunt, J. (2009). Mental health and academic success in college. *B.E. Journal of Economic Analysis & Policy, 9*(1), 1–37.

Fazel, S., Doll, H., & Langstrom, N. (2008). Mental disorders among adolescents in juvenile detention and correctional facilities: A systematic review and metaregression analysis of 25 surveys. *Journal of the American Academy of Child and Adolescent Psychiatry, 47*(9), 1010–1019. doi:10.1097/chi.0b013e31817eecf3.

Federal Drug Administration. (2015). *FDA approved drug products*. Retrieved from http://www.accessdata.fda.gov/scripts/cder/drugsatfda/index.cfm.

Fite, P. J., Rubens, S. L., Preddy, T. M., Raine, A., & Pardini, D. A. (2014). Reactive/proactive aggression and the development of internalizing problems in males: The moderating effect of parent and peer relationships. *Aggressive Behavior, 40*(1), 69–78. doi:10.1002/ab.21498.

Freeman, A. J., Youngstrom, E. A., Michalak, E., Siegel, R., Meyers, O. I., & Findling, R. L. (2009). Quality of life in pediatric bipolar disorder. *Pediatrics, 123*, 446–452. doi:10.1542/peds.2008-0841.

Fristad, M. A., & MacPherson, H. A. (2014). Evidence-based psychosocial treatments for child and adolescent bipolar spectrum disorders. *Journal of Clinical Child & Adolescent Psychology, 43*(3), 339–355. doi:10.1080/15374416.2013.822309.

Gearing, R. E., & Mian, E. A. (2005). An approach to maximizing treatment adherence of children and adolescents with psychotic disorders and major mood disorders. *Canadian Journal of Child and Adolescent Psychiatry Review, 14*(4), 106–113.

References

Geller, B., Bolhofner, K., Craney, J. L., Williams, M., DelBello, M. P., & Gundersen, K. (2000). Psychosocial functioning in a prepubertal and early adolescent bipolar disorder phenotype. *Journal of the American Academy of Child and Adolescent Psychiatry, 39*(12), 1543–1548. doi:10.1097/00004583-200012000-00018.

Goldstein, B. I., & Bukstein, O. G. (2010). Comorbid substance use disorders among youth with bipolar disorder: Opportunities for early identification and prevention. *The Journal of Clinical Psychiatry, 71,* 348–358. doi:10.4088/JCP.09r05222gry.

Goldstein, T. R., Birmaher, B., Axelson, D., Ryan, N. D., Strober, M. A., Gill, M. K. ... Keller M. (2005). History of suicide attempts in pediatric bipolar disorder: Factors associated with increased risk. *Bipolar Disorders, 7,* 525–535. doi:10.1111/j.1399-5618.2005.00263.x.

Goldstein, N., Olubadewo, O., Redding, R., & Lexcen, F. (2005). Mental health disorders. In K. Heilbrun, N. E. S. Goldstein, & R. E. Redding (Eds.), *Juvenile delinquency: Prevention, assessment, and intervention.* Oxford: Oxford University Press.

Guyer, A. E., McClure, E. B., Adler, A. D., Brotman, M. A., Rich, B. A., Kimes, A. S., et al. (2007). Specificity of facial expression labeling deficits in childhood psychopathology. *Journal of Child Psychology and Psychiatry, 48,* 863–871. doi:10.1111/j.1469-7610.2007.01758.x.

Hart, S. R., Brock, S. E., & Jeltova, I. (2014). *Identifying, assessing, and treating bipolar depression at school.* New York: Springer.

Henin, A., Biederman, J., Mick, E., Hirshfeld-Becker, D., Sachs, G., Wu, Y., ... Nierenberg, A. (2007). Childhood antecedent disorders to bipolar disorder in adults: A controlled study. *Journal of Affective Disorders, 99,* 51–57.

Hoeve, M., McReynolds, L. S., & Wasserman, G. A. (2013). The influence of adolescent psychiatric disorder on young adult recidivism. *Criminal Justice and Behavior, 40,* 1368–1382. doi:10.1177/0093854813488106.

Horn, K., Roessner, V., & Holtmann, M. (2011). Neurocognitive performance in children and adolescents with bipolar disorder: A review. *European Child & Adolescent Psychiatry, 20,* 433–450. doi:10.1007/s00787-011-0209-x.

Horwitz, S. M., Demeter, C. A., Pagano, M. E., Youngstrom, E. A., Fristrad, M. A., et al. (2010). Longitudinal assessment of manic symptoms (LAMS) study: Background, design, and initial screening results. *Journal of Clinical Psychiatry, 71*(11), 1511–1517. doi:10.4088/JCP.09m05835yel.

Hysenbegasi, A., Hass, S. L., & Rowland, C. R. (2005). Impact of depression on the academic productivity of university students. *The Journal of Mental Health Policy and Economics, 8,* 145–151.

Individuals With Disabilities Education Act, 20 U.S.C. § 1400 (2004)

Jacobson, C. M., & Mufson, L. (2012). Interpersonal psychotherapy for depressed adolescents adapted for self-injury (IPT-ASI): Rationale, overview, and case summary. *American Journal of Psychotherapy, 66,* 349–374.

Johnston, H. F., & Fruehling, J. J. (2008). Pharmacological approaches with children and adolescents. In R. J. Morris & T. R. Kratochwill (Eds.), *The practice of child therapy* (4th ed., pp. 207–248). New York, NY: Lawrence Erlbaum Associates.

Joshi, G. G., & Wilens, T. (2009). Comorbidity in pediatric bipolar disorder. *Child and Adolescent Psychiatric Clinics of North America, 18,* 291–319. doi:10.1016/j.chc.2008.12.005.

Jucksch, V., Salbach-Andrae, H., Lenz, K., Goth, K., Dopfner, M., & Poustka, F., ... Holtmann, M. (2011). Severe affective and behavioural dysregulation is associated with significant psychosocial adversity and impairment. *Journal of Child Psychology and Psychiatry, 52*(6), 686-695. doi:10.1111/j.1469-7610.2010.02322.x

Kato, T. (2008). Molecular neurobiology of bipolar disorder: A disease of 'mood-stabilizing neurons'? *Trends in Neurosciences, 31,* 495–503. doi:10.1016/j.tins.2008.07.007.

Kaslow, N. J., Clark, A. G., & Sirian, L. M. (2008). Childhood depression. In R. J. Morris & T. R. Kratochwill (Eds.), *The practice of child therapy* (4th ed., pp. 29–92). NY: Lawrence Erlbaum Associates.

Kazdin, A. E., & De Los Reyes, A. (2008). Conduct disorder. In R. J. Morris & T. R. Kratochwill (Eds.), *The practice of child therapy* (4th ed., pp. 207–248). NY: Lawrence Erlbaum Associates.

Keenan-Miller, D., & Miklowitz, D. J. (2011). Interpersonal functioning in pediatric bipolar disorder. *Clinical Psychology: Science and Practice, 18*, 342–356. doi:10.1111/j.1468-2850.2011.01266.x.

Kerner, B., Lambert, C. G., & Muthén, B. O. (2011). Genome-wide association study in bipolar patients stratified by co-morbidity. *PLoS One, 6*, 1–10. doi:10.1371/journal.pone.0028477.

Kinscherff, R. (2012). *A primer for mental health practitioners working with youth involved in the juvenile justice system*. Washington, DC: Technical Assistance Partnership for Child and Family Health.

Kofler, M. J., McCart, M. R., Zajac, K., Ruggiero, K. J., Saunders, B. E., & Kilpatrick, D. G. (2011). Depression and delinquency covariation in an accelerated longitudinal sample of adolescents. *Journal of Consulting and Clinical Psychology, 79*, 458–469. doi:10.1037/a0024108.

Kolb, B., & Whishaw, I. Q. (2008). *Fundamentals of human neuropsychology* (6th ed.). New York: Macmillan.

Kovacs, M., Kovacs, M., & Pollack, M. (1995). Bipolar disorder and comorbid conduct disorder in childhood and adolescence. *Journal of the American Academy of Children and Adolescent Psychiatry, 34*, 526–529.

Kowatch, R. A., Youngstrom, E. A., Danielyan, A., & Findling, R. L. (2005). Review and meta-analysis of the phenomenology and clinical characteristics of mania in children and adolescents. *Bipolar Disorder, 7*, 483–496.

Leahy, R. L. (2007). Bipolar disorder: Causes, contexts, and treatments. *Journal of Clinical Psychology: In Session, 83*, 417–424. doi:10.1002/jclp.20360.

Leibenluft, E. (2011). Severe mood dysregulation, irritability, and the diagnostic boundaries of bipolar disorder in youth. *American Journal of Psychiatry, 168*(2), 129–142.

Lofthouse, N., & Fristad, M. A. (2008). Bipolar disorders. In G. G. Bear & K. M. Minke (Eds.), *Children's needs III: Development, prevention, and intervention* (pp. 211–224). Bethesda, MD: National Association of School Psychologists.

Loeber, R., & Keenan, K. (1994). Interaction between conduct disorder and its comorbid conditions: Effects of age and gender. *Clinical Psychology Review, 14*(6), 497–523. doi:10.1016/0272-7358(94)90015-9.

Lorberg, B., Wilens, T. E., Martelon, M., Wong, P., & Parcell, T. (2010). Reasons for substance use among adolescents with bipolar disorder. *The American Journal on Addictions, 19*, 474–480. doi:10.1111/j.1521-0391.2010.00077.x.

Lundy, S. M., Silva, G. E., Kaemingk, K. L., Goodwin, J. L., & Quan, S. F. (2010). Cognitive functioning and academic performance in elementary school children with anxious/depressed and withdrawn symptoms. *The Open Pediatric Medical Journal, 14*, 1–9. doi:10.2174/1874309901004010001.

Mallett, C. A., Stoddard-Dare, P. A., & Seck, M. M. (2009). Predicting juvenile delinquency: The nexus of childhood maltreatment, depression, and bipolar disorder. *Criminal Behavior and Mental Health, 19*(4), 235–246. doi:10.1002/cbm.737.

March, J., Silva, S., Petrycki, S., Curry, J., Wells, K., Fairbank, J., … Severe, J. (2004). Fluoxetine, cognitive-behavioral therapy, and their combination for adolescents with depression: Treatment for Adolescents With Depression Study (TADS) randomized controlled trial. *JAMA: The Journal of the American Medical Association, 292*(7), 807-820. doi:10.1001/jama.292.7.807

March, J., Silva, S, Petrycki, S., Curry, J., Wells, K., Fairbank, J., … Severe, J. (2007). The treatment for adolescents with depression study (TADS): Long-term effectiveness and safety outcomes. *Archives of General Psychiatry, 64*(10), 1132-1143. doi:10.1001/archpsyc.64.10.1132

Margulies, D. M., Weintraub, S., Basile, J., Grover, P. J., & Carlson, G. A. (2012). Will disruptive mood dysregulation disorder reduce false diagnosis of bipolar disorder in children? *Bipolar Disorders, 14*(5), 488–496. doi:10.1111/j.1399-5618.2012.01029.x.

Masi, G., Perugi, G., Toni, C., Millepiedi, S., Mucci, M., Bertini, N., et al. (2006). Attention-deficit hyperactivity disorder—bipolar comorbidity in children and adolescents. *Bipolar Disorders, 8*, 373–381. doi:10.1111/j.1399-5618.2006.00342.x.

Mattis, S., Papolos, D., Luck, D., Cockerham, M., & Thode, H. C. (2011). Neuropsychological factors differentiating treated children with pediatric bipolar disorder from those with attention-deficit/hyperactivity disorder. *Journal of Clinical and Experimental Neuropsychology, 33*(1), 74–84.

McClure-Tone, E. B. (2010). Social cognition and cognitive flexibility in bipolar disorder. In D. J. Miklowitz & D. Cicchetti (Eds.), *Understanding bipolar disorder: A developmental psychopathology perspective* (pp. 331–369). New York, NY: Guilford Press.

McIntyre, R., Konarski, J., Wilkins, K., Soczynska, J., & Kennedy, S. (2006). Obesity in bipolar disorder and major depressive disorder: Results from a national community health survey on mental health and well-being. *Canadian Journal of Psychiatry, 51*, 274–280.

McReynolds, L. S., Schwalbe, C. S., & Wasserman, G. A. (2010). The contribution of psychiatric disorder to juvenile recidivism. *Criminal Justice and Behavior, 37*(2), 204–216. doi:10.1177/0093854809354961.

Miklowitz, D., Axelson, D., Birmaher, B., Taylor, D. O., Schneck, C. D., Beresford, C. A., et al. (2008). Family-focused treatment for adolescents with bipolar disorder. *Archives of General Psychiatry, 65*(9), 1053–1061.

Moor, S., Crowe, M., Luty, S., Carter, J., & Joyce, P. R. (2012). Effects of comorbidity and early age of onset in young people with bipolar disorder on self harming behavior and suicide attempts. *Journal of Affective Disorders, 136*, 1212–1215. doi:10.1016/j.jad.2011.10.018.

Mufson, L. H., Dorta, K. P., Wickramaratne, P., Nomura, Y., Olfson, M., & Weissman, M. M. (2004). A randomized effectiveness trial of interpersonal psychotherapy for depressed adolescents. *Archives of General Psychiatry, 61*, 577–584.

National Institute of Mental Health. (2014). *Depression in children and adolescents fact sheet.* Bethesda, MD: Author.

Nicholson, R. A., & Kugler, K. E. (1991). Competent and incompetent criminal defendants: A quantitative review of comparative research. *Psychological Bulletin, 109*(3), 355–370. doi:10.1037//0033-2909.109.3.355.

Nieto, R. G., & Castellanos, F. X. (2011). A meta-analysis of neuropsychological functioning in patients with early onset schizophrenia and pediatric bipolar disorder. *Journal of Clinical Child and Adolescent Psychology, 40*, 266–280. doi:10.1080/15374416.2011.546049.

Obeidallah, D. A., & Earls, F. J. (1999). *Adolescent girls: The role of depression in the development of delinquency: Summary of research.* Washington, DC: U.S. Department of Justice, Office of Justice Programs, National Institute of Justice.

Reichart, C. G., & Nolen, W. A. (2004). Earlier onset of bipolar disorder in children by antidepressants or stimulants? An hypothesis. *Journal of Affective Disorders, 78*, 81–84. doi:10.1016/S0165-0327(02)00180-5.

Reinemann, D., Stark, K., Molnar, J., & Simpson, J. (2006). Depressive disorders. In G. G. Bear & K. M. Minke (Eds.), *Children's needs III: Development, prevention, and intervention* (pp. 199–210). Bethesda, MD: National Association of School Psychologists.

Renou, S., Hergueta, T., Flament, M., Mouren-Simeoni, M. C., & Lecrubier, Y. (2004). Diagnostic structured interviews in child and adolescent's psychiatry. *Encephale, 30*, 122–134. doi:10.1016/S0013-7006(04)95422-X.

Rich, B. A., Vinton, D. T., Roberson-Nay, R., Hommer, R. E., Berghorst, L. H., McClure, E. B., et al. (2006). Limbic hyperactivation during processing of neutral facial expressions in children with bipolar disorder. *Proceedings of the National Academy of Sciences, 103*(23), 8900–8905. doi:10.1073/pnas.0603246103.

Roybal, D. J., Chang, K. D., Chen, M. C., Howe, M. E., Gotlib, I. H., & Singh, M. K. (2011). Characterization and factors associated with sleep quality in adolescents with Bipolar I disorder. *Child Psychiatry and Human Development, 42*, 724–740.

Schubert, C. A., Mulvey, E. P., & Glasheen, C. (2011). Influence of mental health and substance use problems and criminogenic risk on outcomes in serious juvenile offenders. *Journal of the American Academy of Child and Adolescent Psychiatry, 50*(9), 925–937. doi:10.1016/j.jaac.2011.06.006.

Section 504 of the Rehabilitation Act of 1977, Pub. L. No. 93-112, § 87, Stat. 394 (1973).

Saveanu, R. V., & Nemeroff, C. B. (2012). Etiology of depression. Genetic and environmental factors. *Psychiatry Clinics of North America, 35*(1), 51–71.

Shelton, D. J., & Kirwan, C. B. (2013). A possible negative influence of depression on the ability to overcome memory interference. *Behavioural Brain Research, 256*, 20–26. doi:10.1016/j.bbr.2013.08.016.

Staton, D., Volness, L. J., & Beatty, W. W. (2008). Diagnosis and classification of pediatric bipolar disorder. *Journal of Affective Disorders, 105*, 205–212. doi:10.1016/j.jad.2007.05.015.

Stoddard-Dare, P. S., Mallett, C.A., & Boitel, C. (2011). Association between mental health disorders and juveniles' detention for a personal crime. *Child and Adolescent Mental Health 16*(4), 208-213. doi:10.1111/j.1475-3588.2011.00599.x

Stouthamer-Loeber, M., Loeber, R., Wei, E., Farrington, D. P., & Wikström, P. O. H. (2002). Risk and promotive effects in the explanation of persistent serious delinquency in boys. *Journal of Consulting and Clinical Psychology, 70*(1), 111–123.

Stringaris, A. (2013). Editorial: The new DSM is coming—It needs tough love. *Journal of Child Psychology and Psychiatry, 54*(5), 501–502. doi:10.1111/jcpp.12078.

Sullivan, A. E., & Miklowitz, D. J. (2010). Family functioning among adolescents with bipolar disorder. *Journal of Family Psychology, 24*, 60–67. doi:10.1037/a001813.

Takeda, Y. (2000). Aggression in relation to childhood depression: A study of Japanese 3rd–6th graders. *Japanese Journal of Developmental Psychology, 11*(1), 1–11.

Teplin, L. A., Abram, K. M., McClelland, G. M., Dulcan, M. K., & Mericle, A. A. (2002). Psychiatric disorders in youth in juvenile detention. *Archives of General Psychiatry, 59*(12), 1133–1143. doi:10.1001/archpsyc.59.12.1133.

U.S. Department of Education. (2014). *Thirty-sixth annual report to Congress on the implementation of the Individuals with Disabilities Education Act*. Washington, DC: Author.

Weersing, V. R., & Brent, D. A. (2013). Treating depression in adolescents using individual cognitive-behavioral therapy. In J. R. Weisz & A. E. Kazdin (Eds.), *Evidence-based psychotherapies for children and adolescents* (2nd ed.). New York: Guilford Press.

Weersing, V. R., Iyengar, S., Kolko, D. J., Birmaher, B., & Brent, D. A. (2006). Effectiveness of cognitive behavioral therapy for adolescent depression: A benchmarking investigation. *Behavior Therapy, 37*, 36–48.

Wilens, T. E., Adler, L. A., Adams, J., Sgambati, S., Rotrosen, J., Sawtelle, R., … Fusillo, S. (2008). Misuse and diversion of stimulants prescribed for ADHD: A systematic review of the literature. *Journal of the American Academy of Child and Adolescent Psychiatry, 47*, 21–31.

Wozniak, J., Biederman, J., Kiely, K., Ablon, J. S., Faraone, S. V., & Mundy, E. (1995). Mania-like symptoms suggestive of childhood-onset bipolar disorder in clinically referred children. *Journal of the American Academy of Child and Adolescent Psychiatry, 34*, 867–876.

Youngstrom, E. A., Findling, R. L., Youngstrom, J. K., & Calabrese, J. R. (2005). Toward an evidence-based assessment of pediatric bipolar disorder. *Journal of Clinical Child and Adolescent Psychology, 34*, 433–448. doi:10.1207/s15374424jccp3403_4.

Youngstrom, E. A., Birmaher, B., & Findling, R. L. (2008). Pediatric bipolar disorder: Validity, phenomenology, and recommendations for diagnosis. *Bipolar Disorders, 10*, 194–214. doi:10.1111/j.1399-5618.2007.00563.x.

Zara, G., & Farrington, D. P. (2013). Assessment of risk for juvenile compared with adult criminal onset implications for policy, prevention, and intervention. *Psychology, Public Policy, and Law, 19*(2), 235. doi:http://dx.doi.org/10.1037/a0029050

Zuckerman, M. (1999). *Vulnerability to psychopathology: A biosocial model*. Washington, DC: American Psychological Association.

Chapter 11
Anxiety and Trauma-Related Disorders

While fear and anxiety are normal experiences across the life-span, these symptoms qualify as a mental health disorder when they become developmentally inappropriate and/or the fear or anxiety is excessive and out of proportion to situations, subsequently interfering with the child's or adolescent's functioning. In general, anxiety-related disorders have been found to be prevalent in the juvenile offender population, with estimates being considerably higher than those reported in the general child and adolescent population (e.g., Teplin et al. 2002).

While studies have shown a high prevalence of anxiety-related disorders among the juvenile delinquency population, few, if any, differentiate between types of anxiety disorders or history of abuse or neglect to determine the degree to which trauma history contributes to the high rates of anxiety reported among juvenile offenders. This is important to consider given that while both generalized anxiety disorders and trauma-related disorders typically have a common symptomatology involving high anxiety, the presentation of other behavioral difficulties, thoughts, and feelings on the part of youth, as well as the treatment emphases for these disorders, are often different (Saigh et al. 2008). In this regard, Chen, Voisin, and Jacobson (2013) indicated that the majority of youth offenders have been exposed to violence, abuse, or trauma during childhood; therefore, it would not be unexpected that trauma history could be an important contributing factor to the anxiety that these youth experience.

Generalized Anxiety Disorder

There are a variety of anxiety disorders discussed in the DSM-5, with the type of anxiety disorder being directly related to the feared setting, event, or activity. Specific types of anxiety disorders include separation anxiety disorder, selective mutism, specific phobia, social anxiety disorder, panic disorder, agoraphobia, and generalized anxiety disorder (APA, 2013). While obsessive-compulsive disorder was previously referred to as an anxiety disorder, the DSM-5 now considers this in its own category of disorders. Each specific type of anxiety disorder has its own diagnostic criteria and recommended treatment plan. For example, separation anxiety disorder includes the specification that the person's significant anxiety be caused by the separation from caregivers, while in the case of social anxiety disorder, the significant anxiety is caused by various social situations and events. The most common anxiety disorder among youth is generalized anxiety disorder (GAD), with its prevalence being approximately 1 % of the child and adolescent general population. It occurs more often in females than males, with approximately two-thirds of those diagnosed being female (APA, 2013).

The DSM-5 diagnostic criteria for GAD include the following:

(a) Excessive anxiety and worry that occur more often than not for at least a six-month period, with the anxiety being about a variety of events or activities (versus a specific event, setting or activity as in specific phobia or social anxiety disorder). Children and adolescents with generalized anxiety often fear failure and are critical of their performance in school, sports, or other areas. Their worries are often largely irrational and out of proportion with events in their life. This may be observed with the youth chronically worrying about his or her family relationships despite no apparent difficulties, fear of family members dying (despite there being no factual evidence that this will happen), irrational concern that the youth himself or herself is sick or will become chronically ill, fear that he or she will end up in prison after committing a relatively minor offense, or ongoing concern about future life events that are relatively unpredictable and/or unlikely to occur.
(b) The child or adolescent struggles to control the worry.
(c) The worry is associated with restlessness, fatigue, difficulty concentrating, irritability, muscle tensions, and/or sleep disturbance (APA, 2013).

In order for a youth to qualify for a diagnosis of GAD, the symptoms need to cause significant impairment in important areas of functioning, such as their ability to be successful at school or maintain social relationships. For example, a teenager with a diagnosis of GAD may be highly anxious about school performance or relationships with peers, and subsequently develop irrational fears of attending school and/or even refuse to go. This may result in truancy violations and related disciplinary actions.

Youth who meet the criteria for this diagnosis typically have a long history of worry, nervousness, or anxiousness. The specific causes for GAD are relatively unknown, but research suggests that it is likely due to a combination of genetic factors, temperament, and environmental influences (APA, 2013). A review of childhood anxiety disorders by Beesdo, Knappe, and Pine (2009), for example, found that youth with anxiety disorders are more likely to have parents or immediate family members with anxiety, they are more likely to be sensitive to criticism and feedback from others starting in early childhood, and they are more likely to experience stressful life events that can increase anxiety or even be in environments that model/reinforce anxiety symptoms.

The actual implications of an anxiety disorder will vary considerably depending on the specific symptoms, but it would not be uncommon to observe academic difficulties, as these youth may struggle with test-taking anxiety, refuse to turn in homework unless they are assured it is perfect (and, therefore, have missing assignments and poor grades), or refuse to attend school if the anxiety is extreme (Kendall, Furr, & Podell, 2010). Social difficulties can also occur if the youth is too anxious to participate in extracurricular activities, spend time with friends away from parents, or otherwise form relationships with peers (Beesdo et al. 2009). In addition, GAD is highly comorbid with other internalizing disorders, particularly depressive disorders (APA, 2013).

In regard to treatment of GAD, there are currently no well-established, evidence-based interventions in youth. However, there are some studies that suggest that CBT may be an effective approach to treating anxiety disorders in children (Silverman, Pina, & Viswesvaran, 2008). The goal of CBT is to target somatic, cognitive, and behavioral aspects of GAD, and treatment components may include psychoeducation about anxiety, teaching coping skills to manage physical symptoms related to anxiety, as well as cognitive restructuring to address irrational thoughts that lead to generalized anxiety (Kendall, Furr, & Podell, 2010). Many CBT programs are conducted in an individual therapy setting; however, there is some research that suggests that a family or group CBT-based program can also be effective in treating GAD in children and adolescents (e.g., Silverman et al. 2008; Wood, Piacentini, Southam-Gerow, Chu, & Sigman, 2006).

While CBT has been shown to be effective in treating GAD, for youth with moderate to severe symptoms, it may be the case that medication may also be necessary to treat symptoms (Southam-Gerow, Kendall, & Weersing, 2001). While currently there are not any FDA-approved medications for GAD, research studies have found medications to be helpful in treating symptoms (e.g., Kodish, Rockhill, & Varley, 2011; Rynn, Siqueland, & Rickels, 2001). That being said, even with medication and treatment, remission of GAD is relatively low, and many youth with this anxiety disorder go on to struggle with anxiety into adulthood (Silverman et al. 2008).

Generalized Anxiety Disorder and Juvenile Delinquency

While research has suggested that anxiety disorders themselves are overrepresented in the juvenile delinquency population (e.g., Teplin et al. 2002), the prevalence of GAD specifically among juvenile offenders is difficult to ascertain. Most studies have a general category of "anxiety disorders" that include diagnoses such as post-traumatic stress disorder (PTSD), largely based on the fact that previous editions of the DSM considered PTSD an anxiety disorder—although in the DSM-5, it is included in a separate category known as trauma-related disorders (APA, 2013). Given the research that suggests there is a high prevalence of PTSD in juvenile delinquents (e.g., Kerig, Moeddel, & Becker, 2010; Wilson et al. 2013), it is difficult to determine whether the suggested high rates of anxiety disorders among juvenile delinquents are due to GAD, specific anxiety disorders, or PTSD.

Nevertheless, given that research has found that most mental health disorders are overrepresented in the juvenile offender population in comparison to the general population, it would not be unexpected that GAD would also be elevated in this population. In this regard, some researchers have reported that those youth who experience high levels of anxiety and distress are more likely to display lower levels of self-restraint, which then increases their risk of delinquency (Loeber, Stouthamer-Loeber, & White, 1999). Others have found positive relationships between anxiety levels and antisocial behavior as well as severity of offending (e.g., Monahan, Goldweber, Meyer, & Cauffman, 2012; Parker, Morton, Lingefelt, & Johnson, 2005; Sareen, Stein, Cox, & Hassard, 2004). On the other hand, Monahan et al. (2012) suggested that anxiety itself does not independently increase a youth's risk for delinquency, but rather it serves as a moderating factor in that it increases a youth's risk when the youth also has risk factors such as negative attitude and poor peer relationships.

Given the available literature, if a particular juvenile offender is found to have a GAD, it would be important to take this disorder into consideration when interacting and working with the youth during the various phases of the juvenile court process and when determining appropriate treatment programming for the youth. For example, a youth having GAD may have difficulty while in detention and separated from his or her familiar caregivers. The presence of high levels of anxiety could also negatively impact the youth's ability to comply with rules or requests from juvenile court staff if the youth is placed in detention and struggles to adjust to a highly populated setting in which he or she has little control of belongings, routines, and interactions. He or she may also have difficulty communicating with an attorney or other court personnel and may appear as aloof, withdrawn, or disinterested when, in fact, the youth is too anxious to readily engage with others.

Implications on Functioning. While there are no significant cognitive impairments associated with GAD that would be expected to directly affect competency, there are often social difficulties that may interfere with a youth's ability to adequately interact with his attorney. In addition, a youth with a diagnosis of GAD may have difficulty fully complying with probation or other court requirements. For example, if school attendance is a requirement for probation and the youth offender has a diagnosis of GAD, he or she may appear to be defiant or actively violating conditions of release when the refusal is more related to the presence of debilitating anxiety. Instead, this youth may benefit from participating in a small, alternative school setting or even an online grade-equivalent education program.

Another instance in which a youth offender with GAD could have difficulty complying with a condition of his or her probation is in a situation where the youth is required to attend group counseling for substance abuse or anger management. In this type of group setting, the youth might become agitated because of the perception that others are evaluating his or her participation. Or the youth might even skip required sessions since the anticipatory anxiety associated with attending sessions is so high that avoidance of the session is a safer alternative for the youth.

In our opinion, if it is known that a youth offender has GAD, he or she may be better served by receiving individual programs and services, with the goal to gradually fade in group programming or services. If GAD is suspected in a youth, then a comprehensive psychological or psychiatric evaluation would be helpful in determining specific impairments related to the anxiety disorder and in identifying appropriate interventions and recommendations to the court regarding the processing of the case based on the presence of the GAD.

Trauma and Stressor-Related Mental Health Disorders

The Case of Brianna

Brianna was a 17-year-old juvenile offender awaiting adjudication for a referral that included probation violation, heroin possession, and possession of a deadly weapon. Brianna had first been arrested at age 15 for drug charges, and she had six subsequent referrals for drug-related offenses and one for domestic violence at home. Her pending offense was her most serious, primarily because she was in possession of an illegal firearm. She also had several probation violations, which typically occurred for not following curfew, staying out overnight (sometimes for more than one day), not attending school as required, or not checking in with her probation officer. Brianna's mother had expressed concern to the court that she was unable to control Brianna in the home setting, describing Brianna's behavior as erratic, defiant, and angry. The mother also expressed concern that she felt Brianna was engaging in serious drug use. Brianna had attended court-ordered and intensive outpatient substance abuse treatment as well as group anger management classes, with no improvement in behavior or reduction in substance use.

According to her mother, Brianna was a typically developing child and adolescent until age 15, when her uncle molested her over a period of three months. Brianna attended individual therapy for approximately three months after the abuse was reported; however, this was stopped after she began engaging in substance use and had her first interaction with the juvenile justice system (and was referred for substance abuse treatment and anger management). At the trial review for her pending charges, Brianna was court ordered for a psychological evaluation by the judge presiding over her case, as the judge was concerned about Brianna's history of sexual abuse and whether it may be related to her substance abuse and delinquency.

A comprehensive psychological evaluation was conducted, during which it became clear that Brianna's sexual abuse history did appear to be a significant contributing factor to her behavior and legal difficulties. Brianna endorsed many significant symptoms of a trauma-related disorder, including having nightmares, flashbacks, high levels of anxiety, and depressive symptoms. She had also reportedly begun using substances soon after the abuse began as a self-medicated way of coping with these symptoms, particularly the anxiety. She began abusing prescription painkillers and engaging in recreational use of methamphetamine at age 16, during which time her behavior at home became more erratic (typically while under the influence or experiencing withdrawal symptoms), and she began skipping school while under the influence and leaving at night to use drugs.

Brianna also admitted that she had begun engaging in prostitution as a means to pay for and obtain drugs. She admitted that she had been involved in many dangerous situations as a result of her exchanging sexual favors for drugs, including an instance a month before her most recent arrest in which she alleged that she was raped while under the influence. Upon telling a friend of the incident, they decided to go and threaten the man who had allegedly raped her. It was on that night that she and her friend went to threaten the man with a gun when Brianna was stopped by a police officer and found in possession of the weapon and of heroin.

A psychological evaluation report was provided to the courts, which recommended that Brianna be considered for inpatient treatment at a residential treatment center that could offer both intensive substance abuse treatment as well as trauma-focused cognitive behavior therapy to help her cope with her trauma history and symptoms of PTSD. While in many respects it appeared that Brianna's behaviors and offenses were related to a substance use disorder and/or a disruptive behavior disorder, it actually appeared to the psychologists that the symptoms and related behaviors associated with her PTSD were a large contributing factor to her misbehaviors yet it had never been addressed in court-ordered treatment.

As mentioned earlier, there is a high prevalence of maltreatment history among delinquents. Maltreatment may include physical, sexual, or emotional neglect or abuse. Studies have estimated that between 26 and 60 % of court-involved youth have a history of maltreatment (e.g., Bender, 2010; Sedlak & McPherson, 2010). In addition, many of these youth have been exposed to violence in the home or community. While the majority of youth who experience maltreatment or violence do *not* become involved in the juvenile justice system (e.g., Kelley, Thornberry, & Smith, 1997; Smith, Ireland, & Thornberry, 2005), there is a large number of youth offenders with a history of maltreatment or exposure to violence. In this regard, studies have reported that youth offenders with this history may begin offending at an earlier age (Widom, 1989), and they often have a history of more serious offenses and increased court involvement (e.g., Lemmon, 1999; Loeber & Farrington, 2001; Yun, Ball, & Lim, 2011). Youth with a history of maltreatment and trauma are also at an increased risk of substance abuse problems and mental health difficulties (e.g., Hawkins et al. 2010; Kilpatrick et al. 2003).

Specific mental health disorders related to a history of trauma and childhood stressors such as exposure to violence and abuse in the home include *PTSD, acute stress disorder, adjustment disorder*, and *reactive attachment disorder*. These mental health disorders can lead to a variety of atypical maladaptive behaviors, social relationship difficulties, and disruptive behaviors and, in our opinion, should be taken into consideration when working with a youth offender or when the youth is being processed through the juvenile court system.

Post-Traumatic Stress Disorder

PTSD is a mental health disorder that occurs after an individual witnesses or experiences a highly stressful, traumatic event. Discussions related to PTSD have been popularized in the media based on the difficulties experienced by various military personnel who were in combat. Books, television news programs, and movies have portrayed the difficulties these individuals experience when they return home, with high levels of anger, low frustration tolerance, increased suicidal ideation, and increases in aggressiveness often being observed. Children and adolescent often experience similar difficulties and are also more likely to develop disruptive, disrespectful, or destructive behaviors (NIMH, 2014).

The DSM-5 identifies several criteria that must be present in order for an individual to qualify for a diagnosis of PTSD:

(a) Exposure to serious threat, death, or sexual violence. Exposure can include directly experiencing the traumatic event, witnessing it occurring, or learning about it happening to a close family member or friend. For example, in the case of a juvenile offender having PTSD, traumatic events may take the form of a youth experiencing physical, emotional, or sexual abuse. The youth may also be exposed to a home environment that includes frequent domestic violence, or he or she may live in a neighborhood that has high levels of gang violence or crime. These youth may be more likely to be involved in a gang, have family members in a gang, or associate with peers who engage in high-risk or gang-related behavior that exposes the youth to a greater chance of friends or family experiencing a traumatic death. Juvenile offenders involved in drug use may also be at a greater risk of experiencing a traumatic event, such as a female being taken advantage of or abused sexually in exchange for drugs.
(b) Distressing symptoms occur after the traumatic event. These symptoms may include recurrent, distressing memories, nightmares, flashbacks, or high levels of stress when faced with cues or symbols related to the event.
(c) Persistent avoidance of stimuli *associated* with the traumatic event. For example, the youth may avoid certain locations or situations that remind them of the event.
(d) Negative changes in one's thoughts or mood after the traumatic event. This may be observed with an increase in depressed mood, low frustration tolerance, high irritability, or suicidal ideation.
(e) Increased arousal and reactivity after the event, which may include angry outbursts with little provocation, self-destructive or reckless behavior, or hypervigilance (APA, 2013). In the case of a youth offender having PTSD, increased arousal and reactivity may be manifested by may suddenly engaging in more extreme or high-risk drug use, being more susceptible to peer pressure, an increase in illegal acts, or becoming more aggressive (APA, 2013).

To meet the criteria for PTSD, the symptoms must last longer than one month and cause significant impairment. If symptoms are present but it has been less than one month, an individual may instead qualify for acute stress disorder. Once these symptoms continue past a month's period, however, the diagnosis then becomes PTSD.

According to the National Institute of Mental Health (Merikangas et al. 2010), approximately 4 % of youth may meet the criteria for PTSD, though research has found PTSD to be more common among juvenile offenders than other adolescent populations, of upward of 32–52 % of delinquents (e.g., Kerig et al. 2010; Wilson et al. 2013). This may be due to a variety of reasons, including the fact that these youth are more likely to be from impoverished, low socioeconomic families which, in turn, have higher rates of domestic violence and abuse/neglect, are living in at-risk neighborhoods with more exposure to violence, and are involved in gang activity.

The literature suggests that not all children and adolescents who are exposed to a serious traumatic event will develop PTSD (e.g., Saigh et al. 2008). In this regard, a number of factors have been identified that may increase one's risk of, or resiliency against, developing PTSD. For example, risk factors associated with developing PTSD include the person having little social support after the serious traumatic event, having additional external stressors in one's life, or having a history of mental illness. Resiliency or protective factors include having immediate social support after the traumatic event, general ongoing social support in daily functioning, and having coping strategies to deal with the trauma (Brewin, Andrews, & Valentine, 2000). In addition, research has begun examining biological risk factors for developing PTSD, looking at brain imaging, physiology, and genetics to determine changes in the body after one is exposed to a traumatic event. While the research is still limited, early evidence suggests that there may be some genetic and biological differences in individuals who develop PTSD (e.g., De Bellis, Hooper, Woolley, & Shenk, 2009; NIMH, 2014).

Implications on Functioning. As mentioned above, some studies have reported an association between brain functioning and PTSD. Specifically, research has identified relationships between PTSD and areas of the brain such as the amygdala, hippocampus, and prefrontal cortex (e.g., Bremner, 2006; Etkin & Wager, 2007; Suvak & Barrett, 2011). The exact relationship is not yet understood, but in general there appears to be evidence that individuals with PTSD have an abnormally large amygdala, which is the area of the brain responsible for processing emotion; irregular functioning in the hippocampal region, which is the area associated with memory formation; and under-responding of the prefrontal cortex, which is the area of the brain associated with executive functioning and behavioral regulation (Suvak & Barrett, 2011). What is not understood, however, is whether interplay of these regions could put certain individuals at a greater risk of developing PTSD once exposed to a traumatic event or whether these could be changes in brain functioning that occur after one is exposed to a traumatic event. Deficits in cognitive functioning have also been found to be associated with PTSD, specifically in the areas of attention and executive functioning (e.g., Beers & De Bellis, 2002; Polak, Witteveen, Reitsma, & Olff, 2012).

Academic difficulties have also been found among youth with PTSD. For example, studies have reported that these students often have a lower grade point average, miss more days of school, and perform more poorly on standardized achievement tests (e.g., Delaney-Black et al. 2002; Nickerson, 2009). When examining implications of PTSD, the majority of the research has focused on the emotional and behavioral difficulties commonly experienced by children and adolescents having PTSD, with the type and severity of these difficulties being exacerbated by multiple exposures to trauma (Silvern & Griese, 2012). Studies have also suggested that children and adolescents with PTSD are at a greater risk for social difficulties (Schwartz & Proctor, 2000), often present with other internalizing disorders, such as depressive disorders and high levels of anxiety, and are at an increased risk of substance abuse (e.g., Finkelhor, Ormrod, & Turner, 2007; Kilpatrick et al. 2003; Silvern & Griese, 2012).

In addition to the internalizing difficulties, youth with PTSD have been found to be more inclined toward aggressive behaviors, and they are more likely to develop disruptive and externalizing behaviors (Silvern & Griese, 2012) that could place them at an increased risk of being involved with the juvenile justice system.

Treatment. The most common treatments for PTSD and stress-related disorders include psychologically based therapies and medication management (see, for example, Saigh et al. 2008; Johnston & Fruehling, 2008); however, Johnston and Fruehling (2008) indicate that "As a general rule, medication treatments should only be considered for those symptoms that have not responded adequately to non-drug interventions such as psychotherapy and systematic desensitization" (p. 467). In addition, evidence has been found for the benefits of both individual and group psychotherapies (Silverman et al. 2008). The most common individual therapy modality that has been found to be beneficial in treating PTSD is CBT (Saigh et al. 2008). The types of CBT that have been found to be beneficial include:

(a) *Exposure therapy*. This type of therapy exposes the individual to their fear or trauma they experiences while they are in a safe place. The exposure can occur by proxy through mental imagery or writing, or it could include in vivo exposure in which the adolescent visits the location where the traumatic event occurred. Exposure therapy helps the individual confront the trauma and then utilize coping skills to cope with the related feelings, ultimately working toward reducing the fears and traumatic thoughts related to the PTSD-causing event.
(b) *Cognitive restructuring*. This is a core component of CBT which helps the client make sense of the negative memories or subsequent feelings related to the traumatic event.
(c) *Stress inoculation training*. This type of CBT utilizes a variety of methods to help a person gain coping skills to reduce anxiety related to the traumatic memories, feelings, and cognitions (Saigh et al. 2008).

CBT used to treat symptoms of PTSD is often referred to as "trauma-focused cognitive behavior therapy," as it addresses problems specifically associated with the traumatic event that led to the use of CBT (Cohen, Mannarino, & Deblinger, 2013). In general, this trauma-focused CBT helps to teach the client about trauma and the related effects, helps the client better understand his or her reactions and related thoughts and feelings, and teaches the client coping skills to deal with his or her anger, fear, or other feelings related to the PTSD symptoms that are being experienced. Group CBT maintains a similar focus but is conducted in a group setting (Cohen et al. 2013).

With regard to medication treatment, Johnston and Fruehling (2008) indicate that "…the pharmacological treatment of this disorder is complex and must be tailored specifically to each individual child" (p. 467). There are no FDA-approved medications for PTSD, but medication may be used to treat related symptoms such as anxiety or depressive feelings (APA, 2013). Regardless of treatment modality, early identification and treatment will be important in terms of the long-term prognosis for people having this disorder.

Adjustment Disorder

Adjustment disorder is a mental health diagnosis given when an individual has been exposed to some type of environmental stressor and is having difficulty adjusting or responding successfully to the stressful experience. The environmental stressor could range from such mild stressors as moving to a different state, home or changing schools, to more significant stressors such as divorce of parents, death of a family member, or witnessing a violent or traumatic event such as a murder. In these latter situations, the key difference between adjustment disorder and an acute traumatic disorder or PTSD is that the symptoms of adjustment disorder are typically considered much milder and transient in nature (APA, 2013). Specifically, the diagnosis of adjustment disorder *cannot* be given if the individual qualifies for any other related mental health disorder (e.g., major depressive disorder, PTSD, GAD), or the symptoms that result from a stressor are not merely an exacerbation of another mental health disorder. The DSM-5 provides additional diagnostic criteria for adjustment disorder, including:

(a) Emotional and behavioral symptoms develop within three months in response to an identifiable stressor, with these symptoms being out of proportion to the severity of the stressor.
(b) The emotional and behavioral symptoms do not persist for more than 6 months.
(c) The emotional and behavioral symptoms cause significant impairment in functioning but do not meet the criteria for another mental health disorder (APA, 2013)

The DSM-5 identifies several emotional and behavioral symptoms that may exist, including depressed mood, anxious mood, and/or conduct problems. In children and adolescents, symptoms of adjustment disorder are likely to manifest themselves with increased irritability or mood difficulties, increased defiance or arguing, or other behavior problems at home or school (APA, 2013). However, as noted above, these impairments and symptoms cannot be severe enough as to qualify for another mental health disorder. Therefore, while the symptoms must be significant enough to cause some impairment in functioning, they will likely be much less significant than those observed in mental health disorders such as major depressive disorder, GAD, or oppositional defiance disorder.

A major criticism of this diagnosis is the vagueness in the diagnostic criteria (Patra & Sarkar, 2013). Emotional reactions to stressful events are developmentally appropriate in many situations; therefore, it can become controversial regarding determining the conditions under which a response to a stressful event is considered sufficiently atypical or impairing that it results in a diagnosis of adjustment disorder. Because of this, reliability and validity of the disorder has been demonstrated to be weak (Patra & Sarkar, 2013), and there is no standard evidence-based treatment protocol for adjustment reaction. Not surprisingly, prevalence and incidence rates for adjustment reaction are also variable, with lifetime estimates ranging from 5 to 21 % (APA, 2013). With regard to the juvenile offender population, there are no estimates available regarding the prevalence of this disorder. This is not necessarily because adjustment disorder is rare among juvenile delinquents but, from our point of view, researchers have chosen to study more reliable and valid diagnostic categories when examining mental health disorders among juvenile offenders.

Since a diagnosis of adjustment disorder implies a less serious form of mental health disorder, it would be expected that the behaviors, thoughts, and feelings of a youth having this disorder would, in turn, have much less of an impact on his or reaction to the juvenile court processing procedures. However, given that adjustment disorder is often a precursor for later mental health difficulties (APA, 2013), it is our belief that it would be important to monitor the daily functioning of any youth offender who has received this diagnosis since he or she is at a greater risk of developing more serious mental health problems.

Reactive Attachment Disorder

Reactive attachment disorder (RAD) is a disorder that begins in early childhood. The prominent feature of RAD is the absence of attachments between a child and caregiver/guardian, with this occurring after a child experiences gross neglect, abuse, or separation from caregivers during early childhood (i.e., before three years of age). In order to be diagnosed with RAD, the abuse/neglect and symptoms must have begun during early childhood and prior to five years of age (APA, 2013). The extreme neglect in care can be a result of severe social deprivation, frequent changes in caregivers that limit the opportunity to form a close attachment, or spending time in a setting that does not allow for frequent social and interpersonal interactions with caregivers. In addition to early social neglect, the DSM-5 provides the following diagnostic criteria for RAD:

(a) A pattern of inhibited, emotionally withdrawn behavior toward caregivers, with a child rarely seeking comfort when upset or rarely responding when comforted by others when the child is distressed.
(b) Chronic emotional or social difficulties during which a child is minimally responsive to others, has limited positive affect, or has unexplained episodes of irritability, sadness, or fearfulness even when in nonthreatening, secure environments (APA, 2013).

In the text revision of the fourth edition of the *Diagnostic and Statistical Manual of Mental Disorders* (DSM-IV; APA, 2000), two subtypes of RAD were identified: the *inhibited/withdrawn subtype* and *social/disinhibited subtype*. Individuals having the inhibited/withdrawn subtype demonstrated significant social isolation and inability to form relationships with others, while those having the social/disinhibited subtype acted indiscriminately with strangers, had poor social boundaries, or sought out excessive physical contact (e.g., O'Connor & Zeanah, 2003; Zeanah & Gleason, 2015). However, in the DSM-5 (APA, 2013), those children with a social/disinhibited pattern of behavior have been assigned a separate mental disorder, namely, *disinhibited social engagement disorder* (DSED; APA, 2013). This section does not specifically address DSED given that it is a new diagnosis with little, if any, research literature available. Rather, the majority of research available, particularly with delinquents, focuses on the general category of RAD which included both inhibited and disinhibited subtypes.

RAD has gained increasing attention in the mental health literature over the past 20–25 years, with diagnoses increasing as the adoption rates of children from orphanages worldwide increased in the 1990s. Much of the early awareness in the 1990s was negative, with some people making comments about these children as having poor empathy and/or antisocial tendencies (e.g., Lederer, 2008; Thomas, 1997; Thomas, Thomas, & Thomas, 2002). More contemporary professionals and researchers attribute many of the bizarre or atypical behaviors related to RAD as being associated with anxiety that is related to the lack of early attachment and normative social skills development (e.g., Stryker, 2013). In this regard, there are a variety of atypical characteristics, disruptive behaviors, and social difficulties associated with RAD. The types of atypical behaviors vary considerably, but observational reports include the hoarding of food (e.g., hiding perishable food in a closet or under a bed), irritability, poor emotional regulation, running away without cause, acting impulsively, being aggressive toward others, fire setting, stealing meaningless objects from family members, cruelty toward animals, poor empathy, and/or inability to form meaningful relationships with peers or adults (e.g., Glowinski, 2011; Hall & Geher, 2003; Reber, 1996).

Even in severe cases of neglect, RAD is relatively uncommon and estimated to occur in less than 10 % of severe neglect cases (e.g., APA, 2013; Gleason et al. 2011). It presently remains unclear regarding the reasons why some children with a history of severe abuse and/or neglect have positive long-term success while others have significant difficulties, but it has been suggested that the reason is likely related to the level and severity of neglect experienced initially as well as to protective factors such as temperament or therapeutic support that was provided following the severe neglect (e.g., Van Den Dries, Juffer, Van Ijzendoorn, Bakermans-Kranenburg, & Alink, 2012; Zeanah & Smyke, 2014). Research has also increasingly demonstrated that RAD may be associated with functional and structural differences in the brain, including underdeveloped brain structures (e.g., Corbin, 2007). Evidence of ongoing neurological difficulties is supported by the fact that symptoms of RAD often exist even after a child is placed in a supportive, functional environment and given access to positive social relationships (e.g., Kemph & Voeller, 2008; Lake, 2005).

RAD is rare within the general child and adolescent population. While the risk factors associated with RAD suggest that those with the disorder may be at a greater risk for juvenile delinquency, there is little available data regarding the prevalence of RAD among the youth offender population. This may be related to the fact that this diagnosis is typically provided during early childhood and may not be available in a youth offender's mental health records or it may be related to the misdiagnosis of a youth's presenting symptoms. However, given the prevalence of a history of maltreatment, abuse, and/or neglect in the juvenile delinquency population, we believe that it is important for professionals working with these youth to have an understanding of RAD.

Implications on Functioning. In general, children and adolescents having RAD have significant difficulties functioning in their daily environment, even after they have been removed from the causes of the maltreatment. These children are more likely to need special education services and have more mental health problems than their typically developing peers (e.g., Rutter et al. 2007; Zeanah & Gleason, 2015). They also have ongoing social and behavior problems that can last into adolescence and adulthood (Gleason et al. 2011). These long-lasting difficulties may be related to a variety of factors, one being the fact that structural changes have been found in the brains of children with RAD. For example, studies have found reduced gray and white matter volumes (e.g., Sheridan, Fox, Zeanah, McLaughlin, & Nelson, 2012) and disruptions in the amygdala and prefrontal cortex (e.g., Govindan, Behen, Helder, Makki, & Chugani, 2009). These findings are associated with deficits in executive functioning deficits (e.g., Gleason et al. 2011; Pears, Bruce, Fisher, & Kim, 2010).

The social difficulties observed in youth having RAD have been compared to those observed in children with ASD, in that these youth often lack social reciprocity, poor empathy and ability to understand the emotions of others, and limited ability to form relationships and interact appropriately with others (Gleason et al. 2011). Significant behavioral difficulties are also often observed in youth having RAD, with them being at a greater risk of developing oppositional defiance disorder, conduct disorder, and demonstrating other antisocial traits (Hornor, 2008). These youth have also been noted to be more hyperactive and aggressive than their typical peers (Lyons-Ruth, Bureau, Riley, & Atlas-Corbett, 2009). In addition, Hall and Geher (2003) using behavior and personality questionnaires completed by parents found that children with RAD had significantly more behavioral problems than those not having RAD. They also found that children with RAD rated themselves as lower in regard to empathy and higher on self-monitoring of their surroundings. These children were also found to have greater social difficulties, more somatic complaints, and attention problems and be more likely to engage in delinquency than youth without RAD.

Treatment. Removal from pathogenic care and placement in a supportive, secure setting where attachments can be developed is the first step of treatment for youth having RAD (Smyke et al. 2012). For those youth who continue to display disruptive behaviors and atypical behaviors following the provision of supportive care, the most popular psychological intervention is attachment-based therapies which are based on the notion that disruptive and atypical behaviors associated with RAD are directly the result of anger associated with poor attachments (Hanson & Spratt, 2000). However, little research exists at present to support the efficacy of these therapies, with some writers suggesting that they could actually do more harm than good if they exacerbate problematic relationships (e.g., Barth, Crea, John, Thoburn, & Quinton, 2005; Hanson & Spratt, 2000).

Other therapies discussed in the literature include parent-child interaction therapy, behavior management, and social skills training programs (e.g., Buckner, Lopez, Dunkel, & Joiner, 2008; O'Connor, Spagnola, & Byrne, 2012); however, evidence supporting the efficacy of these treatments is limited. Moreover, some researchers have suggested that the treatment prognosis for these youth is weak and full recovery difficult if the pathogenic care experienced by the youth extends beyond infancy or early childhood, since considerable changes take place in brain development after early childhood (e.g., Kemph & Voeller, 2008; Vanderwert, Marshall, Nelson, Zeanah, & Fox, 2010).

Trauma and Stressor-Related Disorders in the Juvenile Justice System

Trauma and stressor-related disorders, in general, are overrepresented among the juvenile delinquency population. For example, while it is estimated that approximately 4 % of children and adolescents in the general population meet the criteria for PTSD (Kilpatrick et al. 2003), studies have found that 32 to 52 % of incarcerated juvenile delinquents may meet the criteria for PTSD (e.g., Kerig et al. 2010; Wilson et al. 2013). Rosenberg et al. (2014) examined the relationship between trauma history, mental health functioning, and delinquency and found that 45.7 % of their sample of 350 delinquent youth met the criteria for PTSD, with this being significantly correlated with depression and substance abuse. Not surprisingly, this study found that a greater number of traumatic events were associated with a higher level of impairment.

There are a variety of theories that attempt to explain this relationship between trauma and offense history. For example, social learning theory posits that youth learn from what is modeled and subsequently may learn to accept violence and delinquency as a part of everyday life (Monks et al. 2009). As described in Chap. 4, social disorganization theory and general strain theory also attempt to explain delinquency, in part, by the exposure these youth have to violence and abuse (e.g., Agnew, 1992; Sampson & Lauritsen, 1994; Shaw & McKay, 1942).

The high incidence of trauma-related disorders in this population is largely attributed to the fact that many of these youth have been exposed to violence, abuse, or trauma during childhood (Chen et al. 2013). For example, in their study of 264 detained youth, Ford, Hartman, Hawke, and Chapman (2008) found that 48 % of their sample had experienced traumatic loss, 38 % had experienced a significant accident or disaster-related trauma, and 30 % had experienced childhood abuse or family violence. Stimmel, Cruise, Ford, and Weiss (2014) found that 86 % of their sample of youth offenders had been exposed to at least one traumatic event, with those meeting criteria for PTSD having a greater number of emotional and behavioral problems.

While the causal relationship between juvenile delinquency and mental health disorders is difficult to fully understand, there does appear to be evidence that exposure to trauma and/or violence can increase the likelihood of a youth engaging in disruptive or illegal acts. For example, research has found that children who witness violence are more likely to have internalizing *and* externalizing symptoms and engage in disruptive behaviors (e.g., Ludwig & Warren, 2009; Mrug & Windle, 2010). There is also some evidence provided by Sharf, Kimonis, and Howard (2014) to suggest that early exposure to traumatic events is related to conduct problems and callous-unemotional traits, which are often associated with conduct disorder and antisocial personality disorder.

Researchers have also reported an association between offense history and trauma-related disorders, with juvenile offenders with these disorders having a greater number of offenses, more severe offenses, and more offenses against persons (e.g., Eitle & Turner, 2002; Ford, Chapman, Connor, & Cruise, 2012). In this regard, Smith, Leve, and Chamberlain (2006) examined a sample of 88 delinquent females and found a positive association between PTSD diagnosis and the severity and number of offenses. Becker and Kerig (2011) examined the prevalence and impact of PTSD in a sample of 83 detained males between 12 and 17 years of age and found that 95 % of the sample had experienced trauma to some degree and 20 % met the diagnostic criteria for PTSD. In terms of the relationship between PTSD and offending, Becker and Kerig also found a significant relationship between severity of symptoms and number of arrests and offense severity. In addition, Patchin, Huebner, McCluskey, Varano, and Bynum (2006) found that youth offenders are more likely to carry a weapon, assault others, and engage in criminal activity into adulthood.

The symptoms associated with trauma-related disorders are heterogeneous and vary depending on the stressor or traumatic event; therefore, it is difficult to determine specific difficulties youth with these disorders may have while being processed through the juvenile justice system. Given that these youth have a greater likelihood of emotional instability, irritability, and aggressiveness (e.g., Mrug & Windle, 2010), it would be expected that they may have a greater risk of negative interactions at the time of arrest, detainment, or when communicating with court personnel. During the hearing processes, therefore, it is our opinion that it would be important to take into consideration a youth's trauma history when determining appropriate programming, placement, and court requirements. The fact that these youth are at a greater risk of reoffending cannot be ignored, but neither can the fact that they have poor social support systems and probably have not received the therapeutic interventions necessary to address their respective trauma-related symptoms.

A determination should also be made whether the types of problematic behaviors presented by these youth are related to a trauma or stress-related disorder rather than to antisocial functioning, particularly if these youth have never before been provided any opportunities for treatment. In the case of Brianna, for example, while she demonstrated many symptoms of a disruptive behavior disorder such as oppositional defiant disorder or conduct disorder, symptoms of PTSD appeared to be a primary contributing factor to her substance abuse and delinquency. Brianna had received some court-related interventions (i.e., substance abuse treatment and anger management); however, none of these had addressed her PTSD.

Directly related to the case of Brianna, assuming no significant developmental or learning disabilities are present, it would be expected that these youth would have the intellectual ability to participate in most court programming; however, if a youth's trauma history and related symptoms are major contributing factors to his or her delinquency, then not addressing the trauma and related behaviors within individual or group trauma-focused therapy may result in other interventions (e.g., anger management, substance abuse programs, or behavior modification programs) being ineffective.

Impact on Risk and Risk Assessment

There appears to be a strong association between trauma-related disorders and juvenile delinquency, particularly when these disorders are related to a history of maltreatment or a diagnosis of PTSD. In regard to *risk of dangerousness*, the research appears to indicate that youth with PTSD are at a greater risk of violence toward others and demonstrating more callous or unemotional personality styles. This does not imply that these youth are more antisocial in nature, but rather that they may be more inclined to display trauma-related symptoms such as angry outbursts, irritability, or reckless behavior, which could be misconstrued as indicators of conduct disorder (e.g., Bertram & Dartt, 2009; Ovaert, Cashel, & Sewell, 2003). Ford, Chapman, Mack, and Pearson (2006) have named the trauma-related symptoms being displayed by these youth via callousness or indifference as *survival coping theory*.

In terms of GAD, while there is a relationship between anxiety-related disorders and juvenile offending, these youth do *not* have early indicators of antisocial personality characteristics; rather, their disruptive behaviors are more likely related to severe anxiety that should be treated accordingly instead of attributing their behaviors as a disruptive behavior disorder. The same seems to be the case for youth having an adjustment disorder. The risk of dangerousness, therefore, for youth having GAD or adjustment disorder is, in our opinion, lower than it is for those having PTSD.

The evidence regarding the level of *sophistication and maturity* in youth having anxiety and trauma-related disorders is less clear, in that there is little research available that assists professionals in differentiating whether the aggressive and disruptive behaviors and/or illegal acts that are demonstrated by these youth are premeditated or reactive in nature. Level of sophistication and maturity, therefore, may be difficult to determine for youth having these disorders.

In terms of *treatment amenability*, there are two primary factors that would need to be considered. First, it is important to consider whether there is a comorbid disruptive behavior diagnosis present. Disruptive behavior disorders have a weak prognosis in regard to treatment amenability and are likely to exacerbate the frequency of socially unacceptable behaviors and illegal acts. The second consideration is whether the youth with these disorders, for example, are currently being treated for their disorder using evidence-based methods. For GAD, use of evidence-based interventions by trained clinicians would be important in any rehabilitation or court program that focuses on the reduction or elimination of future offending. With respect to trauma-related disorders, each youth having this disorder should be carefully evaluated given the serious implications that the behaviors associated with this disorder can have on how the youth offender responds to court intervention and the effectiveness of these interventions. For example, as expressed by Bailey, Smith, Huey, McDaniel, and Babeva (2014) in their case discussion on the treatment of gang-related youth with a history of PTSD, not addressing PTSD symptoms can lead to inaccurate perceptions of the youth not being actively involved in treatment and lead to unfavorable outcomes. As noted above, there are no evidence-based treatments available for RAD, therefore it is difficult to ascertain or make assumptions regarding their relative treatment amenability in the juvenile justice system.

Competency

Issues related to the impact of GAD on competency are similar to that for mood disorders. Specifically, there are no significant cognitive or social impairments inherently associated with GAD that would be expected to prevent understanding, participating, or collaborating during a trial. Rather, any issues related to competency would need to be evaluated on a case-by-case basis depending on the type and severity of the GAD or other serious anxiety disorder, as well as on the presence of any comorbid conditions that could contribute to impairment. For example, youth with severe anxiety may have considerable difficulty working cooperatively with their attorney and participating in the court process. Similarly, youth having trauma-related disorders need to be evaluated on an individual basis to determine if they have the cognitive ability and emotional regulation to fully participate in their legal defense and their trail. For example, a youth dealing with PTSD could experience flashbacks, paranoia, or other related symptoms during the court process that would significantly interfere with his or her ability to fully and rationally participate in his or her trial.

Remediation for youth unable to participate in their trial is likely to rest largely on the type and consistency of intervention used to treat, for example, their GAD or trauma-related disorder. Specifically, an individual experiencing severe anxiety would likely need to participate in an intensive individual therapy program that may also include medication. While with an appropriate treatment, it would be expected that restoration could be obtained in a reasonable amount of time, the length, intensity, and type of treatment being used should be carefully considered.

References

Agnew, R. (1992). Foundation for generalism strain theory of crime and delinquency. *Criminology, 30*, 47–87. doi:10.1111/j.17459125.1992.tb01093.x.

American Psychiatric Association. (2013). *Diagnostic and statistical manual for mental disorders* (5th ed.). Washington, DC: Author.

Bailey, C. E., Smith, C., Huey, S. J., Jr., McDaniel, D. D., & Babeva, K. (2014). Unrecognized posttraumatic stress disorder as a treatment barrier for a gang-involved juvenile offender. *Journal of Aggression, Maltreatment & Trauma, 23*(2), 199–214. doi:10.1080/10926771.2014.872748.

Barth, R. P., Crea, T. M., John, K., Thoburn, J., & Quinton, D. (2005). Beyond attachment theory and therapy: Towards sensitive and evidence-based interventions with foster and adoptive families in distress. *Child & Family Social Work, 10*(4), 257–268. doi:10.1111/j.1365-2206.2005.00380.x.

Becker, S. P., & Kerig, P. K. (2011). Posttraumatic stress symptoms are associated with the frequency and severity of delinquency among detained boys. *Journal of Clinical Child and Adolescent Psychology, 40*(5), 765–771. doi:10.1080/15374416.2011.597091.

Beers, S. R., & De Bellis, M. D. (2002). Neuropsychological function in children with maltreatment-related posttraumatic stress disorder. *American Journal of Psychiatry, 159*(3), 483–486. doi:10.1176/appi.ajp.159.3.483.

Beesdo, K., Knappe, S., & Pine, D. S. (2009). Anxiety and anxiety disorders in children and adolescents: Developmental issues and implications for DSM-V. *Psychiatric Clinics of North America, 32*(3), 483–524. doi:10.1016/j.psc.2009.06.002.

Bender, K. (2010). Why do some maltreated youth become juvenile offenders? A call for further investigation and adaptation of youth services. *Children Youth Services Review, 32*(2), 466–473. doi:10.1016/j.childyouth.2009.10.022.

Bertram, R. M., & Dartt, J. L. (2009). Post traumatic stress disorder: A diagnosis for youth from violent, impoverished communities. *Journal of Child and Family Studies, 18*(3), 294–302. doi:10.1007/s10826-008-9229-7.

Bremner, J. D. (2006). Traumatic stress: Effects on the brain. *Dialogues in Clinical Neuroscience, 8*(4), 445–461.

Brewin, C. R., Andrews, B., & Valentine, J. D. (2000). Meta-analysis of risk factors for posttraumatic stress disorder in trauma-exposed adults. *Journal of Consulting and Clinical Psychology, 68*(5), 748–766. doi:10.1037/0022-006x.68.5.748.

Buckner, J. D., Lopez, C., Dunkel, S., & Joiner, T. E. (2008). Behavior management training for the treatment of reactive attachment disorder. *Child Maltreatment, 13,* 289–297.

Chen, P., Voisin, D. R., & Jacobson, K. C. (2013). Community violence exposure and adolescent delinquency: Examining a spectrum of promotive factors. *Youth & Society.* doi:10.1177/0044118X13475827.

Cohen, J. A., Mannarino, A. P., & Deblinger, E. (2013). *Trauma-focused CBT for children and adolescents: Treatment applications.* New York, NY: Guilford Press.

Corbin, J. R. (2007). Reactive attachment disorder: A biopsychosocial disturbance of attachment. *Child Adolescent Social Work Journal, 24*(6), 539–552. doi:10.1007/s10560-007-0105-x.

De Bellis, M. D., Hooper, S. R., Woolley, D. P., & Shenk, C. E. (2009). Demographic, maltreatment, and neurobiological correlates of PTSD symptoms in children and adolescents. *Journal of Pediatric Psychology, 35*(5), 570–577. doi:10.1093/jpepsy/jsp116.

Delaney-Black V., Covington C., Ondersma S.J., Nordstrom-Klee, B., Templin, T., Ager, J., ... & Sokol, R.J. (2002). Violence exposure, trauma, and IQ and/or reading deficits among urban children. *Archives of Pediatrics & Adolescent Medicine, 156*(3), 280-285. doi:10.1001/archpedi.156.3.280.

Eitle, D., & Turner, R. J. (2002). Exposure to community violence and young adult crime: The effects of witnessing violence, traumatic victimization, and other stressful life events. *Journal of Research in Crime and Delinquency, 39*(2), 214–237. doi:10.1177/002242780203900204.

Etkin, A., & Wager, T. D. (2007). Functional neuroimaging of anxiety: A meta-analysis of emotional processing in PTSD, social anxiety disorder, and specific phobia. *American Journal of Psychiatry, 164,* 1476–1488. doi:10.1176/appi.ajp.2007.07030504.

Finkelhor, D., Ormrod, R., & Turner, H. (2007). Poly-victimization: A neglected component in child victimization. *Child Abuse & Neglect, 31*(1), 7–26. doi:10.1016/j.chiabu.2006.06.008.

Ford, J. D., Chapman, J., Connor, D. F., & Cruise, K. R. (2012). Complex trauma and aggression in secure juvenile justice settings. *Criminal Justice and Behavior, 39*(6), 694–724. doi:10.1177/0093854812436957.

Ford, J. D., Chapman, J., Mack, J. M., & Pearson, G. (2006). Pathway from traumatic child victimization to delinquency: Implications for juvenile and permanency court proceedings and decisions. *Juvenile and Family Court Journal, 57*(1), 13–26. doi:10.1111/j.1755-6988.2006.tb00111.x.

Ford, J. D., Hartman, K., Hawke, J., & Chapman, J. F. (2008). Traumatic victimization, posttraumatic stress disorder, suicidal ideation, and substance abuse risk among juvenile justice-involved youth. *Journal of Child and Adolescent Trauma, 1*(1), 75–92. doi:10.1080/19361520801934456.

Gleason, M. M., Fox, N. A., Drury, S., Smyke, A. T., Egger, H. L., Nelson, C. A., ... Zeanah, C. H. (2011). The validity of evidence-derived criteria for reactive attachment disorder: Indiscriminately social/disinhibited and emotionally withdrawn/inhibited types. *Journal of the American Academy of Child and Adolescent Psychiatry, 50*(3), 216–231. doi:10.1016/j.jaac.2010.12.012.

Glowinski, A. L. (2011). Reactive attachment disorder: An evolving entity. *Journal of the American Academy of Child & Adolescent Psychiatry, 50*(3), 210–212. doi:10.1016/j.jaac.2010.12.013.

References

Govindan, R. J., Behen, M. E., Helder, E., Makki, M. I., & Chugani, H. T. (2009). Altered water diffusivity in cortical association tracts in children with early deprivation identified with Tract-Based Spatial Statistics (TBSS). *Cerebral Cortex, 20*(3), 561–569. doi:10.1093/cercor/bhp122.

Hall, S., & Geher, G. (2003). Behavioral and personality characteristics of children with reactive attachment disorder. *Journal of Psychology: Interdisciplinary and Applied, 137*(2), 145–162. doi:10.1080/00223980309600605.

Hanson, R. F., & Spratt, E. G. (2000). Reactive attachment disorder: What we know about the disorder and implications for treatment. *Child Maltreatment, 5*(2), 137–145. doi:10.1177/1077559500005002005.

Hawkins, A. O., Danielson, C. K., de Arellano, M. A., Hanson, R., Ruggiero, K., Smith, D. W., ... Kilpatrick, D. G. (2010). Ethnic/racial differences in the prevalence of injurious spanking and other child physical abuse in a national survey of adolescents. *Child Maltreatment, 15*(3), 242-249. doi:10.1177/1077559510367938.

Hornor, G. (2008). Reactive attachment disorder. *Journal of Pediatric Health Care, 22*(4), 234–239. doi:10.1016/j.pedhc.2007.07.003.

Johnston, H. F., & Fruehling, J. J. (2008). Pharmacological approaches with children and adolescents. In R. J. Morris & T. R. Kratochwill (Eds.), *The practice of child therapy* (4th ed., pp. 207–248). NY: Lawrence Erlbaum Associates.

Kelley, B. T., Thornberry, T. P., & Smith, C. A. (1997). *In the wake of childhood maltreatment*. Washington, DC: National Institute of Justice.

Kemph, J. P., & Voeller, K. K. S. (2008). Reactive attachment disorder in adolescence. *Adolescent Psychiatry, 30*, 159–180.

Kendall, P. C., Furr, J. M., & Podell, J. L. (2010). Child-focused treatment of anxiety. In J. R. Weisz & A. E. Kazdin (Eds.), *Evidence-based psychotherapies for children and adolescents* (2nd ed., pp. 45–60). New York, NY: Guilford Press.

Kerig, P. K., Moeddel, M. A., & Becker, S. P. (2010). Assessing the sensitivity and specificity of the MAYSI-2 for detecting trauma among youth in juvenile detention. *Child and Youth Care Forum, 40*(5), 345–362. doi:10.1007/s10566-010-9124-4.

Kilpatrick, D. G., Ruggiero, K. J., Acierno, R., Saunders, B. E., Resnick, H. S., & Best, C. L. (2003). Violence and risk of PTSD, major depression, substance abuse/dependence, and comorbidity: Results from the National Survey of Adolescents. *Journal of Consulting and Clinical Psychiatry, 71*(4), 692–700. doi:10.1037/0022-006x.71.4.692.

Kodish, I., Rockhill, C., & Varley, C. (2011). Pharmacotherapy for anxiety disorders in children and adolescents. *Dialogues in Clinical Neurosciences, 13*, 439–452.

Lake, P. M. (2005). Recognizing reactive attachment disorder. *Behavioral Health Management, 25*(5), 41–44.

Lederer, A. (2008). *Taming the wild child: From living Hell to living well*. Bloomington, IN: iUniverse.

Lemmon, J. H. (1999). How child maltreatment affects dimensions of juvenile delinquency in a cohort of low-income urban males. *Justice Quarterly, 16*(2), 357–376. doi:10.1080/07418829900094171.

Loeber, R., & Farrington, D. P. (2001). The significant concern of child delinquency. In R. Loweber & D. P. Farrington (Eds.), *Child delinquents: Development, intervention, and service needs* (pp. 1–22). Thousand Oaks, CA: Sage.

Loeber, R., Stouthamer-Loeber, M., & White, H. R. (1999). Developmental aspects of delinquency and internalizing problems and their association with persistent juvenile substance use between ages 7 and 18. *Journal of Clinical Child Psychology, 28*(3), 322–332. doi:10.1207/s15374424jccp280304.

Ludwig, K. A., & Warren, J. S. (2009). Community violence, school-related protective factors, and psychosocial outcomes in urban youth. *Psychology in the Schools, 46*(10), 1061–1073. doi:10.1002/pits.20444.

Lyons-Ruth, K., Bureau, J. F., Riley, C. D., & Atlas-Corbett, A. F. (2009). Socially indiscriminate attachment behavior in the strange situation: Convergent and discriminant validity in relation to caregiving risk, later behavior problems, and attachment insecurity. *Development and Psychopathology, 21*(2), 355–367. doi:10.1017/s0954579409000376.

Merikangas K. R., He J., Burstein M., Swanson S. A., Avenevoli S., Cui L., … Swendsen J. (2010). Lifetime prevalence of mental disorders in U.S. adolescents: Results from the National Comorbidity Study-Adolescent Supplement (NCS-A). *Journal of the American Academy of Child & Adolescent Psychiatry, 49*(10), 980-989. doi:10.1016/j.jaac.2010.05.017.

Monahan, K. C., Goldweber, A., Meyer, K., & Cauffman, E. (2012). Anxiety and antisocial behavior the moderating role of perceptions of social prominence among incarcerated females. *Youth & Society, 44*(1), 76–94. doi:10.1177/0044118x10396634.

Monks, C. P., Smith, P. K., Naylor, P., Barter, C., Ireland, J. L., & Coyne, I. (2009). Bullying in different contexts: Commonalities, differences and the role of theory. *Aggression and Violent Behavior, 14*(2), 146–156. doi:10.1016/j.avb.2009.01.004.

Mrug, S., & Windle, M. (2010). Prospective effects of violence exposure across multiple contexts on early adolescents' internalizing and externalizing problems. *Journal of Child Psychology & Psychiatry, 51*, 953–961. doi:10.1111/j.1469-7610.2010.02222.x.

National Institute of Mental Health. (2014). *Depression in children and adolescents fact sheet*. Bethesda, MD: Author.

Nickerson, A. (2009). *Identifying, assessing, and treating PTSD at school*. New York: Springer.

O'Connor, T. G., Spagnola, M., & Byrne, J. G. (2012). Reactive attachment disorder and severe attachment disturbances. In M. Hersen & P. Sturmey (Eds.), *Handbook of evidence-based practice in clinical psychology* (Child and adolescent disorders, Vol. 1, pp. 433–454). Hoboken, NJ: Wiley.

O'Connor, T. G., & Zeanah, C. H. (2003). Attachment disorders: Assessment strategies and treatment approaches. *Attachment & Human Development, 5*(3), 223–244. doi:10.1080/146167303 10001593974.

Ovaert, L. B., Cashel, M. L., & Sewell, K. W. (2003). Structured group therapy for posttraumatic stress disorder in incarcerated male juveniles. *American Journal of Orthopsychiatry, 73*, 294–301. doi:10.1037/0002-9432.73.3.294.

Parker, J. S., Morton, T. L., Lingefelt, M. E., & Johnson, K. S. (2005). Predictors of serious and violent offending by adjudicate male adolescents. *North American Journal of Psychology, 7*, 407–417.

Patchin, J. W., Huebner, B. M., McCluskey, J. D., Varano, S. P., & Bynum, T. S. (2006). Exposure to community violence and childhood delinquency. *Crime & Delinquency, 52*(2), 307–332. doi:10.1177/0011128704267476.

Patra, B. N., & Sarkar, S. (2013). Adjustment disorder: Current diagnostic status. *Indian Journal of Psychological Medicine, 35*(1), 4–9. doi:10.4103/0253-7176.112193.

Pears, K. C., Bruce, J., Fisher, P. A., & Kim, H. (2010). Indiscriminate friendliness in maltreated foster children. *Child Maltreatment, 15*(1), 64–75. doi:10.1177/1077559509337891.

Polak, A. R., Witteveen, A. B., Reitsma, J. B., & Olff, M. (2012). The role of executive function in posttraumatic stress disorder: A systematic review. *Journal of Affective Disorders, 141*(1), 11–21. doi:10.1016/j.jad.2012.01.001.

Reber, K. (1996). Children at risk for reactive attachment disorder: Assessment, diagnosis, and treatment. *Progress: Family Systems Research and Therapy, 5*(3), 83–98.

Rosenberg, H. J., Vance, J. E., Rosenberg, S. D., Wolford, G. L., Ashley, S. W., & Howard, M. L. (2014). Trauma exposure, psychiatric disorders, and resiliency in juvenile-justice-involved youth. *Psychological Trauma: Theory, Research Practice, and Policy, 6*(4), 430–437. doi:10.1037/a0033199.

Rutter, M., Colvert, E., Kreppner, J., Beckett, C., Castle, J., Groothues C., … Sonuga-Barke, E.J. (2007). Early adolescent outcomes for institutionally-deprived and non-deprived adoptees. I: Disinhibited attachment. *Journal of Child Psychology and Psychiatry, 48*(1), 17–30. doi:10.1111/j.1469-7610.2006.01688.x.

Rynn, M. A., Siqueland, L., & Rickels, K. (2001). Placebo-controlled trial of sertraline in the treatment of children with generalized anxiety disorder. *American Journal of Psychiatry, 158*, 2008–2014.

Saigh, P. A., Lee, K. S., Ward, A., Westphal, E. L., Wilson, K., & Fairbank, J. A. (2008). Posttraumatic stress disorder in children and adolescents: History, risk, and cognitive behavioral treatments. In R. J. Morris & T. R. Kratochwill (Eds.), *The practice of child therapy* (4th ed., pp. 433–454). NY: Lawrence Erlbaum Associates.

Sampson, R. J., & Lauritsen, J. L. (1994). Violent victimization and offending: Individual-, situational-, and community-level risk factors. In A. J. Reiss & J. A. Roth (Eds.), *Understanding and preventing violence* (Vol. 3). Washington, DC: National Academy Press.

Sareen, J., Stein, M. B., Cox, B. J., & Hassard, S. T. (2004). Understanding comorbidity of anxiety disorders with antisocial behavior: Findings from two large community surveys. *The Journal of Nervous and Mental Disease, 192*(3), 178–186. doi:10.1097/01.nmd.0000116460.25110.9f.

Schwartz, D., & Proctor, L. J. (2000). Community violence exposure and children's social adjustment in the school peer group: The mediating roles of emotion regulation and social cognition. *Journal of Consulting and Clinical Psychology, 68*(4), 670. doi:10.1037//0022-006x.68.4.670.

Sedlak, A., & McPherson, K. S. (2010). *Conditions of confinement: Findings from the survey of youth in residential placement.* Washington, DC: U.S. Department of Justice, Office of Justice Programs, Office of Juvenile Justice and Delinquency Prevention. doi:10.1037/e553962010-001.

Sharf, A., Kimonis, E. R., & Howard, A. (2014). Negative life events and posttraumatic stress disorder among incarcerated boys with callous-unemotional traits. *Journal of Psychopathology and Behavioral Assessment, 36*(3), 401–414. doi:10.1007/s10862-013-9404-z.

Shaw, C. R., & McKay, H. D. (1942). *Juvenile delinquency in urban areas.* Chicago, IL: University of Chicago Press.

Sheridan, M. A., Fox, N. A., Zeanah, C. H., McLaughlin, K. A., & Nelson, C. A. (2012). Variation in neural development as a result of exposure to institutionalization early in childhood. *Proceedings of the National Academy of Sciences, 109*, 12927–12932. doi:10.1073/pnas.1200041109.

Silverman, W. K., Pina, A. A., & Viswesvaran, C. (2008). Evidence-based psychosocial treatments for phobic and anxiety disorders in children and adolescents: A review and meta-analyses. *Journal of Clinical Child & Adolescent Psychology, 37*(1), 105–130. doi:10.1080/15374410701817907.

Silvern, L., & Griese, B. (2012). Multiple types of child maltreatment, posttraumatic stress, dissociative symptoms, and reactive aggression among adolescent criminal offenders. *Journal of Child & Adolescent Trauma, 5*(2), 88–101. doi:10.1080/19361521.2012.671799.

Smith, C. A., Ireland, T. O., & Thornberry, T. P. (2005). Adolescent maltreatment and its impact on young adult antisocial behavior. *Child Abuse & Neglect, 29*, 1099–1119.

Smith, D. K., Leve, L. D., & Chamberlain, P. (2006). Adolescent girls' offending and health-risking sexual behavior: The predictive role of trauma. *Child Maltreatment, 11*(4), 346–353. doi:10.1177/1077559506291950.

Smyke, A. T., Zeanah, C. H., Gleason, M. M., Drury, S. S., Fox, N. A., Nelson, C. A., & Guthrie, D. G. (2012). A randomized controlled trial of foster care vs. institutional care for children with signs of reactive attachment disorder. *American Journal of Psychiatry, 169*(5), 508–514. doi:10.1176/appi.ajp.2011.11050748.

Southam-Gerow, M. A., Kendall, P. C., & Weersing, V. R. (2001). Examining outcome variability: Correlates of treatment response in a child and adolescent anxiety clinic. *Journal of Clinical Child Psychology, 30*, 422–436.

Stimmel, M. A., Cruise, K. R., Ford, J. D., & Weiss, R. A. (2014). Trauma exposure, posttraumatic stress disorder symptomatology, and aggression in male juvenile offenders. *Psychological Trauma: Theory, Research, Practice, and Policy, 6*(2), 184–191. doi:10.1037/a0032509.

Stryker, R. (2013). Violent children and structural violence: Re-signaling 'RAD Kids' to inform the social work professions. *Children and Youth Services Review, 35*, 1182–1188. doi:10.1016/j.childyouth.2013.04.005.

Suvak, M. K., & Barrett, L. F. (2011). Considering PTSD from the perspective of brain processes: A psychological construction approach. *Journal of Traumatic Stress, 24*(1), 3–24. doi:10.1002/jts.20618.

Teplin, L. A., Abram, K. M., McClelland, G. M., Mericle, A. A., Dulcan, M. K., & Washburn, J. J. (2002). *Psychiatric disorders of youth in detention.* D.C. Office of Juvenile Justice and Delinquency Prevention: Washington.

Thomas, N. (1997). *When love is not enough: A guide to parenting children with RAD*. Glenwood Springs, CO: Families by Design Publishing.

Thomas, N., Thomas, T., & Thomas, B. (2002). *Dandelion on my pillow, butcher knife beneath*. Glenwood Springs, CO: Families by Design Publishing.

Widom, C. S. (1989). Does violence beget violence? A critical examination of the literature. *Psychological Bulletin, 106*(1), 3. doi:10.1037/0033-2909.106.1.3.

Wilson, H. W., Berent, E., Donenberg, G. R., Emerson, E. M., Rodriguez, E. M., & Sandesara, A. (2013). Trauma history and PTSD symptoms in juvenile offenders on probation. *Victims & Offenders, 8*(4), 465–477. doi:10.1080/15564886.2013.835296.

Wood, J. J., Piacentini, J. C., Southam-Gerow, M., Chu, B. C., & Sigman, M. (2006). Family cognitive behavioral therapy for child anxiety disorders. *Journal of the American Academy of Child and Adolescent Psychiatry, 45*, 314–321.

Van Den Dries, L., Juffer, F., Van Ijzendoorn, M. H., Bakermans-Kranenburg, M. J., & Alink, L. R. A. (2012). Infants' responsiveness, attachment, and indiscriminate friendliness after international adoption from institutions or foster care in China: Application of Emotional Availability Scales to adoptive families. *Development and Psychopathology, 24*(1), 49–64. doi:10.1017/s0954579411000654.

Vanderwert, R. E., Marshall, P. J., Nelson, C. A., Zeanah, C. H., & Fox, N. A. (2010). Timing of intervention affects brain electrical activity in children exposed to severe psychosocial neglect. *PLoS One, 5*(7), 1–5. doi:10.1371/journal.pone.0011415.

Yun, I., Ball, J. D., & Lim, H. (2011). Disentangling the relationship between child maltreatment and violent delinquency: Using a nationally representative sample. *Journal of Interpersonal Violence, 26*(1), 88–110. doi:10.1177/0886260510362886.

Zeanah, C. H., & Gleason, M. M. (2015). Annual research review: Attachment disorders in early childhood—Clinical presentation, causes, correlates, and treatment. *Journal of Child Psychology and Psychiatry, 56*(3), 207–222. doi:10.1111/jcpp.12347.

Zeanah, C. H., & Smyke, A. T. (2014). Attachment disorders and severe deprivation. In M. Rutter, D. Bishop, D. Pine, S. Scott, J. Stevenson, E. Taylor, & A. Thapar (Eds.), *Rutter's child and adolescent psychiatry*. London: Blackwell.

Chapter 12
Externalizing Disorders

Externalizing disorders are likely the most researched mental health disorder in the juvenile delinquency population, largely because the disruptive, impulsive, and/or aggressive behaviors that are associated with externalizing disorders are the same as those commonly reported for juvenile offenders. While internalizing disorders represent those mental health disorders in which the primary symptoms such as a person's thoughts, feelings, and beliefs reside largely within the person, externalizing disorders are those in which the primary symptoms are manifested by the person's outward behaviors and related actions (e.g., Achenbach, 1978; Campbell, Shaw, & Gilliom, 2000). In general, children and adolescents with internalizing disorders often think or act in a manner that directly and negatively impacts themselves, while those with externalizing disorders often act out toward their environment in a manner that violates social rules of conduct and involves negative acts against others and/or property. In addition, youth manifesting externalizing disorders are more likely to have behavioral difficulties at home, school, and/or within the community and are more likely to become involved with the juvenile justice system than youth who do not have externalizing disorders (Gresham, 2015).

Disorders commonly considered to be externalizing disorders include attention deficit hyperactivity disorder (ADHD), oppositional defiant disorder (ODD), conduct disorder (CD), and intermittent explosive disorder (IED). Since ODD and CD have considerable overlap and both have a significant direct and negative impact on a youth's surrounding environment, these two disorders have been commonly grouped together under the category of "disruptive behavior disorders."

Attention Deficit Hyperactivity Disorder

ADHD is one of the most frequently studied psychological disorders of childhood and adolescence (DuPaul & Barkely, 2008), with the diagnosis of this disorder increasing exponentially since the 1990s (Visser et al., 2014). Consistent with this, the number of prescriptions written for ADHD medications has also risen over 300% in the past 10 years, leading many to question whether ADHD has been overdiagnosed in the general child and adolescent population (Hinshaw & Scheffler, 2014). In this regard, some writers have suggested that active, energetic children who have difficulty adjusting to a traditional school setting are being misidentified as having an attentional disorder, while others have taken the position that the prevalence of ADHD has increased because of the greater awareness of this disorder and its subtypes on the part of parents and various professionals (e.g., Hinshaw & Scheffler, 2014; Willcutt et al., 2009). Presently, the DSM-5 estimates that approximately 5% of children and adolescents have ADHD (APA, 2013), while data released by the American Academy of Child and Adolescent Psychiatry (Visser et al., 2014) found that approximately 11% of children and adolescents have been diagnosed with ADHD.

The most prominent characteristics associated with ADHD are a persistent pattern of inattentiveness and/or hyperactivity and impulsivity. As with other child and adolescent mental health disorders discussed in this book, the symptoms associated with this disorder must be severe enough that they interfere with a youth's daily functioning. The DSM-5 identifies the following symptoms as being consistent with *inattentiveness*:

(a) Failure to pay attention to details or making careless mistakes in work
(b) Difficulty sustaining attention during tasks
(c) Not appearing to listen when spoken to directly
(d) Not following through on instructions or failing to finish required work
(e) Having difficulty with organization and managing tasks or belongings
(f) Struggling to engage in tasks that require sustained focus and effort, such as homework or lengthy work projects
(g) Frequently losing important things (e.g., homework, keys, glasses)
(h) Being easily distracted
(i) Being forgetful in daily activities (APA, 2013).

The following symptoms are listed as diagnostic examples of *hyperactivity* and *impulsivity*:

(a) Excessive fidgeting
(b) Having difficulty remaining seated when it is expected
(c) Restlessness and running or climbing around in inappropriate environments or situations
(d) Difficulty engaging quietly in leisure activities
(e) Being "on the go" and having difficulty sitting still for extended periods of time
(f) Talking excessively
(g) Blurting out answers
(h) Having difficulty waiting in line or waiting for his or her turn
(i) Interrupting or intruding on others' conversations or activities (APA, 2013).

Symptoms of inattentiveness and hyperactivity/impulsivity must be present in an individual before 12 years of age, and they must occur in *at least two settings* (e.g., home and school, home and the community, or the school and the community) (APA, 2013).

The DSM-5 identifies three subtypes of ADHD: (1) *ADHD (predominantly inattentive presentation)*, which is diagnosed if an individual meets at least six characteristics of inattentiveness but has no excessive hyperactivity or impulsivity present (this subtype was often referred to in the past as "attention deficit disorder" or ADD); (2) *ADHD (predominantly hyperactive/impulsive presentation)*, which is diagnosed if an individual meets at least six hyperactive/impulsive characteristics listed above; and (3) *ADHD (combined presentation)* if both symptoms of inattention and hyperactivity/impulsivity are met (APA, 2013).

The diagnosis of ADHD is typically made by a psychologist or physician, such as a pediatrician or psychiatrist. Determining whether a youth presents with ADHD typically includes a variety of procedures. A detailed behavior history is often first obtained from the youth's parents or guardians to determine when the inattention, hyperactivity, or impulsive behavior symptoms began and to what degree they are currently interfering with the youth's daily functioning. In addition, because the DSM-5 criteria require that symptoms be present in at least two settings, multiple sources of information are often sought-out, such as from parents and teachers plus the youth himself or herself, to confirm the presence of the symptoms in more than one setting. Although the diagnosis of ADHD can be made through these latter clinical interviews and review of the youth's background history, best practice procedures suggest the use of *both* clinical interview and objective measures, such as the use of behavior rating scales or standardized measures of attention (Barkley, 2014).

The DSM-5 indicates that symptoms of ADHD must be present prior to age 12; however, many children are first diagnosed in elementary school as this is when symptoms of inattentiveness and hyperactivity become most prominent and interrupt the learning process at school. While the developmental course of ADHD varies from individual to individual, reports indicate that many parents observe hyperactivity and excessive motor activity during the toddler years, with inattentiveness becoming more prominent during late childhood and adolescence (APA, 2013).

Etiology

In the 1990s there was a surge of research examining the relationship between diet and symptoms of ADHD, particularly studies related to excessive sugar consumption. However, despite an early popular belief that increased sugar consumption can lead to hyperactivity and ADHD in children, empirical research has *not* found any difference in the behaviors of children who consumed increased amounts of sugar (e.g., Wolraich, Wilson, & White, 1995). Researchers, however, have found a large placebo effect, with parents reporting higher levels of hyperactivity and behavior problems when they thought their children were receiving large amounts of sugar (Hoover & Milich, 1994).

More contemporary research suggests that ADHD is largely neurodevelopmental in nature, with there being a strong genetic component. For example, while no specific genes have yet been identified, research has found a high incidence of

ADHD in first-degree relatives (Faraone & Beiderman, 2013). A large body of research has also focused on the neural mechanisms related to ADHD. While this area of research is still growing in terms of its understanding of the neurology of ADHD, there is considerable evidence to support that individuals with ADHD have brains that differ in structure and/or function from those who do not have ADHD. For example, research has found that the brain of youth with ADHD matures more slowly than that of youth without ADHD, particularly in brain regions associated with attention, planning, and higher-level thinking (Shaw et al., 2007). Other studies have found that the cortex of the brain develops more slowly in youth having ADHD (Shaw et al., 2012), and there has been some evidence of abnormal growth in the corpus callosum, which is the structure that allows the two halves of the brain to communicate (Gilliam et al., 2011).

Most notably, research in cognitive neuroscience has consistently found impairments or dysfunction in areas of the prefrontal cortex in youth with ADHD (e.g., Barkley, 1997; Pennington & Ozonoff, 1996; Schultz, Tremblay, & Hollerman, 2000; Seidman, Valera, & Makris, 2005; Willcutt, Doyle, Nigg, Faraone, & Pennington, 2005). The prefrontal cortex is an area of the brain largely responsible for executive functioning, or those processes including impulse control, attention, flexible thinking, problem solving, planning, and organization (Pennington, 2002). Areas of the prefrontal cortex also regulate decision-making, emotional regulation, delayed gratification, and learning from previous mistakes.

A variety of environmental factors have also been identified as risk factors for ADHD. For example, there is an increased incidence of a history of child abuse and neglect in youth having ADHD and an increased incidence in those youth exposed to drugs or alcohol in utero. There has also been a positive correlation observed between lead exposure and ADHD (e.g., APA, 2013; Millichap, 2008; Nomura, Marks, & Halperin, 2010). Given the variety of symptoms associated with ADHD, this suggests that there may not be one specific cause of this disorder but, rather, a variety of causal factors (e.g., Fair, Bathula, Nikolas, & Nigg, 2012, Nigg, Goldsmith, Sachek, 2004).

Implications on Functioning

Cognitive and Academic Implications. ADHD is commonly associated with deficits in cognitive functioning, particularly in the area of executive functioning or, as mentioned earlier, the processes used to regulate behavior and attention. There are a variety of executive functions that have been associated with the diagnosis of ADHD, including planning, organization, cognitive flexibility, and problem solving. However, the most empirically supported deficit areas include *working memory*, which is essentially one's ability to retain and process information needed to complete tasks or follow directions (e.g., Martinussen, Hayden, Hogg-Johnson, & Tannock, 2005), and *impulse control and sustained attention* (e.g., Coghill, Hayward, Rhodes, Grimmer, & Matthews, 2014; Willcutt et al., 2005). Recent research findings have further suggested that specific subtypes of ADHD can be identified based on the neuropsychological and cognitive assessment results obtained with respect to a youth's executive functioning deficits (Fair et al., 2012), but it is important to note that these results are correlative and not causal and, therefore, not all youth with ADHD will display deficits (Fair et al., 2012).

One of the most common reasons that children and adolescents are referred for evaluation and treatment of ADHD is because of academic difficulties (Loe & Feldman, 2007), with research suggesting that anywhere from 50% to 80% of students with ADHD have difficulty succeeding academically in school (DuPaul & Stoner, 2014). The academic difficulties expressed by students with ADHD are significant enough that some researchers have suggested that this is the mediating factor in the link between ADHD and juvenile delinquency (Defoe, Farrington, & Loeber, 2013), given that academic difficulties are frequently identified in youth offenders.

Academic impairments in youth with ADHD are often broad-based, with these youth manifesting poor grades, low scores on standardized achievement tests, higher rates of retention, and increased risk for school dropout (DuPaul & Stoner, 2014). Youth with ADHD also often have difficulty staying on task in the school environment and have more difficulty accurately completing classwork, homework, or other school-related work. In addition, these youth have difficulty paying attention to classroom instructions, may have a tendency to rush through their work and not check the accuracy of their work, and have poor academic motivation which can lead to poor grades (e.g., APA, 2013; Imeraj et al., 2013; Volkow et al., 2010). Academic deficits have been observed as young as preschool (DuPaul, McGoey, Eckert, & VanBrakle, 2001) and these difficulties typically exist through high school and college (e.g., Landberg, et al., 2011; Massetti et al., 2008). Not surprisingly, students with ADHD are less likely to enroll in college (Kuriyan et al., 2013) and those who do attend college are more likely to experience difficulties completing their course work and not completing their college degree program (Weyandt et al., 2013).

In addition to the symptoms of ADHD making classroom performance more difficult for youth having this diagnosis, research has suggested that 30% to 50% of youth with ADHD have comorbid learning disabilities (e.g., DuPaul & Stoner, 2014; DuPaul, Gormley, & Laracy, 2014). However, whether ADHD causes a SLD in these youth or the presence of a SLD in these youth causes ADHD is unclear.

Social-Emotional and Behavioral Implications. Social difficulties are common among children and adolescents having ADHD, with these youth having difficulties making friends and maintaining these friendships over time (Normand et al., 2013). These social relationship difficulties may be due to a variety of factors. For example, the specific symptoms reflective of ADHD may make it difficult to develop positive relationships, as these youth may appear annoying to their peers since they are often observed interrupting others, talking excessively, or being disruptive during class or other school-related activities (e.g., Hoza et al., 2005; McQuade & Hoza, 2014). In addition, there is some evidence to suggest that youth with ADHD have low social awareness. Studies have reported that youth having ADHD rated their peers as liking them more than their peers actually endorsed liking them (Mrug et al, 2009) and had poor social awareness in how they interpreted social cues (Andrade et al., 2012) or identified the emotions of others (Uekermann et al., 2010). Consistent with these findings, Landau and Milich (1988) asked children with ADHD to shift between roles of a host and a guest in a mock TV talk show game. They found that while the typically developing children had no difficulty transitioning between the social roles, the youth with ADHD had difficulty and, in general, failed to modulate their behavior between the roles. In addition to having poor social awareness and difficulty making friends, it has been estimated that between 50% and 80% of youth having ADHD have been bullied or rejected by their peers (e.g., Hoza, 2007; Wiener & Mak, 2009).

Symptoms such as irritability, low frustration tolerance, labile mood, and poor regulation of emotions are also frequently associated with ADHD (Barkley, 2014). In addition, there is not only a high comorbidity with a SLD, but also with other mental health disorders. For example, the DSM-5 (APA, 2013) indicates that approximately 50% of children with the diagnosis of ADHD (combined presentation) also meet the criteria for a disruptive behavior disorder. Adolescents having ADHD have also been found to be more likely to engage in risky behaviors (e.g., Whalen, Jamner, Henker, Delfino, & Lozano, 2002) and associate with a "problematic" peer group (e.g., Bagwell, Molina, Pelham, & Hoza, 2001), with each of these maladaptive behaviors possibly being exacerbated with the presence of a comorbid disruptive behavior disorder diagnosis. Interestingly, as research has advanced in the area of cognitive neuroscience and related areas, studies have increasingly found similar biological markers, neurological pathways, and neuropsychological consistencies among youth having various externalizing disorders, which may partially explain the high comorbidity among these disorders (Johnson, 2015). It is also not surprising, therefore, that many juvenile offenders are diagnosed as having ADHD and/or externalizing disorders.

As mentioned above, youth having ADHD are more inclined to engage in high risk-taking and sensation-seeking behaviors. For example, adolescents with ADHD are nearly four times as likely to have an automobile accident within their first five years of driving and are more likely to get speeding tickets or be involved in other traffic violations (e.g., Barkley, 2000; Woodward, Fergusson, & Horwood, 2000). These youth also have more injuries than their typically developing peers, being more inclined to have emergency room visits and inpatient hospital stays (Leibson, Katusic, Barbaresi, Ransom, & O'Brien, 2001). In addition, these youth are at an increased risk of substance abuse compared to their peers (Robb, 2008).

Treatment of ADHD

ADHD is considered a neurodevelopmental disorder, meaning that the symptoms begin early in life and are related to impairments in the brain (APA, 2013). There is no "cure" for ADHD, although a variety of treatments are available to reduce the frequency and severity of the symptoms (e.g., DuPaul & Barkley, 2008).

A variety of treatment procedures have been suggested in the literature for youth having ADHD, including various modalities of individual therapy, parent training, and medication. The most effective treatments for ADHD include medication, home-based and/or school-based behavior therapy procedures, or a combination of medication and behavioral therapies (e.g., DuPaul & Barkley, 2008). However, as DuPaul and Barkley (2008) point out, "[t]he comprehensive treatment of children with ADHD is a long-term process that should not be undertaken by the uninitiated"(p. 178).

While the use of medications does not "cure" ADHD, they do control the symptoms while they are being taken by the youth. Medication can also help improve focus and regulate hyperactivity and impulsivity which, in turn, can lead to better school work, better self-regulated behaviors, and increased prosocial activity. In this regard, research has found medications to be effective, particularly when they are regularly monitored and adjusted to fit the needs of the youth (e.g., MTA Cooperative Group, 1999; Scheffler, Brown, Fulton, Hinsaw, Levine, & Stone, 2009).

Parent training programs based on behavior therapy principles and procedures are effective for treating ADHD (e.g., Evans, Owens, & Bunford, 2014). These treatment programs teach parents not only basic principles of behavioral management but also strategies for improving communication and helping parents develop more structured, organized environments for their child or adolescent (Barkley, 2013). Parent training follows a manualized curriculum and typically occurs in an individual or group setting over the course of several weeks. The behavior therapy procedures typically focus on various management strategies that can be implemented at home or in the classroom (DuPaul & Barkley, 2008).

Given that social skill deficits are also common among youth having ADHD, social skills training is a common intervention strategy. Social skills training can include such areas as helping children learn social rules or norms such as waiting in line, not interrupting others, learning to read facial the expressions of others, or responding appropriately to others (Jacobs, 2002). However, while social skills training is commonly used for children with ADHD, there is little research to support any long-term changes in these youth in their interpersonal interactions in various settings (e.g., DuPaul & Barkley, 2008; Evans et al., 2014).

One of the most comprehensive studies on the treatment of ADHD is known as the Multimodal Treatment Study of Children with Attention Deficit Hyperactivity Disorder (MTA; MTA Cooperative Group, 1999). This study compared four different treatment modalities with 579 children having ADHD, including 1) medication only, in which a child saw a physician once per month; 2) behavioral intervention only, in which up to 35 individual therapy sessions and an intensive training program was implemented; 3) a combination of medication and behavioral intervention; and 4) routine community care during which parents saw a physician from a community mental health center once or twice a year. Treatment was implemented over a 14-month period, and results found that the biggest improvements were observed in those children who received combination treatment (medication + behavioral therapy). The second most effective was medication only, closely followed by those receiving only behavioral interventions. Those receiving community-only treatment saw considerable less improvement in functioning. These results were obtained regardless of comorbid difficulties such as disruptive behavior disorders.

A three-year follow-up of the MTA study found that many improvements in functioning were sustained though rates of delinquency and substance abuse remained high regardless of treatment modality (Molina et al., 2009). Interestingly, while it was initially one of the most effective treatment modalities, long-term benefits of medication were not sustained at the three-year follow-up. The researchers concluded that this was due, in part, to the fact that those who had been only taking medication were more likely to stop, whereas those who were receiving behavioral-only treatment were more likely to learn life skills and also later begin medication. During an eight-year follow-up, however, researchers found little relationship between initial treatment and long-term functioning (e.g., Molina et al, 2009). In this regard, they found that initial treatment did not predict later functioning. Instead, these researchers stated that early ADHD symptom trajectory was most prognostic of long-term outcomes. Specifically, those with the most severe behavioral problems initially and greater environmental risk factors (e.g., low family support and low socioeconomic status) had the worst long-term prognosis regardless of initial treatment (Molina et al., 2009).

Disruptive Behavior Disorders

As previously mentioned, disruptive behavior disorders include such externalizing disorders as ODD and CD. While ODD and CD are two distinct mental health disorders in the DSM-5, there is considerable overlap and many research studies combine these disorders when examining the etiology, treatment, and related implications of the disorders. These two disorders are also frequently combined in studies focused on juvenile delinquency.

Oppositional Defiant Disorder

ODD is a disruptive behavior disorder largely characterized by a persistent pattern of negative, hostile, defiant, and disobedient behaviors toward others (APA, 2013). Parents or teachers may complain that a particular youth acts as though social rules and related norms do not apply to him or her, or the youth does what he or she pleases regardless of societal norms. While defiance, rule-breaking, and argumentativeness are behaviors common, for example, in all adolescents to some degree, these behaviors are considered to be developmentally inappropriate when they begin to significantly interfere with the youth's functioning. For example, the defiance and arguing may be to a degree to which a particular child or adolescent is frequently being suspended from school or causing significant family disruption and fighting. In addition to having a significant impact on the youth or others in the youth's immediate environment, the DSM-5 requires that a youth present with at least four of the following symptoms for a period of at least six months:

(a) Frequently losing his or her temper
(b) Being easily annoyed

(c) Often being angry and resentful toward others
(d) Frequently arguing with authority figures or adults
(e) Actively defying or refusing to comply with rules or requests from authority figures. In the case of a youth offender, this may include not following classroom rules, refusing to comply with established rules while in detention, breaking curfew, or not following probation
(f) Purposely annoying others
(g) Blaming others for his or her mistakes and not taking responsibility for misbehaviors. For example, a youth offender may blame his or her father for his or her arrest because the father alerted the probation officer that the youth was not complying with probation rules
(h) Being spiteful or vindictive toward others, such as destroying a sibling's favorite item or ruining a parent's garden (APA, 2013).

Conduct Disorder

CD is the behavior disorder most widely associated with juvenile delinquents, with this disorder being characterized by a pattern of behavior that violates the rights of others. While the symptoms of CD typically decrease as an individual transitions into adulthood, the presence of CD in adolescence is a requirement for an adult diagnosis of antisocial personality disorder (APA, 2013). CD is thought to appear in approximately 4% of the population (APA, 2013), with it being more common in males than females, primarily for the childhood-onset subtype (APA, 2013). While both males and females can be diagnosed with CD, the presentation of symptoms has been found to be different for males than females. Specifically, while males are more likely to have engaged in violent or aggressive behaviors, females are more likely to display rule-breaking behaviors such as lying, truancy, running away, substance use, and prostitution (APA, 2013).

According to the DSM-5 (APA, 2013), there are four main groups of behaviors that individuals with CD may display. These categories include:

(a) *Aggression to people or animals.* This category can include explicit aggressive behaviors toward others, violent activity such as forced sexual activity, or armed robbery. It can also include less physically aggressive but still cruel behaviors such as bullying, threatening, or intimidating others. Offenses that would meet this criterion include school bullying, fighting, rape, assault, and (rarely) homicide.
(b) *Destruction of other's property*, which can include fire setting, vandalizing property, throwing rocks through windows, or other destructive behaviors.
(c) *Deceitfulness or theft*, which includes behaviors such as breaking into a house, building, or car, manipulating others, lying, or shoplifting.
(d) *Serious violation of rules.* This category applies to other statutory offenses such as running away from home, staying overnight without permission, or skipping school (APA, 2013).

In order for a youth to be diagnosed as having CD, at least three different disruptive behaviors (from any of the four main categories) must be present over a period of at least one year, and they must significantly impair functioning. The DSM-5 identifies two subtypes of CD, including *childhood onset*, which is diagnosed when symptoms began occurring before age 10, and *adolescent onset* when symptoms do not occur until after age 10. Childhood onset is typically associated with a poorer prognosis, particularly for long-term outcomes. For example, children diagnosed with childhood onset are more likely to have symptoms that continue into adulthood (APA, 2013).

Etiology of Disruptive Behavior Disorders

Similar to most mental health disorders, no specific cause for disruptive behavior disorders has been identified. Rather, there are likely several variables that contribute to the development of CD or ODD and, not surprisingly, many of these are similar to common characteristics observed across the juvenile delinquency population. For example, Murray and Farrington (2010) conducted a broad literature review of studies examining the etiology of CD and identified several important risk factors associated with the development of this disorder. These included impulsivity, low average intelligence, academic difficulties, poor parenting strategies, family discord, a history of abuse, low socioeconomic status, and exposure to crime (via criminal activity in the neighborhoods of youth, by peers, and/or by family members). Other studies have found maladaptive parenting practices and family discord to be correlated with ODD in youth, as well as low socioeconomic status (e.g., Bornovalova, Blazei, Malone, McGue, & Iacono, 2013; Burke, et al., 2002; Martel, Nikolas, Jernigan, Friderici, & Nigg, 2012).

Though evidence is limited, there is some research to suggest that there may be biological influences on the development of disruptive behavior disorders. For example, research suggests that a child's temperament, such as his or her inflexibility or intense and reactive way of responding, may be associated with the development of ODD (Burke et al., 2002). Adolescents with ODD have also been found to have lower heart rates and skin conductance activity, reduced basal cortisol reactivity, and abnormalities in the prefrontal cortex and amygdala (Burke et al., 2002). Neurological differences have also been suggested, with some structural and functional differences in brain areas associated with emotional regulation and processing being noted. In this regard, Crowley and colleagues (2010) compared neural activity in adolescents having CD versus those without CD and found decreased activity in areas of the brain associated with decision-making, as well as differences in areas associated with reward and punishment, which the authors posited may be related to the risk-taking behaviors often associated with youth having CD. Functional differences have also been observed in areas of the brain associated with emotional regulation, with decreased emotional responses observed (e.g., Beauchaine, Gatzke-Kopp, & Mead, 2007; Bellani, Garzitto, & Brambilla, 2012). In those who demonstrate callous behavior and low empathy, studies have found reduced activity in the amygdala when showing distressed faces (e.g., Jones, Laurens, Herba, Barker, & Viding, 2009; Viding et al., 2012).

Research has further reported that the risk of being diagnosed as having CD is higher in those youth with a parent or sibling who has also been diagnosed with CD. While no specific genetic markers have been identified, it has been suggested that there may be genetic variations in individuals with versus without CD (Grigorenko et al., 2010), with these variations influencing various neurotransmitters such as dopamine and serotonin, which have been associated with behavior regulation (e.g., Rogeness & McClure, 1996; Thapar, Holmes, Poulton, & Harrington, 1999). Consistent with this, Rhee and Waldman (2009) conducted a meta-analysis and determined that nearly 41% of the variance in youth being diagnosed as having CD could be attributed to genetic factors.

While it can be difficult to differentiate between specific environmental and genetic influences, research with twins has suggested that parents with antisocial tendencies are more likely to have children with disruptive behavior disorders, independent of environmental factors. Bornovalova and colleagues (2013) conducted a study of 1,255 families with same-sex twin pairs to determine the effects of antisocial traits in parents, ineffective parenting practices, and marital problems on the development of disruptive behavior disorders. A positive relationship was found with all variables, suggesting that both environmental and biological influences may contribute to the development of disruptive behavior disorders.

Taking a variety of causal factors into consideration, there are several theories that attempt to explain the development of CD. One such theory is the *hostile attribution bias theory*, which relies on the notion that individuals with CD are more likely to misperceive the actions and intentions of others as being hostile or threatening and, in turn, the person with CD responds in a threatening or aggressive way (e.g., APA, 2013; Dodge, Price, Bachorowski, & Newman, 1990). Another theory, the *social-information processing model* (e.g., Crick & Dodge, 1994; Lemerise & Arsenio, 2000), indicates that it is a combination of cognitive distortions (such as hostile attributions) and impaired cognitive processes that result in youth having poor social interactions and negative relationships and interactions with others. The *coercive parent-child interaction theory*, on the other hand, suggests that a major contributing factor to escalated disruptive behaviors is poor communication and exchanges between parent and child and inconsistent discipline practices that result in more negative interactions and a cyclical pattern of increased communication and parenting difficulties (Patterson, 1982, 2002).

While many theories focus on psychological and environmental factors, Dodge (2009) presents a *diathesis-stress model* to explain the etiology of disruptive behavior disorders. This theory emphasizes a gene-environment interaction effect, in which disruptive behaviors result from neural, autonomic, and information-processing system interactions. Specifically, the model proposes that individuals have a genetic predisposition toward having negative responses to stimuli and interactions, which when placed in a situation of high environmental stressors can result in maladaptive, psychopathological responses (i.e., disruptive behaviors).

Implications on Functioning

Cognitive and Academic. While some have suggested that youth having disruptive behavior disorders are more likely to have lower levels of intelligence than their typical peers, evidence to support this position is limited (e.g., Frazier, Demaree, & Youngstrom, 2004; Lynham & Henry, 2001). There is more convincing evidence, however, to indicate that these youth are more commonly experiencing deficits in executive functioning skills and language. Language difficulties, for example, have been linked for many years to behavior problems, disruptive behavior disorders, and juvenile delinquency (e.g., Silva, Williams, & McGee, 1987; Lynham, Moffitt, & Stouthamer-Loeber, 1993; St. Clair, Pickles, Durkin, & Conti-Ramsden, 2011; Stevenson, McCann, Watkin, Worsfold, & Kennedy, 2010; Yew & O'Kearney, 2012; Conti-Ramsden, 2013).

There is also consistent evidence that suggests children and adolescents with disruptive behavior disorders show deficits in executive functioning commensurate with those related to ADHD (e.g., Barnett, Maruff, & Vance, 2009; van Goozen et al., 2004). In this regard, a meta-analysis by Schoemaker, Mulder, Devokic, and Matthys (2013) found that children with disruptive behavior disorders showed executive functioning deficits in working memory, impulse control, and flexible thinking, which are all common areas of weakness in children with ADHD. As mentioned previously, however, research has also shown that there is a high comorbidity between ADHD and ODD/CD, so these deficits may, in fact, be related to ADHD rather than disruptive behavior disorder.

Evidence regarding an association between cognitive functioning and disruptive behavior disorders is somewhat limited; however, there is clear evidence that these youth have difficulty academically. In fact, the academic pattern of youth with disruptive behavior disorders is very similar to that reported for many juvenile offenders (Pardini, 2008). These latter youth frequently struggle with reading, demonstrate poor academic performance, and are more likely to have a history of truancy, suspensions, expulsions, and school dropout (e.g., Sayal, Washbrook, &Propper, 2015).

There is also considerable overlap between risk factors for disruptive behavior problems, juvenile delinquency, and academic underachievement, making it difficult to formulate a causal relationship between academic failure and disruptive behavior disorders. For example, in a study by DeFoe, Farrington, and Loeber (2013) examining the relationship between juvenile delinquency, hyperactivity, academic achievement, depression, and low socioeconomic status, the researchers found that academic achievement was directly related to ADHD and socioeconomic status which, in turn, predicted conduct problems and juvenile delinquency. Sayal and colleagues (2015), however, studied the long-term academic outcomes of children who presented with disruptive behaviors at six years of age and were later diagnosed with ADHD or a disruptive behavior disorder. While the academic difficulties associated with disruptive behavior disorders were not as significant as those with ADHD, results of this long-term study did find that disruptive behavior disorders were associated with significant academic difficulties regardless of ADHD history.

Social-Emotional and Behavioral Implications. Children and adolescents with ODD and CD have an increased difficulty in social interaction types of behaviors (Pardini & Fite, 2010); however, there is little evidence to suggest that these difficulties are due to factors such as poor social awareness or limited social skills like in those youth having ADHD. Rather, these latter social interaction difficulties with peers, adults, and family members are likely due to the tendencies of these youth to act in angry, irritable, and argumentative interactional styles (e.g., APA, 2013; Burke, Pardini, & Loeber, 2008). Therefore, it is not surprising that youth having a disruptive behavior disorder are at a greater risk of being arrested and becoming involved in the juvenile justice system (Pardini & Fite, 2010). In addition, Burke and colleagues (2008) found that those youth with an early diagnosis of ODD were at a greater risk of developing childhood-onset CD and later engage in antisocial behaviors. However, while ODD may be comorbid with CD, youth having ODD will not necessarily develop adolescent onset CD (Nock et al., 2007).

Youth with disruptive behavior disorders are also at an increased risk of developing internalizing mental health disorders such as depression or anxiety, but these other disorders may be secondary to the difficulties caused by the presence of their disruptive behavior disorder (e.g., Kessler et al., 2012; Loeber et al., 2000, Nock, Kazdin, Hiripi, & Kessler, 2007).

Treatment of Disruptive Behavior Disorders

Disruptive behavior disorders are difficult to treat. A variety of interventions have been proposed for the treatment of ODD and CD, including individual psychotherapy, anger management, boot camps, social skills training, family therapy, community-based procedures, residential treatment programs, and medication, but there is limited research to support many of these treatment approaches (Kazdin & De Los Reyes, 2008). In this regard, Litschge, Vaughn, and McCrea (2009) examined 26 meta-analyses that reviewed over 2,000 studies on the treatment of disruptive behavior disorders and found variable levels of effectiveness for a variety of interventions. Specifically, these researchers found behavioral and cognitive behavioral interventions to be moderately effective, as were family-based and multimodal therapies. In general, they noted that programs that aggregate groups of youth with conduct problems were less effective, parent-centered programs were more effective than child-focused programs, social skills training was appropriate and helpful for many youth, and many commonly supported treatments such as boot camp-type programs were not effective.

Evidence-based intervention research further suggests that child-focused treatments are limited in their effectiveness, while interventions are effective that focus on the parent and family unit and include a variety of components such as parent management training, skills building, and multisystemic family therapy (e.g., Burke et al., 2002; Capaldi & Eddy, 2015; Garland, Hawley, Brookman-Frazee, & Hurlburt, 2008; Sprague & Thyer, 2003). Parent management training is similar in scope to that used with ADHD. For youth with disruptive behavior disorders, this form of treatment focuses on teaching parents or caregivers techniques to improve the efficacy of their parenting skills (Kazdin, 2005). The overall goal is to improve the child-parent relationship in order to reduce the child's oppositional behavior, while working toward building prosocial behaviors and communication strategies (Feldman & Kazdin, 1995). For example, parents may be taught strategies to promote positive social interaction behaviors by utilizing techniques such as positive reinforcement procedures where praise is provided for desired behaviors rather than punishment methods for undesirable behaviors (e.g., Kazdin, 2005). Parent management training is one of the few treatments shown to be effective in treating disruptive behavior disorders (e.g., Costin & Chambers, 2007; Eyberg, Nelson, & Boggs, 2008; Hamilton & Armando, 2008; Ollendik et al., 2015).

Multisystemic therapy (MST) is another empirically supported intervention for youth with disruptive behavior disorders (Henggeler, Schoenwald, Borduin, Rowland, & Cunningham, 2009). Based on the assumption that youth having disruptive behavior disorders are embedded within multiple systems that include, for example, family, peers, school, neighborhood, and community, effective treatment necessitates an approach that addresses a youth's interactions within each of these systems and subsystems within each system (e.g., Kazdin & De Los Reyes, 2008). This approach, therefore, involves a family-oriented therapy that is designed to be implemented in the natural environment. It is a home-based method that lasts approximately four months and is intended to target multiple factors in the youth's social network that may be contributing to his or her disruptive behaviors. There are several goals of MST, including improving parent discipline strategies, improving family communication, decreasing the youth's association with delinquent peers, improving school performance, and improving engagement in prosocial activities and support systems.

While individual therapy has limited support for youth having disruptive behavior disorders, CBT may be used with these youth in an attempt to decrease negative and hostile thinking, while also working to improve their social skills. Although CBT has limited evidence to support its effectiveness (Kazdin & De Los Reyes, 2008), some writers have suggested that this youth-focused therapy can be beneficial when working with older youth, particularly if parent training strategies are also implemented (e.g., Eyberg, Nelson, & Boggs, 2008).

A key consideration in the treatment of disruptive behavior disorders is that behavior problems are more likely to be frequent and severe when a particular youth has a greater number of risk factors present. This, in turn, will require that a multimodal treatment program be implemented over the long-term. Limited short-term success, therefore, should not necessarily be considered a treatment failure for youth receiving long-term multimodal treatment. Instead, such short-term limited success should, from our point of view, be construed as an indication that the treatment regimen needs to continue for a longer period of time with regular future treatment outcome assessment (TOA) periods identified using objective measures to evaluate treatment effectiveness relative to previous TOA periods. The results found during these latter TOA periods should also serve as a stimulus for discussion by the treatment team regarding whether certain aspects of the multimodal treatment approach need to be modified or additions made to the treatment regimen.

Intermittent Explosive Disorder

Intermittent explosive disorder (IED) is commonly referred to as an "impulse control disorder," as it is a disorder most recognizable by the impulsive, aggressive outbursts that occur with relatively little (or no) warning or provocation (APA, 2013). The DSM-5 provides the following diagnostic criteria for intermittent explosive disorder:

(a) A recurring pattern of impulsive outbursts that are characterized by either temper tantrums or physical outbursts, which may result in physical assault or destruction of property.
(b) The intensity of the outbursts and related aggressiveness is largely out of proportion to the precipitating event.
(c) The outbursts are impulsive and serve no readily identifiable purpose (e.g., intimidation) (APA, 2013).

These outbursts must cause significant impairment in functioning and occur frequently (approximately twice per week or less if they result in significant assault or property damage) (APA, 2013).

The lifetime prevalence of IED has been estimated to range between 1.6% to 7.3% (e.g., Coccaro, Posternak, & Zimmerman, 2005; Coccaro, Schmidt, Samuels, & Nestadt, 2004; Kessler et al., 2006), with the wide range in percentages likely due to the broad diagnostic criteria, since no temporal guidelines are presented regarding when the outbursts need to occur. Interestingly, despite the evidence suggesting that the symptoms of IED typically can begin in childhood or adolescence (e.g., Coccaro et al., 2004; Kessler et al., 2006), few studies have examined the prevalence of this disorder specifically in different age groups of youth, and very little research exists that examines the functional implications of this disorder. This is of concern since the limited research findings that are available suggest that IED may be more prevalent among youth than earlier thought. For example, the National Comorbidity Survey–Adolescent was a large nationwide survey conducted across households that examined mental health and behavioral functioning of over 6,000 adolescents. Results found that almost two-thirds of the sample had a history of at least one aggressive outburst that involved violence or threats of violence, and 7.8% met the criteria for IED (McLaughlin et al., 2012).

Etiology and Treatment

In regard to risk factors associated with IED, there is some evidence to suggest that this disorder may be more common in families with several children and single-parent households (McLaughlin et al., 2012). A familial relationship has also been suggested, with studies finding that first-degree relatives (i.e., parent, son, daughter, or sibling) are at an increased risk of being diagnosed as having IED (e.g., Coccaro, 2010; McLaughlin et al., 2012). Research has also found that individuals with a history of trauma are at an increased risk of developing IED (APA, 2013).

For example, in a study of adults, Nickerson, Aderka, Bryant, and Hofmann (2012) examined a large sample of trauma-exposed persons and found that IED was associated with trauma exposure in childhood, PTSD, and anxiety. However, in order to more fully understand IED, more systematic research is needed with children and adolescents.

In regard to biological risk factors, research has found that IED may be related to structural and functional abnormalities in the brain. Specifically, it has been suggested that there may be irregularities in areas of the brain that regulate arousal and impulse control (Ploskin, 2013), which can contribute to the impulsive, explosive outbursts in seemingly insignificant situations. There has also been some evidence to suggest that the impulsive, aggressive outbursts may be related to differences in serotonin, a neurotransmitter in the brain that is important for mood balance (Ploskin, 2013).

Treatment approaches for youth having IED typically involve a combination of therapy and medication. CBT is a commonly used procedure, in which the focus is on helping a youth learn which situations trigger the explosive outbursts and then helping him or her learn more prosocial ways to recognize the feelings associated with this and then manage his or her anger (e.g., McCloskey, Noblett, Deffenbacher, Gollan, & Coccaro, 2008). There are no medications specific to IED; however, a variety of medications have been helpful in treating the outbursts, including antidepressant, antianxiety, and mood stabilizing medications (e.g., Jones, Arlidge, Gilliham, Reagu, van den Bree, & Taylor, 2011).

Implications on Functioning

As noted above, the majority of research related to IED focuses on adults. Little is available that examines specifically the impact on functioning that the disorder has on children and adolescents, but the majority of the research available with adults has found that this disorder can have severe social and emotional implications, as the presence of explosive outbursts can cause relationship difficulties, family difficulties, employment difficulties, and even legal difficulties (Coccaro, 2003).

IED has also been found to be comorbid with other mental health disorders, specifically depression, anxiety, and substance use disorders. For example, a nationwide survey conducted by McLaughlin and colleagues (2012) found that 63.9% of adolescents with IED also met the criteria for another mental health disorder. Anxiety or fear-related disorders were the most common comorbid disorder, followed by depressive disorders and substance use disorders. The presence of another disruptive behavior disorder is also considered a significant risk factor for developing IED (APA, 2013).

In regard to behavioral difficulties, children and adolescents having IED typically have a very low frustration tolerance and are likely to become irritable and upset with very minimal frustration. As described above in the DSM-5 diagnostic criteria, the angry outbursts can include verbal or physical aggression, and this aggression may be directed toward property (e.g., hitting walls) or people (e.g., hitting people). While there is no timeframe specified in the DSM-5, qualitatively these outbursts may last less than 30 minutes and are most identifiable by the fact that they are not premeditated and have no identifiable purpose. In addition, youth displaying these outbursts may be more likely to have difficulties at school and/or at home and become involved in the juvenile justice system given the impact that these rages and outbursts can have on their environment.

Externalizing Disorders and Juvenile Delinquency

The prevalence of juvenile offenders having disruptive behavior disorders is quite high. While 5 to 10% of the general population has been diagnosed with ADHD (APA, 2013), studies have found that nearly 50% of juvenile delinquents may qualify for a diagnosis of ADHD. Similarly, while disruptive behavior disorders are estimated to occur in 1 to 10% of the general population (APA, 2013), rates of ODD and CD may be 50% to 75% of the juvenile delinquency population (e.g., Teplin, Abram, McClelland, Dulcan, & Mericle, 2002; U.S. Department of Justice, 2006). While youth having IED are also at an increased risk of legal involvement, the prevalence of this disorder among delinquents is largely unknown at this time. Given the high prevalence rates, it is clear that youth having externalizing disorders present an increased risk regarding becoming involved with the juvenile justice system. The presence of these disorders also increases the likelihood that these youth will engage in a variety of offense types and at varying levels of severity. In addition, as described below, juvenile offenders who have externalizing disorders will also be more likely to re-offend (McReynolds, Schwalbe, &Wasserman, 2010).

There are several considerations that need to be taken into account when working with youth who present with externalizing disorders. First, it is important to understand what specific externalizing disorder has been diagnosed. While externalizing disorders are related to an increased risk of becoming involved with the juvenile justice system, youth having ADHD have more developmental and neurological causal vectors associated with the disorder than do the other disorders. In addition, youth having a diagnosis of ADHD appear to be more amenable to treatments protocols, and their respective disruptive behaviors are more likely related to impulsivity and sensation seeking than premeditation and antisocial traits and thinking (e.g., Barkley, 1997; 2014. Conversely, a disorder such as CD may be more related to antisocial traits and thinking and, therefore, present a greater risk for committing illegal acts and being arrested.

When a juvenile offender receives a diagnosis of a disruptive behavior disorder, we believe that it would be important to ensure that the disruptive behaviors shown by the youth are not also related to a comorbid diagnosis of ADHD or IED. Given the prevalence of ADHD among juvenile offenders (Teplin et al., 2002), if a youth appears to have difficulties with attention, hyperactivity, or impulsivity, a psychological or psychiatric evaluation may be warranted to determine which, if any, contributing factors may be present in order to establish an appropriate treatment protocol for the youth.

Impact on Risk and Risk Assessment

While the evidence presented in this book clearly indicates a relationship between juvenile delinquency and disability, externalizing disorders appear to have the strongest relationship with juvenile offending and are the most prevalent disorders among this population. The evidence seems clear that youth having a disruptive behavior disorder are at a greater risk of juvenile delinquency and more severe offending, particularly since impulsive, aggressive, and/or rule-breaking behaviors are diagnostic criteria for these disorders. For example, McReynolds and colleagues (2010) conducted a study with 915 youth to determine if mental health disorders were associated with rates of recidivism. Approximately half of the youth included in this study had one mental health disorder, and the results showed that the presence of a disruptive behavior disorder more than doubled a juvenile offender's risk for recidivism. In addition, these youth were more likely to offend at an early age and have a history of more severe offenses. Internalizing disorders were not related to recidivism unless they were comorbid with an externalizing disorder.

While disruptive behavior disorders diagnoses are clearly common among the juvenile offender population, this is not to imply that the category of "disruptive behavior disorders" should be construed as nothing more than an alternative label for "youth offenders" or "juvenile delinquents." Instead, from our point of view, youth who manifest the symptoms of any of the disruptive behavior disorders should be considered to be at risk for committing illegal acts and becoming involved in the juvenile justice system. In addition, juveniles with these diagnoses should be expected to be at risk for re-offending unless a long-term, multimodal treatment program is implemented. Intervention will need to occur across professional discipline settings—including, for example, psychology, psychiatry, special education, vocational education, and social work services—and be carried out by professionals who are well trained and licensed or certified in their particular professional discipline.

All youth with externalizing disorders have an increased *risk of dangerousness*. This risk intensity, however, may vary depending on the type of externalizing disorder that is manifested. Specifically, impulse control disorders such as ADHD and IED are less likely to be related to premeditated, antisocial thinking. In regard to ADHD, the impulsivity may result in poorly planned acts that are also illegal, while in the case of youth having IED, the impulsivity may result in aggressiveness and property being destroyed or people being harmed. On the other hand, youth having such disruptive behavior disorders as ODD or CD have the capacity of premeditation and, therefore, will plan their respective aggressive and/or disruptive acts which could also result in property destruction and/or harm to others. Although all youth offenders who also have an externalizing disorder are potentially dangerous in the short-term, those having ADHD and IED may have a lower level of dangerousness in the long-term if they are provided with an evidence-based treatment program. Those youth having CD and ODD will take longer to treat successfully.

Another important consideration when examining risk would be when the youth began to initiate his or her externalizing disorders, since research has suggested that those who begin engaging in these behaviors later in adolescence are less of a long-term risk (Moffitt, 1993). These "late starters" are more likely to manifest deviant behavior that is influenced by a negative peer group, have disruptive behaviors that are shorter in duration, have higher levels of social skills, and not present with as many risk factors such as cognitive impairments or family difficulties (Patterson, 2002). Those with "childhood-onset difficulties" such as childhood-onset conduct disorder are more likely to continue having difficulties and engage in offending later in life.

With regard to the *sophistication and maturity* of the youth, particular attention needs to be paid to the type of externalizing disorder presented. This is particularly true for ADHD, which is a disorder largely characterized by impulsivity. The level of impulsivity should be carefully considered in light of the executive functioning deficits that occur in these youth. Implementing sophisticated illegal acts typically requires a high level of thinking and decision-making, which is less likely to be the case if ADHD is the primary diagnosis for a youth offender. While a youth having IED will also manifest impulse control difficulties, it is noteworthy to mention that this disorder is highly comorbid with other mental health disorders (particularly, ODD or CD). Therefore, the level of sophistication and maturity may be influenced by the presence of these other mental health disorders. In regard to disruptive behavior disorders, manipulative and seemingly antisocial behaviors are more common with these disorders (APA, 2013), which can increase their level of sophistication and maturity in youth offending.

Treatment amenability may be one of the most important considerations when working with youth having externalizing disorders given that there is a considerable difference in the expected improvement in functioning in a youth having ADHD in comparison to a youth having CD. ODD and CD are frequently cited as disorders that have a low probability of treatment effectiveness (Litschge et al., 2009), whereas treatments for ADHD have been found to be effective if provided appropriately (DuPaul & Barkley, 2008). The MTA study, however, that examined treatment modalities for ADHD found that regardless of treatment modality, the prevalence of delinquency in children with ADHD remained high. Specifically, researchers found that while 7.4% of the general youth sample became involved in delinquent behavior, 27.1% of youth with ADHD became engaged in delinquency (Molina et al., 2009). This implies that while ADHD is more amenable to treatment, the impact that the treatment has on decreasing juvenile offending is yet unclear.

Competency

Competency is determined by evaluating two different capacities: the degree of reasonable understanding a youth has in regard to the court process, as well as the youth's ability to sufficiently participate in the court trial and collaborate with his or her attorney. Competence to stand trial assumes that a youth has both a factual *and* rational understanding of the juvenile justice system and court process. There is no strong evidence to suggest that youth with externalizing disorders have specific cognitive impairments that may impact their ability to understand and learn from their environment. These youth may have executive functioning deficits that can contribute to them being more impulsive and have difficulty thinking long-term, and juvenile delinquents, in general, have been found to have lower IQs, but there are no cognitive impairments specific to externalizing disorders that would necessitate careful consideration when determining whether a youth with one of these disorders has the ability to have a reasonable understanding of the court process.

Similarly, while the presence of language difficulties should be evaluated given the increased risk of these difficulties in this population, there are no inherent deficits in youth with externalizing disorders that would necessitate extra consideration in how well they can participate in their trial. Rather, it would be more important for those working with the youth to understand that many of them are likely to perceive their arrest and the juvenile court process in a hostile manner, misinterpret social interaction situations, and display negative behaviors while interacting with court personnel. In addition, for youth offenders having ADHD who are detained throughout the adjudication process and not treated with medication and/or behavior management procedures, it would be expected that they may have more difficulty complying with the requirements in their environment which typically involve following strict rules and relying heavily on the youth being able to self-regulate.

In summary, while youth with externalizing disorders are at a greater risk of behavioral difficulties during court hearings and the adjudication process, there is no indication that these youth are at a greater risk for being incompetent to stand trial. If competency is not found, the most important consideration for restoration will likely be the type of program and instruction used when trying to restore competency. Language-dependent programs may be more difficult, and these youth may have more difficulty fully participating in a group setting given their tendency toward social interaction difficulties, impulsiveness, and disruptive behaviors that may interfere with the learning process.

References

Achenbach, T. M. (1978). The child behavior profile: Boys aged 6-11. *Journal of Consulting and Clinical Psychology, 46*(3), 478–488. doi:10.1037//0022-006x.46.3.478.

American Psychiatric Association. (2013). *Diagnostic and Statistical Manual for Mental Disorders, (DSM-5®)*. American Psychiatric Pub.

Andrade, B. F., Waschbusch, D. A., Doucet, A., King, S., MacKinnon, M., McGrath, P.J., … Corkum, P. (2012). Social information processing of positive and negative hypothetical events in children with ADHD and conduct problems and controls. *Journal of Attention Disorders, 16*, 491-504. doi:10.1177/1087054711401346.

Bagwell, C. L., Molina, B. G., Pelham, W. E., & Hoza, B. (2001). Attention-deficit hyperactivity disorder and problems in peer relations: Predictions from childhood to adolescence. *Journal of the American Academy of Child and Adolescent Psychiatry, 40*, 1285–1291. doi:10.1097/00004583-200111000-00008.

Barkley, R. A. (1997). Behavioral inhibition, sustained attention, and executive functions: Constructing a unified theory of ADHD. *Psychological Bulletin, 121*(1), 65–94. doi:10.1037//0033-2909.121.1.65.

Barkley, R. A. (2000). *Taking charge of ADHD: The complete authoritative guide for parents.* New York: Guilford Press.

Barkley, R. A. (2013). *Defiant children: A clinician's manual for assessment and parent training* (3rd ed.). New York: Guilford Press.

Barkley, R. A. (2014). Emotional dysregulation is a core component of ADHD. In R. A. Barkley (Ed.), *Attention-deficit hyperactivity disorder: A handbook for diagnosis and treatment.* New York: Guilford Press.

Barnett, R., Maruff, P., & Vance, A. (2009). Neurocognitive function in attention-deficit-hyperactivity disorder with and without comorbid disruptive behaviour disorders. *Australian and New Zealand Journal of Psychiatry, 43*(8), 722–730. doi:10.1080/00048670903001927.

Beauchaine, T. P., Gatzke-Kopp, L., & Mead, H. K. (2007). Polyvagal theory and developmental psychopathology: Emotion dysregulation and conduct problems from preschool to adolescence. *Biological Psychology, 74*(2), 174–184. doi:10.1016/j.biopsycho.2005.08.008.

Bellani, M., Garzitto, M., & Brambilla, P. (2012). Functional MRI studies in disruptive behaviour disorders. *Epidemiology and Psychiatric Sciences, 21*(1), 31–33. doi:10.1017/s2045796011000692.

Bornovalova, M. A., Blazei, R., Malone, S. H., McGue, M., & Iacono, W. G. (2013). Disentangling the relative contribution of parental antisociality and family discord to child disruptive disorders. *Personality Disorders: Theory, Research, and Treatment, 4*(3), 239. doi:10.1037/a0028607

Burke, J. D., Loeber, R., & Birmaher, B. (2002). Oppositional defiant disorder and conduct disorder: A review of the past 10 years, part II. *Journal of the American Academy of Child and Adolescent Psychiatry, 41*(11), 1275–1293. doi:10.1097/01.CHI.0000024839.60748.E.

Burke, J. D., Pardini, D. A., & Loeber, R. (2008). Reciprocal relationships between parenting behavior and disruptive psychopathology from childhood through adolescence. *Journal of Abnormal Child Psychology, 36*(5), 679–692. doi:10.1007/s10802-008-9219-7.

Campbell, S. B., Shaw, D. S., & Gilliom, M. (2000). Early externalizing behavior problems: Toddlers and preschoolers at risk for later maladjustment. *Development and psychopathology, 12*(03), 467–488. doi:10.1017/s0954579400003114.

Capaldi, D. M., & Eddy, J. M. (2015). Oppositional defiant disorder and conduct disorder. In T. P. Gullotta, R. W. Plant, & M. Evans (Eds.), *Handbook of Adolescent Behavioral Problems: Evidence-Based Approaches to Prevention and Treatment, (Rev. ed. 2)* (pp. 265–286). New York: Springer.

Coccaro, E. (2003). Intermittent explosive disorder. In E.Coccaro (Ed.), *Aggression: Psychiatric assessment and treatment* (149-166). Boca Raton, FL: CRC Press.

Coccaro, E. F. (2010). A family history study of intermittent explosive disorder. *Journal of Psychiatric Research, 44*(15), 1101–1105. doi:10.1016/j.jpsychires.2010.04.006.

Coccaro, E. F., Posternak, M. A., & Zimmerman, M. (2005). Prevalence and features of intermittent explosive disorder in a clinical setting. *Journal of Clinical Psychiatry, 66*, 1221–1227. doi:10.4088/jcp.v66n1003.

Coccaro, E. F., Schmidt, C. A., Samuels, J. F., & Nestadt, G. (2004). Lifetime and 1-month prevalence rates of intermittent explosive disorder in a community sample. *Journal of Clinical Psychiatry, 65*, 820–824. doi:10.4088/jcp.v65n0613.

Coghill, D. R., Hayward, D., Rhodes, S. M., Grimmer, C., & Matthews, K. (2014). A longitudinal examination of neuropsychological and clinical functioning in boys with attention deficit hyperactivity disorder (ADHD): Improvements in executive functioning do not explain clinical improvement. *Psychological Medicine, 44*(5), 1087–1099. doi:10.1017/s0033291713001761.

Compas, B. E., Benson, M., Boyer, M., et al. (2002). Problem-solving and problem-solving therapies. In M. Rutter & E. Taylor (Eds.), *Child and Adolescent Psychiatry, (Rev. ed. 4)* (pp. 938–948). Oxford: Blackwell.

Conti-Ramsden, G. (2013). Commentary: Increased risk of later emotional and behavioural problems in children with SLI – reflections on Yew and O'Kearney (2013). *Journal of Child Psychology and Psychiatry, 54*(5), 525–526. doi:10.1111/jcpp.12027.

Costin, J., & Chambers, S. M. (2007). Parent management training as a treatment for children with oppositional defiant disorder referred to a mental health clinic. *Clinical Child Psychology and Psychiatry, 12*(4), 511–524. doi:10.1177/1359104507080979.

Crick, N. R., & Dodge, K. A. (1994). A review and reformulation of social information-processing mechanisms in children's social adjustment. *Psychological Bulletin, 115*, 74–101. doi:10.1037//0033-2909.115.1.74.

Crowley, T. J., Dalwani, M. S., Mikulich-Gilbertson, S. K., Du, Y. P., Lejuez, C. W., Raymond, K. M. & Banich, M. T. (2010). Risky decisions and their consequences: Neural processing by boys with antisocial disorder. *PloS One, 5*(9), e12835. doi:10.1371/journal.pone.0012835.

Defoe, I. N., Farrington, D. P., & Loeber, R. (2013). Disentangling the relationship between delinquency and hyperactivity, low achievement, depression, and low socioeconomic status: Analysis of repeated longitudinal data. *Journal of Criminal Justice, 41*(2), 100–107. doi:10.1016/j.jcrimjus.2012.12.002.

Dodge, K. (2009). Mechanisms of gene-environment interaction effects in the development of conduct disorder. *Perspectives on Psychological Science, 4*, 408–414.

Dodge, K. A., Price, J. M., Bachorowski, J., & Newman, J. P. (1990). Hostile attributional biases in severely aggressive adolescents. *Journal of Abnormal Psychology, 99*(4), 385–392.

DuPaul, G. J., & Barkley, R. A. (2008). Attention deficit hyperactivity disorder. In R. J. Morris & T. R. Kratochwill (Eds.), *The practice of child therapy* (4th ed., pp. 143–186). NY: Lawrence Erlbaum Associates.

DuPaul, G. J., Gormley, M. J., & Laracy, S. D. (2013). Comorbidity of LD and ADHD: Implications of DSM-5 assessment and treatment. *Journal of Learning Disabilities, 46*(1), 43–51.

DuPaul, G. J., Gormley, M. J., & Laracy, S. D. (2014). School-Based Interventions for Elementary School Students with ADHD. *Child and adolescent psychiatric clinics of North America, 23*(4), 687–697. doi:10.1016/j.chc.2014.05.003.

DuPaul, G. J., McGoey, K. E., Eckert, T. L., & Van Brakle, J. (2001). Preschool children with attention-deficit/hyperactivity disorder: Impairments in behavioral, social, and school functioning. *Journal of the American Academy of Child & Adolescent Psychiatry, 40*(5), 508–515. doi:10.1177/108705470100500108.

DuPaul, G. J., & Stoner, G. (2014). *ADHD in the schools: Assessment and intervention strategies.* New York: Guilford Publications.

Evans, S. W., Owens, J. S., & Bunford, N. (2014). Evidence-based psychosocial treatments for children and adolescents with attention-deficit/hyperactivity disorder. *Journal of Clinical Child & Adolescent Psychology.* doi:10.1080/15374416.2013.850700.

Eyberg, S. M., Nelson, M. M., & Boggs, S. R. (2008). Evidence-based psychosocial treatments for child and adolescent with disruptive behavior. *Journal of Clinical Child & Adolescent Psychology, 37*(1), 215–237. doi:10.1080/15374410701820117.

Fair, D. A., Bathula, D., Nikolas, M. A., & Nigg, J. T. (2012). Distinct neuropsychological subgroups in typically developing youth inform heterogeneity in children with ADHD. *Proceedings of the National Academy of Sciences, 109*(17), 6769–6774. doi:10.1073/pnas.1115365109.

Faraone, S. V., & Biederman, J. (2013). Neurobiology of attention deficit hyperactivity disorder. In D. S. Charney, J. D. Busbaum, P. Sklar, & E. J. Nestler (Eds.), *Neurobiology of mental Illness* (4th ed.). New York: Oxford University Press. doi:10.1093/med/9780199934959.003.0078.

Frazier, T. W., Demaree, H. A., & Youngstrom, E. A. (2004). Meta-analysis of intellectual and neuropsychological test performance in attention-deficit/hyperactivity disorder. *Neuropsychology, 18*(3), 543–555. doi:10.1037/0894-4105.18.3.543.

Feldman, J., & Kazdin, A. E. (1995). Parent management training for oppositional and conduct problem children. *The Clinical Psychologist, 48*(4), 3–5. doi:10.1037/e555002011-003.

Garland, A. F., Hawley, K. M., Brookman-Frazee, L., & Hurlburt, M. S. (2008). Identifying common elements of evidence-based psychosocial treatments for children's disruptive behavior problems. *Journal of the American Academy for Child and Adolescent Psychiatry, 47*(5), 505 514. doi:10.1097/chi.0b013e31816765c2.

Gilliam, M., Stockman, M., Malek, M., Sharp, W., Greenstein, D., & Shaw, P. (2011). Developmental trajectories of the corpus callosum in attention-deficit/hyperactivity disorder. *Biological Psychiatry, 69*(9), 839–846. doi:10.1016/j.biopsych.2010.11.024.

Gresham, F. M. (2015). *Disruptive behavior disorders: Evidence-based practice for assessment and intervention*. New York: Guilford Press.

Grigorenko, E.L., DeYoung C.G., Eastman, M., Getchell, M., Haeffel, G.J., Klinteberg, B.A., ... Yrigollen, C.M. (2010). Aggressive behavior, related conduct problems, and variation in genes affecting dopamine turnover. *Aggressive Behavior, 36*(3), 158-176. doi:10.1002/ab.20339.

Hamilton, S. S., & Armando, J. (2008). Oppositional defiant disorder. *American Family Physician, 78*(7), 861–866.

Henggeler, S. W., Schoenwald, S. K., Borduin, C. M., Rowland, M. D., & Cunningham, P. B. (2009). *Multisystemic therapy for antisocial behavior in children and adolescents* (2nd ed.). New York: Guilford Press (Rev. ed. 2).

Hinshaw, S. P., & Scheffler, R. M. (2014). *The ADHD explosion: Myths, medications, money, and today's push for performance*. New York: Oxford University Press.

Hoover, D. W., & Milich, R. (1994). Effects of sugar ingestion expectancies on mother-child interactions. *Journal of Abnormal Child Psychology, 22*(4), 501–515. doi:10.1007/bf02168088.

Hoza, B. (2007). Peer functioning in children with ADHD. *Journal of Pediatric Psychology, 32*(6), 655–663. doi:10.1093/jpepsy/jsm024.

Hoza B., Mrug, S., Gerdes, A. C., Hinshaw, S. P., Bukowski, W. M., Gold, J. A., ... Arnold, L. E. (2005). What aspects of peer relationships are impaired in children with attention-deficit/hyperactivity disorder?. *Journal of Consulting and Clinical Psychology, 73*(3), 411-423. doi:10.1037/0022-006x.73.3.411

Imeraj, L., Antrop, I., Sonuga-Barke, E., Deboutte, D., Deschepper, E., Bal, S., & Roeyers, H. (2013). The impact of instructional context on classroom on-task behavior: A matched comparison of children with ADHD and non-ADHD classmates. *Journal of school psychology, 51*(4), 487–498. doi:10.1016/j.jsp.2013.05.004.

Jacobs, B. W. (2002). Individual and group therapy. In M. Rutter & E. Taylor (Eds.), *Child and Adolescent Psychiatry, (Rev. ed. 2)* (pp. 983–997). Oxford: Blackwell.

Johnson, A. C. (2015). Developmental pathways to attention-deficit/hyperactivity disorder and disruptive behavior disorders: Investigating the impact of the stress response on executive functioning. *Clinical Psychology Review, 36*, 1–12. doi:10.1016/j.cpr.2014.12.001.

Jones, R. M., Arlidge, J., Gilliham, R., Reagu, S., van den Bree, M., & Taylor, P. J. (2011). Efficacy of mood stabilizers in the treatment of impulsive or repetitive aggression: Systematic review and meta-analysis. *British Journal of Psychiatry, 198*(2), 93–98. doi:10.1192/bjp.bp.110.083030.

Jones, A. P., Laurens, K. R., Herba, C. M., Barker, G. J., & Viding, E. (2009). Amygdala hypoactivity to fearful faces in boys with conduct problems and callous-unemotional traits. *The American Journal of Psychiatry, 166*, 95–102. doi:10.1176/appi.ajp.2008.07071050.

Kazdin, A. E. (2005). *Parent management training: Treatment for oppositional, aggressive, and antisocial behavior in children and adolescents*. New York: Oxford University Press.

Kazdin, A. E., & De Los Reyes, A. (2008). Conduct disorder. In R. J. Morris & T. R. Kratochwill (Eds.), *The practice of child therapy* (4th ed., pp. 207–248). NY: Lawrence Erlbaum Associates.

Kessler, R. C., Avenevoli, S., McLaughlin, K. A., Green, J. G., Lakoma, M. D., Petukhova, M., ... Merikangas, K. R. (2012). Lifetime co-morbidity of DSM-IV disorders in the US national comorbidity survey replication adolescent supplement (NCS-A). *Psychological Medicine, 42*(9), 1997-2010. doi:10.1017/s0033291712000025.

Kessler, R. C., Coccaro, E. F., Fava, M., Jaeger, S., Jin, R., & Walters, E. E. (2006). The prevalence and correlates of DSM-IV intermittent explosive disorder in the National Comorbidity Survey Replication. *Archives of General Psychiatry, 63*(6), 669–678. doi:10.1001/archpsyc.63.6.669.

Kuriyan, A. B., Pelham Jr., W. E., Molina, B. S., Waschbusch, D. A., Gnagy, E. M., Sibley, M. H., ... Kent, K. M. (2013). Young adult educational and vocational outcomes of children diagnosed with ADHD. *Journal of abnormal child psychology, 41*(1), 27-41. doi:10.1007/s10802-012-9658-z

Landberg, J. M., Molina, B. S. G., Arold, L. E., Epstein, J. N., Altaye, M., Hinshaw, S. P., et al. (2011). Patterns and predictors of adolescent academic achievement and performance in a smaple of children with attention-deficit/hyperactivity disorder (ADHD). *Journal of Clinical Child and Adolescent Psychology, 40*(4), 519–531.

Landau, S., & Milich, R. (1988). Social communication patterns of attention-deficit-disordered boys. *Journal of Abnormal Child Psychology, 16*(1), 69–81. doi:10.1007/bf00910501.

Lemerise, E. A., & Arsenio, W. F. (2000). An integrated model of emotion processes and cognition in social information processing. *Child Development, 71*(1), 107–118. doi:10.1111/1467-8624.00124.

Leibson, C. L., Katusic, S. K., Barbaresi, W. J., Ransom, J., & O'Brien, P. C. (2001). Use and costs of medical care for children and adolescents with and without attention-deficit/hyperactivity disorder. *Journal of the American Medical Association, 285*(1), 60–66.

Litschge, C. M., Vaughn, M. G., & McCrea, C. (2009). The empirical status of treatments for children and youth with conduct problems: An overview of meta-analytic studies. *Research on Social Work Practice, 20*, 21–35. doi:10.1177/1049731508331247.

Loe, I. M., & Feldman, H. M. (2007). Academic and educational outcomes of children with ADHD. *Journal of pediatric psychology, 32*(6), 643–654. doi:10.1093/jpepsy/jsl054.

Loeber, R., Burke, J. D., Lahey, B. B., Winters, A., & Zera, M. (2000). Oppositional defiant and conduct disorder: A review of the past 10 years, part I. *Journal of the American Academy of Child & Adolescent Psychiatry, 39*, 1468–1484. doi:10.1097/00004583-200012000-00007.

Lynham, D., & Henry, B. (2001). The role of neuropsychological deficits in conduct disorders. In J. Hill & B. Maughan (Eds.), *Conduct disorders in childhood and adolescence* (pp. 235–263). New York: Cambridge University Press.

Lynham, D., Moffitt, T., & Stouthamer-Loeber, M. (1993). Explaining the relation between IQ and delinquency: Class, race, test motivation, school failure, or self-control? *Journal of Abnormal Psychology, 102*(2), 187–196. doi:10.1037/0021-843X.102.2.187.

Martel, M. M., Nikolas, M., Jernigan, K., Friderici, K., & Nigg, J. T. (2012). Diversity in pathways to common childhood disruptive behavior disorders. *Journal of Abnormal Child Psychology, 40*, 1223–1236. doi:10.1007/s10802-012-9646-3.

Martinussen, R., Hayden, J., Hogg-Johnson, S., & Tannock, R. (2005). A meta-analysis of working memory impairments in children with attention-deficit/hyperactivity disorder. *Journal of the American Academy of Child and Adolescent Psychiatry, 44*(4), 377–384. doi:10.1097/01.chi.0000153228.72591.73.

Massetti, G. M., Lahey, B. B., Pelham, W. E., Loney, J., Ehrhardt, A., Lee, S. S., & Kipp, H. (2008). Academic achievement over 8 years among children who met modified criteria for attention-deficit/hyperactivity disorder at 4–6 years of age. *Journal of Abnormal Child Psychology, 36*(3), 399–410. doi:10.1007/s10802-007-9186-4.

McCloskey, M. S., Noblett, K. L., Deffenbacher, J. L., Gollan, J. K., & Coccaro, E. F. (2008). Cognitive-behavioral therapy for intermittent explosive disorder: A pilot randomized clinical trial. *Journal of Consulting and Clinical Psychology, 76*, 876–886.

McLaughlin, K. A., Green, J. G., Hwang, I., Sampson, N. A., Zaslavsky, A. M., & Kessler, R. C. (2012). Intermittent explosive disorder in the National Comorbidity Survey Replication Adolescent Supplement. *Archives of General Psychiatry, 69*(11), 1131–1139. doi:10.1001/archgenpsychiatry.2012.592.

McReynolds, L. S., Schwalbe, C. S., & Wasserman, G. A. (2010). The contribution of psychiatric disorder to juvenile recidivism. *Criminal Justice and Behavior, 37*(2), 204–216. doi:10.1177/0093854809354961.

McQuade, J. D., & Hoza, B. (2014). Peer relationships of children with ADHD. In R. A. Barkley (Ed.), *Attention-deficit hyperactivity disorder: A Handbook for diagnosis and treatment* (4th ed., pp. 210–222). New York: Guilford.

Millichap, J. G. (2008). Etiologic classification of attention-deficit/hyperactivity disorder. *Pediatrics, 121*(2), 358–365. doi:10.1542/peds.2007-1332.

Moffitt, T. E. (1993). Adolescence-limited and life-course-persistent antisocial behavior: A developmental taxonomy. *Psychological Review, 100*, 674–701. doi:10.1037//0033-295x.100.4.674.

Molina, B. S. G., Hinshaw, S. P., Swanson, J. M., Arnold, L. E., Vitiello, B., Jensen, P.S., … MTA Cooperative Group. (2009). The MTA at 8 years: Prospective follow-up children treated for combined-type ADHD in a multisite study. *Journal of American Academy of Child and Adolescent Psychiatry, 48*(5), 484-500. doi:10.1097/chi.0b013e31819c23d0

References

Mrug, S., Hoza, B., Gerdes, A. C., Hinshaw, S., Arnold, L., Hechtman, L., & Pelham, W. E. (2009). Discriminating between children with ADHD and classmates using peer variables. *Journal of Attention Disorders, 12*(4), 372–380. doi:10.1177/1087054708314602.

The MTA Cooperative Group. (1999). A 14-month randomized clinical trial of treatment strategies for attention-deficit/hyperactivity disorder. *Archives of General Psychiatry, 56*, 1073–1086. doi:10.1001/archpsyc.56.12.1073.

The MTA Cooperative Group. (2004). National Institute of Mental Health Multimodal Treatment Study of ADHD follow-up: Changes in effectiveness and growth after the end of treatment. *Pediatrics, 113*(4), 762–769. doi:10.1542/peds.113.4.762.

Murray, J., & Farrington, D. P. (2010). Risk factors for conduct disorder and delinquency: Key findings from longitudinal studies. *Canadian Journal of Psychiatry, 55*(10), 633–642.

Nickerson, A., Aderka, I. M., Bryant, R. A., & Hofmann, S. G. (2012). The relationship between childhood exposure to trauma and intermittent explosive disorder. *Psychiatry Research, 197*(1), 128–134. doi:10.1016/j.psychres.2012.01.012.

Nigg, J. T., Goldsmith, H. H., & Sachek, J. (2004). Temperament and attention deficit hyperactivity disorder: The development of a multiple pathway model. *Journal of Clinical Child and Adolescent Psychology, 33*(1), 42–53. doi:10.1207/s15374424jccp3301_5.

Nock, M. K., Kazdin, A. E., Hiripi, E., & Kessler, R. C. (2007). Lifetime prevalence, correlates, and persistence of oppositional defiant disorder: Results from the national comorbidity survey replication. *Journal of Child Psychology and Psychiatry, 48*(7), 703–713. doi:10.1111/j.1469-7610.2007.01733.x.

Nomura, Y., Marks, D. J., & Halperin, J. M. (2010). Prenatal exposure to maternal and paternal smoking on attention deficit hyperactivity disorders symptoms and diagnosis in offspring. *The Journal of Nervous and Mental Disorders, 198*, 672–687. doi:10.1097/nmd.0b013e3181ef3489.

Normand, S., Schneider, B. H., Lee, M. D., Maisonneuve, M. F., Chupetlovska-Anastasova, A., Kuehn, S. M., & Robaey, P. (2013). Continuities and changes in the friendships of children with and without ADHD: A longitudinal, observational study. *Journal of Abnormal Child Psychology, 41*(7), 1161–1175. doi:10.1007/s10802-013-9753-9.

Ollendik, T. H., Greene, R. W., Autstin, K. E., Fraire, M. G., Halldorsdottir, T., … Wolff, J. C. (2015). Parent management training and collaborative & proactive solutions: A randomized control trial for oppositional youth. *Journal of Clinical Child & Adolescent Psychology*. http://dx.doi.org/10.1080/15374416.2015.1004681.

Pardini, D. A. (2008). Empirically supported treatments for conduct disorders in children and adolescents. In J. A. Trafton & W. P. Gordon (Eds.), *Best practices in the behavioral management of health from preconception to adolescence* (Vol. 3, pp. 290–321). Institute for Brain Potential: Los Altos, CA.

Pardini, D. A., & Fite, P. J. (2010). Symptoms of conduct disorder, oppositional defiant disorder, attention-deficit/hyperactivity disorder, and callous-unemotional traits as unique predictors of psychosocial maladjustment in boys: Advancing an evidence base for DSM-V. *Journal of the American Academy of Child & Adolescent Psychiatry, 49*(11), 1134–1144. doi:10.1097/00004583-201011000-00007.

Patterson, G. R. (1982). *Coercive family process*. Eugene, OR: Castalia.

Patterson, G. R. (2002). The early development of family coercive family process. In J. B. Reid, G. R. Patterson, & J. Snyder (Eds.), *Antisocial behavior in children and adolescents: A developmental analysis and model for intervention* (pp. 25–44). Washington, DC: American Psychological Association.

Pelham, W. E., & Fabiano, G. A. (2008). Evidence-based psychosocial treatments for attention-deficit/hyperactivity disorder. *Journal of Clinical Child & Adolescent Psychology, 37*(1), 184–214. doi:10.1080/15374410701818681.

Pennington, B. F. (2002). *The development of psychopathology*. New York: Guilford Press.

Pennington, B. F., & Ozonoff, S. (1996). Executive functions and developmental psychopathology. *Journal of Child Psychology and Psychiatry, 37*(1), 51–87. doi:10.1111/j.1469-7610.1996.tb01380.x.

Petersen, I. E., Bates, J.E., D'Onofrio, B. M., Coyne, C. A., Lansford, J. E., Dodge, K. A., ... Van Hulle, C. A. (2013). Language ability predicts the development of behavior problems in children. *Journal of Abnormal Psychology, 122*(2), 542-557. doi:10.1037/a0031963

Ploskin, D. (2013). What causes intermittent explosive disorder? *Psych Central*. Retrieved June 7, 2015, from http://psychcentral.com/lib/what-causes-intermittent-explosive-disorder/

Rhee, S. H., & Waldman, I. D. (2009). Genetic analysis of conduct disorder and antisocial behavior. In Y. K. Kim (Ed.), *Handbook of behavior genetics* (pp. 455–471). New York: Springer Science + Business Media.

Robb, A. (2008). ADHD and substance use: the importance of integrated treatment. *Beginnings, 11*, 5–7.

Rogeness, G. A., & McClure, E. B. (1996). Development and neurotransmitter-environmental interactions. *Development and Psychopathology, 8*(1), 183–199. doi:10.1017/s0954579400007033.

Rogers, S. J., & Vismara, L. A. (2008). Evidence-based comprehensive treatments for early autism. *Journal of Clinical Child & Adolescent Psychology, 37*(1), 8–38. doi:10.1080/15374410701817808.

Sayal, K., Washbrook, E., & Propper, C. (2015). Childhood behavior problems and academic outcomes in adolescence: Longitudinal population-based study. *Journal of the American Academy of Child and Adolescent Psychiatry, 54*(5), 360–368. doi:10.1016/j.jaac.2015.02.007.

Scheffler, R. M., Brown, T., Fulton, B., Hinshaw, S. P., Levine, P., & Stone, S. I. (2009). Positive association between ADHD medication use and academic achievement during elementary school. *Pediatrics, 123*, 1273–1279.

Schoemaker, K., Mulder, H., Devokic, M., & Matthys, W. (2013). Executive functions in preschool children with externalizing behavior problems: A meta-analysis. *Journal of Abnormal Child Psychology, 41*(3), 457–471. doi:10.1007/s10802-012-9684-x.

Schultz, W., Tremblay, L., & Hollerman, J. R. (2000). Reward processing in primate orbitofrontal cortex and basal ganglia. *Cerebral Cortex, 10*(3), 272–283. doi:10.1093/cercor/10.3.272.

Seidman, L. J., Valera, E. M., & Makris, N. (2005). Structural brain imaging of attention-deficit/hyperactivity disorder. *Biological Psychiatry, 57*(11), 1263–1272. doi:10.1016/j.biopsych.2004.11.019.

Shaw, P., Gornick, M., Lerch, J., Addington, A., Seal, J., Greenstein, D., ... Rapoport, J. L. (2007). Polymorphisms of the dopamine D4 receptor, clinical outcome, and cortical structure in attention-deficit/hyperactivity disorder. *Archives of General Psychiatry, 64*(8), 921-931. doi:10.1001/archpsyc.64.8.921.

Shaw, P., Eckstrand, K., Sharp, W., Blumenthal, J., Lerch, J. P., Greenstein, D., ... Rapoport, J. L. (2007). Attention-deficit/hyperactivity disorder is characterized by a delay in cortical maturation. *Proceedings of the National Academy of Sciences 104*(49), 19649-19654. doi:10.1073/pnas.0707741104.

Shaw, P., Malek, M., Watson, B., Sharp, W., Evans, A., & Greenstein, D. (2012). Development of cortical surface area and gyrification in attention-deficit/hyperactivity disorder. *Biological Psychiatry, 72*(3), 191–197. doi:10.1016/j.biopsych.2012.01.031.

Silva, P. A., Williams, S., & McGee, R. (1987). A longitudinal study of children with developmental language delay at age three: Later intelligence, reading, and behavior problems. *Developmental Medicine & child Neurology, 29*(5), 630–640. doi:10.1111/j.1469-8749.1987.tb08505.x.

Sprague, A., & Thyer, B. A. (2003). Psychosocial treatment of oppositional defiant disorder: A review of empirical outcome studies. *Social Work in Mental Health, 1*(1), 63–72. doi:10.1300/J200v01n01_05.

St. Clair, M. C., Pickles, A., Durkin, K., & Conti-Ramsden, G. (2011). A longitudinal study of behavioral, emotional, and social difficulties in individuals with a history of specific language impairment (SLI). *Journal of Communication Disorders, 44*(2), 186–199. doi:10.1016/j.jcomdis.2010.09.004.

Stevenson, J., McCann, D., Watkin, P., Worsfold, S., & Kennedy, C. (2010). The relationship between language developmental and behaviour problems in children with hearing loss. *Journal of Child Psychology and Psychiatry, 51*(1), 77–83. doi:10.1111/j.1469-7610.2009.02124.x.

References

Teplin, L. A., Abram, K. M., McClelland, G. M., Dulcan, M. K., & Mericle, A. A. (2002). Psychiatric disorders in youth in juvenile detention. *Archives of General Psychiatry, 59*(12), 1133–1143. doi:10.1001/archpsyc.59.12.1133.

Thapar, A., Holmes, J., Poulton, K., & Harrington, R. (1999). Genetic basis of attention deficit and hyperactivity. *The British Journal of Psychiatry, 174*(2), 105–111. doi:10.1192/bjp.174.2.105.

Uekermann, J. J., Kraemer, M. M., Abdel-Hamid, M.M., Schimmelmann, B. G., Hebebrand, J. J., Daum, I. I., … Kis, B. (2010). Social cognition in attention-deficit hyperactivity disorder (ADHD). *Neuroscience and Biobehavioral Reviews, 34*(5), 734-743. doi:10.1016/j.neubiorev.2009.10.009.

U.S. Department of Justice. (2006). *Psychiatric disorders of youth in detention.* Washington, DC: Author.

van Goozen, S. H. M., Cohen-Kettenis, P. T., Snoek, H., Matthys, W., Swaab-Barneveld, H., & van Engeland, H. (2004). Executive functioning in children: A comparison of hospitalized ODD and ODD/ADHD children and normal controls. *Journal of Child Psychology and Psychiatry, 45*(2), 284–292. doi:10.1111/j.1469-7610.2004.00220.x.

Viding, E., Sebastian, C. L., Dadds, M. R., Lockwood, P. L., Cecil, C. A. M., De Brito, S. A., & McCrory, E. J. (2012). Amygdala response to preattentive masked fear in children with conduct problems: The role of callous-unemotional traits. *American Journal of Psychiatry, 169,* 1109–1116. doi:10.1176/appi.ajp.2012.12020191.

Visser, S. N., Danielson, M. L., Bitsko, R. H., Holbrook, J. R., Kogan, M. D., Ghandour, R. M. … Blumberg, S. J. (2014). Trends in the parent-report of health care provider-diagnosed and medicated attention-deficit/hyperactivity disorder: United States, 2003–2011. *Journal of the American Academy of Child and Adolescent Psychiatry, 53,* 34–46.

Volkow, N. D., Wang, G. J., Newcorn, J. H., Kollins, S. H., Wigal, T. L., Telang, F., … Swanson, J. M. (2010). Motivation deficit in ADHD is associated with dysfunction of the dopamine reward pathway. *Molecular Psychiatry, 16*(11), 1147-1154. doi:10.1038/mp.2010.97.

Washbrook, E., Propper, C., & Sayal, K. (2013). Pre-school hyperactivity and attention problems and educational outcomes in adolescence: Prospective longitudinal study. *British Journal of Psychiatry, 203*(4), 265–271. doi:10.1192/bjp.bp.112.123562.

Weyandt, L., DuPaul, G. J., Verdi, G., Rossi, J. S., Swentosky, A. J., Vilardo, B. S., … Carson, K. S. (2013). The performance of college students with and without ADHD: Neuropsychological, academic, and psychosocial functioning. *Journal of Psychopathology and Behavioral Assessment, 35*(4), 421-435. doi:10.1007/s10862-013-9351-8.

Whalen, C. K., Jamner, L. D., Henker, B., Delfino, R. J., & Lozano, J. M. (2002). The ADHD spectrum and everyday life: Experience sampling of adolescent moods, activities, smoking, and drinking. *Child Development, 73*(1), 209–227. doi:10.1111/1467-8624.00401.

Wiener, J., & Mak, M. (2009). Peer victimization in children with attention-deficit/hyperactivity disorder. *Psychology in the Schools, 46*(2), 116–131. doi:10.1002/pits.20358.

Willcutt, E. G., Bidwell, L. C., Hartung, C. M., Santerre-Lemmon, L., Shanahan, M., Barnard, H., et al. (2009). The neuropsychology of ADHD. In K. O. Yeates, M. Douglas, H. G. Taylor, & B. F. Pennington (Eds.), *Pediatric Neuropsychology: Research, Theory, and Practice* (2nd ed., pp. 393–417). New York: Guilford.

Willcutt, E. G., Doyle, A. E., Nigg, J. T., Faraone, S. V., & Pennington, B. F. (2005). A metaanalytic review of the executive function theory of ADHD. *Biological Psychiatry, 57*(11), 1336–1346. doi:10.1016/j.biopsych.2005.02.006.

Wilson, D. B., MacKenzie, D. L., & Ngo, F. T. (2005). *Effects of correctional boot camps on offending: A systematic review.* Washington, D.C.: U.S. Department of Justice.

Wolraich, M. L., Wilson, D. B., & White, J. W. (1995). The effect of sugar on behavior or cognition in children: A meta-analysis. *JAMA, 274,* 1617–1621.

Woodward, L. J., Fergusson, D. M., & Horwood, L. J. (2000). Driving outcomes of young people with attentional difficulties in adolescence. *Journal of the American Academy of Child & Adolescent Psychiatry, 39*(5), 627–634.

Yew, S. G. K., & O'Kearney, R. (2012). Emotional and behavioral outcomes later in childhood and adolescence for children with specific language impairments: Meta-analyses of controlled prospective studies. *Journal of Child Psychology and Psychiatry, 54*(5), 516–524. doi:10.1111/jcpp.12009.

Part IV
Conclusion

Chapter 13
Conclusion

We have tried to assemble in one volume a summary of the research and related scholarly literature that shows that in comparison to the general population, there is an overrepresentation in the juvenile justice system of youth having a disability—including developmental disabilities, learning or emotional disabilities, and/or mental health disorders. In this regard, one of the purposes of this book has been to provide mental health professionals, educational and rehabilitation professionals, court personnel and judges, legal staff, students in training, and others working with juvenile offenders with an overview of the symptoms and related characteristics of the most frequent disabilities found among youth offenders.

This book has also provided information regarding the manner in which the symptoms and related behaviors associated with a youth offender's disability may negatively impact the youth while he or she is being processed through the juvenile justice system. The nature of the disabilities presented by youth offenders is often complex and heterogeneous, so it is difficult to list every way in which a particular youth's disability may impact him or her from the moment of arrest through the various steps in the juvenile court process. We have nevertheless tried to provide the reader with a critical analysis of the various ways in which each type of disability may negatively impact the youth and/or society. In addition, we have tried to provide a discussion of the impact that each type of disability may have on a youth's competency and ability to participate in his or her trial, as well as his or her ability to comply with or benefit from the typical intervention or remediation programs ordered by the court.

We *are not* implying here that a youth's particular disability should be considered a causal factor in his or her juvenile delinquency, since it is evident from the research literature that most youth who have a disability *do not* engage in illegal acts that result in their subsequent arrest and processing through the juvenile court system. Instead, we are suggesting that in comparison to youth offenders who do not have a bona fide disability, the presence of a disability should be taken into consideration by court personnel and judges as a possible mitigating factor associated with the illegal act(s) committed by these youth. In addition, as part of the disposition of a case, we are suggesting that the court consider ordering appropriate evidence-based, educational, developmental, psychological, psychopharmacological, and/or rehabilitative interventions in an attempt to remediate or reduce the various symptoms and related-behaviors associated with the youth's disability.

Moreover, since so many youth offenders have never been diagnosed as having a disability, it seems prudent for the juvenile court system to have a mechanism available for the accurate and timely identification of juvenile offenders who may have a disability. It is our position that such accurate and timely identification has the potential to positively support the juvenile justice system in many ways. For example, if attorneys have an understanding of the social, cognitive, and/or mental health functioning of their juvenile clients, they may be able to better communicate with the youth and, therefore, assist them in regard to how best to represent them in their respective judicial hearings or court trial. In addition, judges who have a solid understanding of the research literature on the relationship between juvenile delinquency and disability, as well as the types of educational and other evidence-based psychosocial, psychopharmacological, and rehabilitative treatments available, can be assisted by this information in making decisions regarding the disposition of certain cases. Court personnel and/or detention staff may also be better able to accommodate detained youth with disabilities by adjusting their procedures and expectations in regard to these youth and modifying, when necessary, the manner in which they communicate with these youth. Finally, a solid understanding of the presence of particular disabilities in juvenile offenders can also help ensure that these youth receive appropriate educational and treatment programs that are tailored to their particular disability, with court staff establishing educational and treatment outcome assessment periods to monitor the effectiveness of the programs and make sure that these programs are meeting the needs of these youth.

Impact of Disability in the Juvenile Justice System

As was discussed in the disability-related chapters, there are many steps in the processing of youth through the juvenile justice system that may be negatively impacted by the presence of a disability in these youth. A diagram of the processing of youth through the juvenile justice system was presented in Chap. 5, with many of the steps that were listed permitting, in our opinion, discretion in many jurisdictions on the part of police and court staff. During these steps, a juvenile's social responsiveness, communication style, and overall demeanor may negatively impact the discretionary decisions made by court personnel that could, in turn, provide a youth with a more lenient or positive outcome regarding his or her case. Examples of steps in which discretion may be exercised are discussed below.

Initial Contact with Law Enforcement

Upon initial police contact, a decision is made by a police officer regarding whether to investigate suspicious acts or behaviors of a youth and whether to arrest the youth. Many of the disabilities discussed in this book have the potential to negatively impact a youth's communication skills, social skills, problem-solving ability, and/or frustration tolerance and impulsivity, which may lead to negative contact with police officers and, therefore, increase the likelihood of the youth being arrested. It is at this initial point of contact that police officers, in general, have discretion and need to be well trained regarding the impact that a disability may have on youth who are in the process of being investigated or arrested.

For example, while it would be expected that a school would be able to effectively handle behaviors related to a student's disability, if police are called for an incident, it would be helpful for a well-trained officer to be informed that the youth has a disability. Subsequently, a police officer who is called to a school to deal with a student having an educational disability needs to know that he or she should first ask school administrators a series of questions, if possible, about (1) the nature of the student's disability, particularly if it is an emotional disability; (2) whether the student has the ability to adequately communicate and understand what is being asked of him or her; and (3) whether the student has a history of physical aggression and impulsivity. Through training in asking these types of questions, such knowledge may assist the officer in deciding on the best method that should be implemented in approaching the student and securing the situation—that is, whether the officer should approach the youth in a cautious and emphatic manner in order to secure the situation and reduce the chances of the youth becoming aggressive versus approaching the youth in a structured and matter-of-fact manner in order to take control and secure the situation.

Instances of police officers having problematic interactions with students having a disability have appeared increasingly in the news media. For example, in *S.R. and L.G. v. Kenton County Sheriff's Office* (2015), the American Civil Liberties Union (ACLU) sued a Kenton County (Kentucky) police department regarding a police officer who was accused of handcuffing an 8-year-old girl and a 9-year-old boy for displaying disruptive behaviors at school, with these behaviors being closely related to each youth's diagnosis of ADHD. The question, therefore, is whether specialized training for police in the nature of children's developmental disabilities, learning and emotional disabilities, and mental health disorders would have resulted in a different approach to taking control of this latter school incident. Ultimately, the effectiveness of such specialized training is an empirical question needing to be systematically studied in terms of outcome and cost-effectiveness.

Diversion

If a youth is a first-time offender or has committed a relatively minor offense, there is discretion, in many instances, on the part of court personnel in allowing for diversion or community service rather than having a formal adjudication hearing. This is another point in which those with an understanding of the relationship between juvenile delinquency and disability may be able to make a better determination regarding what would be a useful intervention for both the youth and the community. For example, if it is known that a youth has a disability that may be related to the type of illegal act committed, this may need to be taken into consideration when determining if a diversion program is appropriate for the youth, as well as which type of diversion program is appropriate. This is particularly important to consider if the youth is having negative social interactions with court personnel, as these negative interactions may be related to the disability rather than to antisocial behavior. A diversion program that is tailored to the youth's disability-based needs may be able to reduce the chances of the youth's further involvement in the juvenile justice system.

Hearing and Trial Reviews

At the time of the judicial hearing or trial, it would be important for a youth offender's attorney, prosecuting attorney, relevant court staff, and the judge to be aware of behaviors and risk factors, as well as a relevant history, which may be indicative of the youth having a disability. At this point, we believe that these court personnel should consider whether a psychological, psychiatric, and/or psychoeducational evaluation should be conducted to determine if the youth has an educational, cognitive, developmental, and/or mental health disability, as well as determine the manner in which the disability is impacting the youth. Based on the research findings presented in this book, we believe that there are several indicators that attorneys, judges, and court personnel could utilize to assist them in deciding whether to request a psychological, psychiatric, or psychoeducational evaluation of a youth offender. In our opinion, the presence of any one indicator below may be sufficient for recommending an evaluation.

- A chronic history of school failure.
- A history of receiving special education services.
- A history of abuse, neglect, or other maltreatment.
- Evidence of a sudden change in the youth's behavior (e.g., from a youth having few or no school-related problems to someone who is suddenly arrested for burglary).
- A history of being seen by a psychiatrist, psychologist, or other mental health professional or a history of placements in residential treatment centers or psychiatric hospitals. In this regard, some mental health problems are often transient in nature (e.g., adjustment disorder or some depressive disorders), while others are more longstanding (e.g., ODD, CD, bipolar disorder, ADHD, and GAD).
- Failure to respond successfully to previous mental health treatment. While failure to respond to mental health counseling or psychotherapy does not necessarily imply that a youth has a disability, it may suggest that it is a mitigating factor. It may also be the case that the previous interventions were not appropriately applied to the youth or that the treatments used were not evidence-based *vis-à-vis* the youth's disability.

For those youth offenders who previously had a psychological, psychiatric, or psychoeducational evaluation, an additional comprehensive evaluation may still be recommended. There are several reasons that may suggest the need for conducting an additional evaluation:

- Children and adolescents are constantly developing and often present with complex, heterogeneous symptoms that are difficult to reliably diagnose. Independent of the level of expertise of the professional who previously evaluated the youth

Impact of Disability in the Juvenile Justice System

and provided a diagnosis, there is the possibility that the diagnosis has changed or the youth has a comorbid diagnosis. From our perspective, if a youth's previous psychological, psychiatric, or psychoeducational report is *more than* 12 months old, then he or she should be re-evaluated. An updated evaluation is also recommended if there appears to be a significant change in a youth's functioning or behaviors since the last evaluation.

- Diagnosing a youth's educational, cognitive developmental, or mental health disability often includes a comprehensive approach that involves parent/guardian interviews; youth interviews; subjective observations; administering objective behavior rating scales to parents, teachers, and the youth; administering standardized intellectual, cognitive, and personality assessment instruments to the youth; and review of the youth's school and medical records. In this regard, if the youth's previous evaluation is based only on a brief intake screening assessment procedure, then it is likely that a new, more comprehensive evaluation should be conducted. In our opinion, diagnoses based on a brief screening procedure may not be able to provide court personnel with a complete description of the strengths and needs of the youth, specific aspects of the diagnosis that are unique to the youth, or of any comorbid diagnoses that are present.
- An updated evaluation is especially recommended if the previous evaluation provided a diagnosis based on, for example, the DSM-IV-TR (APA, 2000), since some of the diagnoses listed in the DSM-IV-TR are no longer listed in the DSM-5 (APA, 2013).

In addition to determining if an additional evaluation is needed, it is at this point in time that attorneys, judges, or other court personnel involved in a case may question a youth offender's competency. Interestingly, despite the fact that the research literature suggests that certain educational, cognitive, developmental, and mental health disabilities may negatively impact a youth offender's ability to think rationally and fully participate in his or her defense or trial, in our experience, relatively few competency evaluations are requested because of these reasons. In addition, most competency evaluations do not include standardized measures of psychological or intellectual functioning (Grisso, 2013). Nevertheless, based on the evidence provided in this book, it would be important for attorneys who represent youth offenders, as well as prosecuting attorneys, judges and other court personnel, to be aware of which types of disabilities in youth offenders may present a greater risk for negatively impacting competency.

Although we recognize that these evaluations are costly and time consuming, the literature suggests that youth offenders having certain disabilities are likely to not be competent to participate with their attorney in their own defense or fully participate in their trial. For example, as we discussed in Chap. 7 in the case of youth having an intellectual disability, we believe that it would be difficult for many of these youth to have *both* a factual and rational understanding of the juvenile justice system and court process.

Since no research literature currently exists that identifies the minimal school grade level, IQ level, or achievement levels in reading, math, and written expression that are necessary for an individual to have a factual and rational understanding of court proceedings—including a complete understanding of the charges against him or her—it seems prudent to recommend a competency evaluation for all youth who have an intellectual disability. Similarly, youth having other developmental disabilities, as well as youth offenders having the types of educational and cognitive disabilities or mental health disorders reviewed in previous chapters, should be considered for a competency evaluation.

We again recognize that there is substantial time involved and costs associated with conducting these competency evaluations; however, given the research findings that have been presented in this book on the cognitive capacity and maturity levels in many youth having a disability, we believe that if the standard for competency established in *Dusky v. United States* (1960) is expected to be applied to youth offenders, then it should be shown to the court that a youth offender who has a disability has "…sufficient present ability to consult with his lawyer with a reasonable degree of rational understanding…" and "…a rational as well as factual understanding of the proceedings against him" (p. 402).

Adjudication and Placement

If it is determined by court personnel that a youth's offense is serious enough that it needs to be referred for a formal hearing, it is at this point in many jurisdictions that it will be at the judge's discretion to determine if adjudication is appropriate and, if so, what court-mandated placement and/or other court requirements are appropriate. In the case of a juvenile offender having a disability, based on the research findings reviewed in this book, we believe that a youth's disability and his or her related cognitive, academic, language, developmental, and emotional functioning should be considered when determining court-mandated placement or other court requirements. While placement in a secure setting of a juvenile delinquent having a disability provides immediate relief of the youth's risk to the community and, perhaps, himself or herself, it does not address the factors that may be contributing to the youth's delinquency and risk of future engagement in illegal acts. By not addressing these contributing factors and initiating a series of systematic intervention programs to ameliorate them, these youth may be at a much higher risk of re-offending and/or becoming involved in the adult criminal court system once they reach 18 years of age.

In this regard, we again recognize the potential high costs and economic hardship on various agencies that will be associated with providing intensive intervention programs, which are also likely to be long-term for youth having certain disabilities. However, these costs and the related extensive (and costly) professional staff time spent with these youth need to be evaluated against the costs to society and the juvenile justice system of the high probability that many of these youth—especially the younger youth—will re-enter the juvenile court system several times in the future or become involved in the adult criminal justice system. Added to the costs of repeated involvement with the legal system are the costs of incarceration and the eventual loss of potentially productive, tax-paying citizens.

If long-term interventions are planned for youth who have a disability, the interventions provided need to be comprehensive and tailored to the youth's disability and his or her level of cognitive, developmental, academic, language, and emotional functioning using evidence-based procedures. In our opinion, if programs are not tailored to a youth offender's disability and do not encompass a systematic program addressing his or her cognitive, developmental, academic, linguistic, and emotional needs, then the chances will be low that the intervention will work and that the youth will not re-offend once released. This, of course, is not to say that all youth who have a disability and who receive a comprehensive and systematic intervention approach will never re-offend; rather, we can only trust that the probability will be lower compared to those who do not receive such comprehensive treatment. Ultimately, this is an empirical question that needs to be answered in a manner similar to the systematic and long-term MTA Cooperative Group (1999) study that was conducted (including subsequent follow-up studies) with youth having ADHD (e.g., Molina et al., 2009). Although the MTA study did not include interventions based on academic, developmental, cognitive, or language functioning and, therefore, cannot be considered a comprehensive approach, per se, it does represent the type of evidence-based research needing to be funded and conducted across emotional, developmental, cognitive, academic, and language functioning of youth having a disability.

Coordinating Services for Youth Offenders Having a Disability

This book is based on our assumption that an understanding of the relationship between juvenile delinquency and disability is important for fulfilling two of the primary purposes of the juvenile justice system: protecting the public and rehabilitating juvenile offenders. We believe that an understanding of the relationship between juvenile delinquency and disability is important for helping to protect the public as we better understand the risk of offending associated with the various disabilities. Research has shown, for example, that some disabilities (e.g., bipolar disorder, IED, PTSD) are related to an increase in violent offending (e.g., Bertram & Dartt, 2009; Stoddard-Dare, Mallett, & Boitel, 2011), particularly when untreated. Research has also consistently demonstrated that the presence of disabilities increases the likelihood of recidivism (e.g., Thompson & Morris, 2013). Therefore, an understanding of the relationship between juvenile delinquency and disability can help court personnel better address significant risk factors for future offending. Related to this, research suggests that providing academic remediation or other interventions can reduce the likelihood of re-offending (Vacca, 2008). Recidivism is an ongoing concern for both youth and adult offenders, and providing effective interventions that can remediate dynamic risk factors of recidivism should lead to a decrease in the likelihood of a youth with a disability from engaging in future illegal acts and, therefore, subsequently protecting the public.

In addition to protecting the public, a major purpose for developing a juvenile justice system separate from the adult criminal justice system was so that it could be *rehabilitative* in nature. We believe that an understanding of the relationship between juvenile delinquency and disability is important toward meeting this goal, since well-informed practitioners can more adequately provide services to these high-risk, high-needs youth. From our point of view, not proactively identifying and treating disabilities in juvenile offenders ignores potential mitigating factors related to a youth's offending and may, therefore, contribute to many traditional court-mandated interventions (e.g., boot camp, group anger management classes) being highly ineffective. In order to be a rehabilitative system, evidence-based interventions need to be implemented, and to be effective, these interventions need to take into consideration a youth's needs and disability.

While we are *not* in support of a juvenile justice system serving as a mental health system for youth with disabilities, the high prevalence of mental health disorders and other educational, cognitive, and developmental disabilities among juvenile offenders cannot be ignored. And, unfortunately, it appears, based on the research literature and our personal experience, that upon having contact with the juvenile justice system, many youth are for the first time being identified as having a developmental, educational, cognitive, or mental health disability. Given this, it is our belief that within the framework of a rehabilitative emphasis, the juvenile court system is in a unique position as *parens patriae* to be able to order and provide comprehensive academic, developmental, language, or mental health assessments, as well as to order and provide related treatment and also connect various systems of care for these youth. The juvenile court system has the ability to cut across traditional professional domains and related boundaries and have contact with a youth's school personnel, speech and language providers, mental health providers, and family members, whereas within other organizational systems—such as the school system or mental health provider system—there are legal restrictions regarding the extent to which professionals within a particular system have the authority to cross such domains.

Courts have slowly taken into consideration the impact that the presence of a disability may have on a youth offender's ability to be competent and participate in court proceedings, which has had a positive impact on how these youth are punished when they are found guilty. However, until mental health practitioners, educators, court professionals, and politicians alike understand the long-term negative impact on society of ignoring the needs of this high-risk, high-needs population, interventions will remain elusive and long-term success will be difficult. Even more concerning is that while the need for services for these youth is clear, what remains less clear is how the court systems will handle this increased need for services, how they will pay for these services, and how they will balance the needs of these youth in conjunction with the safety and security needs of the public. We recognize that there have been significant improvements and advancements over the years in the services provided to youth with disabilities in the juvenile justice system; nevertheless, based on the current state of the juvenile justice system, we can only remain cautiously optimistic that there will be further improvements and advancements.

References

American Psychiatric Association. (2000). *Diagnostic and statistical manual for mental disorders.* Washington, DC: Author (4th ed Text Revision).

American Psychiatric Association. (2013). *Diagnostic and statistical manual for mental disorders* (5th ed.). Washington, DC: Author.

Bertram, R. M., & Dartt, J. L. (2009). Post traumatic stress disorder: A diagnosis for youth from violent, impoverished communities. *Journal of Child and Family Studies, 18*(3), 294–302. doi:10.1007/s10826-008-9229-7.

Dusky v. United States, 362 U.S. 402 (1960).

Grisso, T. (2013). *Forensic evaluation of juveniles* (2nd ed.). Sarasota, FL: Professional Resource Press.

Molina, B. S. G., Hinshaw, S. P., Swanson, J. M., Arnold, L. E., Vitiello, B., Jensen, P.S., ... MTA Cooperative Group. (2009). The MTA at 8 years: Prospective follow-up children treated for combined-type ADHD in a multisite study. *Journal of American Academy of Child and Adolescent Psychiatry, 48*(5), 484-500. doi:10.1097/chi.0b013e31819c23d0.

MTA Cooperative Group. (1999). A 14-month randomized clinical trial of treatment strategies for attention-deficit/hyperactivity disorder. *Archives of General Psychiatry, 56*, 1073–1086. doi:10.1001/archpsyc.56.12.1073.

Stoddard-Dare, P.S., Mallett, C.A., & Boitel, C. (2011). Association between mental health disorders and juveniles' detention for a personal crime. *Child and Adolescent Mental Health 16*(4), 208-213. doi.org/10.1111/j.1475-3588.2011.00599.x

Thompson, K. C., & Morris, R. J. (2013). Predicting recidivism among juvenile delinquents: Comparison of risk factors for male and female offenders. *Journal of Juvenile Justice, 3*, 36–47.

Vacca, J. S. (2008). Crime can be prevented if schools teach juvenile offenders to read. *Children and Youth Services Review, 30*(9), 1055–1062. doi:10.1016/j.childyouth.2008.01.013.

Index

A
Academic impairments, 213
Actuarial assessment, 68
Adaptive functioning, 88
ADHD. *See* Attention deficit hyperactivity disorder (ADHD)
Adjustment disorder
   diagnostic criteria, 196
   DSM-5, 196
   prevalence, 196
Adult criminal justice system, 66
Agnew, R., 46–47
American Academy of Child and Adolescent Psychiatry (AACAP), 167
American Psychiatric Association (APA), 154, 164
Americans with Disabilities Act (ADA), 75, 82
Anomie theory, 46
Anxiety disorder. *See* Obsessive-compulsive disorder
Atkins v. Virginia, 73, 75
Attention deficit hyperactivity disorder (ADHD), 101, 127
   academic difficulties, 213
   adolescents, 214
   behavioral implications, 213–214
   characteristics, 210
   cognitive functioning, 212
   diagnosis, 211
   DSM-5
      hyperactivity and impulsivity, 210
      inattentiveness, 210
      subtypes, 211
      symptoms, 211, 214
   environmental factors, 212
   executive functioning, 212
   learning process, 213
   neuropsychology, 211
   prefrontal cortex, 212
   prevalence, 210
   social difficulties, 213–214
   sugar consumption, 211
   treatment
      behavior therapy, 215
      MTA study, 215–216
      parent training programs, 215
      social skills training, 215
   youth, 214
Auditory Verbal Learning Test, 19
Autism spectrum disorder (ASD)
   absence of the negative, 98
   adolescents, 103
   attention deficits, 101
   case study, 94
   in children, 101, 103
   diagnosis, 102
   DSM-5 criteria
      communication and social deficits, 96
      restricted, repetitive patterns of behavior, interests/activities, 97
   early infantile autism, 96
   etiological factors, 99
   executive functions, 100
   high functioning, 98
   incidence and prevalence, 98
   intellectual disability, 100
   juvenile delinquency
      case analysis, 104, 105
      competency, 106

Autism spectrum disorder(ASD) (*cont.*)
    functional impairments, 104
    illegal acts, 103
    prevalence, 102
    rational understanding, 106
    remediation, 106
    risk assessment, 104
    school environment, 103
    social situations, 103
    sophistication and maturity, 105
    treatment amenability, 105
  language impairments, 101
  limited perspective taking, 98
  treatments, 102

B
Beccaria, C., 42
Behavioral implications, 137–138
Biological theory
  classical theories, 48
  genetic link, 48, 49
  neuropsychological variables, 49
  twin studies, 48
Biopsychosocial theory, 49
Bipolar disorder, 154
  academic difficulties, 174
  ADHD, 175
  anger, 175
  Bipolar I, 171
  Bipolar II, 171
  CBT, 173
  comorbidity, 175
  definition, 171
  depression, 172
  diagnosis, 173–174
  diathesis-stress model, 172
  DSM-5, 172
  executive functioning, 174
  manic episode, 171–175
  medication, 173, 174
  social-emotional and behavioral
      implications, 174–175
  social skills, 175
  treatment, 173–174
Blackstone, W., 56, 57
Blackstone Commentaries, 56

C
CBT. *See* Cognitive behavior therapy (CBT)
Childhood-Onset Fluency Disorder, 108
Classical theory, 42–43
Coercive parent-child interaction theory, 219

Cognitive behavior therapy (CBT), 165, 224
Cognitive functioning, 100–101, 212
Cognitive impairments, 135–136
Communication disorders
  academic difficulties, 111
  behavioral disruptions, 111
  in children, 107
  cognitive effects, 111
  definition, 107
  environmental influences, 110
  genetic influence, 110
  juvenile delinquency
    competency, 114
    justice system, 113
    language impairment, 113
    pragmatic language, 113
    prevalence, 112
    remediation and restoration, 114
    risk assessment, 114
  language disorder, 109
  level of severity, 107
  mental health problems, 112
  prevalence, 108
  social-emotional implications, 111
  speech disorder, 108–109
Comorbidity, 155
Competency, 144, 180, 227–228
  ASD, 106
  communication disorder, 114
  intellectual disability, 93–94
  juvenile justice system, 69–70
Conceptual skills, adaptive functioning, 88
Conduct disorder(CD)
  adolescent onset, 218
  childhood onset, 218
  disruptive behaviors, 217
  prevalence, 217
  symptoms, 217
  youth, 219
Constitutional amendments, 75
Control theory, 47–48
Cook County Juvenile Court, 58

D
Deaf-blindness, 78
Deafness, 78
Deinstitutionalization, 74
Delinquency, 36, 41. *See also* Specific theories
Depression, 32, 36
  academic difficulties, 167
  aggression, 168
  antidepressants, 166
  CBT, 165, 166

Index

cognitive functioning, 167
diagnostic criteria, 167
etiology, 165–166
IPT, 165
major depressive disorder, 164
medication, 166
neurotransmitters, 165
persistent depressive disorder, 164
prevalence, 165
social skill, 166
treatment, 165–166
Depressive disorders, 163–165
Developmental delay, 78
Developmental disability, 88, 94, 107
   ASD (*see* Autism spectrum disorder(ASD))
   communication (*see* Communication disorders)
   intellectual (*see* Intellectual disability)
   prevalence, 87
   symptoms, 87
Diagnostic and Statistical Manual of Mental Disorders Fifth Edition (DSM-5), 121, 124, 125, 128, 131, 134, 154, 164, 167
   ADHD, 210, 211
   ASD, 96
   CD, 217
   IED, 223
   language disorder, 109
   ODD, 216
   speech disorder, 108
Diathesis-stress model, 219
Differential treatment hypothesis, 92
Differential treatment theory, 33
Disability law, 75
   ADA, 82
   Eighth Amendment, 75
   Fourteenth Amendment, 74
   IDEIA (*see* Individuals with Disabilities Education Improvement Act (IDEIA))
   Section 504, 81–82
   survey analysis, 74
Disinhibited social engagement disorder (DSED), 198
Disorganization theory, 45–46
Disproportionate minority representation, 13, 14
Disruptive behavior disorders
   academic pattern, 220
   behavioral implications, 221
   CD (*see* Conduct disorder (CD))
   cognitive functioning, 220
   etiology, 218
   ODD (*see* Oppositional defiant disorder (ODD))
   social interaction, 221
   treatment
      individual therapy, 222
      MST, 222
      multimodal program, 222
      parent management training, 221
      TOA, 222
Diversion program, 241–242
Dodge, K.A., 49, 219
Down Syndrome, 90
Durkheim, E., 46
Dusky v. United States, 244
Dysthymia (*see* Persistent depressive disorder)

E

ED. *See* Emotional disturbance
Education for All Handicapped Children Act (EHA), 76
Educational disability, 35, 121
Eighth Amendment, disability law, 75
Eligible disability
   autism, 77
   deaf-blindness, 78
   deafness, 78
   developmental delay, 78
   ED, 78
   hearing impairment, 78
   intellectual disability, 78
   multiple disabilities, 79
   OHI, 79
   orthopedic impairment, 79
   SLD, 79
   SLI, 79
   TBI, 79
   visual impairment, 80
Emotional disability, 34
   academic difficulties, 136–137
   behavioral implications, 137–138
   cognitive impairments, 135–136
   Competency, 144
   exclusionary criterion, 134
   general education classroom with behavioral support, 139
   juvenile delinquency, 140–142
   prevalence, 135
   residential treatment center, 139
   risk assessment, 142–143
   school-based interventions, 138–140
   self-contained classroom, 139
   social and mental health difficulties, 137
   social maladjustment, 135
   specialized day school, 139
Emotional disturbance (ED), 78, 121

Executive dysfunction hypothesis, 100
Executive functioning skills, 100
Externalizing disorders
    ADHD (*see* Attention Deficit Hyperactivity Disorder (ADHD))
    competency, 227–228
    disruptive behavior disorders (*see* Disruptive behavior disorders)
    IED (*see* Intermittent explosive disorder (IED))
    juvenile delinquency, 225
    recidivism, 226
    risk assessment
        dangerousness, 226
        illegal acts, 226
        sophistication and maturity, 227
        treatment amenability, 227
    symptoms, 209

F

FAPE. *See* Free and appropriate public education (FAPE)
Federal Drug Administration (FDA), 166
Fourteenth Amendment, 60, 74
Free and appropriate public education (FAPE), 121
    IEP, 77
    least restrictive environment, 77
    nondiscriminatory assessment, 76
    parental participation, 77
    procedural due process, 77
    zero reject, 76

G

Generalized anxiety disorder (GAD)
    causes, 188
    diagnosis, 188
    DSM-5 diagnostic criteria, 188
    juvenile delinquency
        PTSD, 189
        risk of, 190
        youth's ability, 190, 191
    treatment, CBT program, 189
Genetic theory, 48

H

Hearing impairment, 78
High functioning, 98
Hirschi, T., 47
Hostile attribution bias theory, 219
House of Refuge, 57

I

Impulse control disorder, 223
Individuals with Disabilities Education Act (IDEA), 35, 166
    autism, 77
    deaf-blindness, 78
    deafness, 78
    developmental delay, 78
    ED, 78
    hearing impairment, 78
    intellectual disability, 78
    multiple disabilities, 79
    OHI, 79
    orthopedic impairment, 79
    SLD, 79
    SLI, 79
    TBI, 79
    visual impairment, 80
Individualized education program (IEP), 77
Individuals with Disabilities Education Improvement Act (IDEIA), 121, 124, 125, 128, 131, 133, 134, 137, 139
    FAPE
        IEP, 77
        least restrictive environment, 77
        nondiscriminatory assessment, 76
        parental participation, 77
        procedural due process, 77
        zero reject, 76
    juvenile correctional settings, 80–81
In re Gault, 58
Intellectual disability
    AAIDD criteria, 88
    adolescents, 89
    ASD, 100
    child's behavior, 89
    cognitive impairments, 88
    etiology, 90
    juvenile delinquency
        case study, 91, 93
        common diversion, 92
        competency, 93–94
        justice system, 92, 93
        learning skills, 94
        meta-analysis, 91
        risk assessment, 93
        theories, 92
    level of severity, 89–90
    prevalence, 91
    signs and symptoms, 89
    treatment, 90
Intellectual functioning (IQ), 88
Intermittent explosive disorder (IED)
    behavioral difficulties, 224

Index

CBT, 224
DSM-5 criteria, 223
impulse control disorder, 223
mental health disorders, 224
prevalence, 223
risk factors, 223

J

Juvenile correctional settings
    ADA, 82–83
    IDEIA, 80–81
    Section 504, 82–83
Juvenile delinquency
    cognitive functioning
        auditory verbal learning test, 19
        biological theory, 18
        executive functioning, 18, 21
        information-processing deficit, 20
        intellectual disability, 18
        IQ, 17
        kaufman assessment battery for children hand movements test, 19
        neuropsychological impairment, 18
        self-reported delinquency scale, 20
        sequential matching memory test, 19
        verbal skills, 20
        WCST, 19
        Wechsler scales of intelligence, 20
    family, 15
    neglect, 15
    prevalence
        age, 10, 11
        ethnicity, 13–14
        female offending, 10
        property offenses, 10
        sex, 12–13
        violent offending, 9, 10
    recidivism
        academic achievement, 23
        age of first offense, 22
        offense history, 22
        sex, 23–24
    school achievement, 16–17
    SES, 14–15
    single-parent households, 15
Juvenile Delinquency Prevention and Control Act, 59
Juvenile Justice and Delinquency Prevention (JJDP), 59
Juvenile justice system
    accurate and timely identification, 240
    adjudication and placement, 244–245
    vs. adult justice system, 66
    case law and statutes
        Breed v. Jones, 60–61
        due process rights, 58
        Eddings v. Oklahoma, 61
        Graham v. Florida, 62
        In re Gault, 58
        In re Winship, 60
        Juvenile Delinquency Prevention and Control Act, 59
        Kent v. United States, 59–60
        Miller v. Alabama, 62
        parens patriae, 58, 59
        Roper v. Simmons, 61
        Schall v. Martin, 61
        Supreme Court decisions, 59
        Thompson v. Oklahoma, 61
    competency, 69–70
    coordinating services, youth offenders, 245–246
    court personnel, 34, 240
    development
        case analysis, 56–57
        Cook County Juvenile Court, 58
        cottage system, 57
        laws of England, 56
        little adults, 56, 57
        reform schools, 57
    diminished capacity, 73
    evaluations and analysis, 242–244
    illegal act, 55
    juvenile delinquent, 55
    multi-state study, 35
    processing of youth, 63–65
    rehabilitative approach, 3
    risk assessment, 68–69
    youth characteristics, 3
    youth disability, 67–70, 240
        case study, 5–6
        cognitive impairments, 7
        common disabilities, 4
        impacts, 5
        research literature, 4

K

Kaufman Assessment Battery for Children Hand Movements Test, 19

L

Labeling theory, 44
Language disorder, 109, 114
Language impairments, 101

Learning disability
    juvenile delinquency, 140–142
    risk assessment, impact, 142–143
Least restrictive environment, 77
Limited perspective taking, 98

M
Math disability
    ADHD, 127
    diagnosis and treatment, 127–128
    etiology, 127
    number sense, 126
    processing speed deficits, 127
    working memory, 127
Mental health disability, 35
Mental health disorders
    causal model, 159
    comorbidity, 155, 156
    diagnostic criteria, 155
    DSM-5, 154
    ethnicity, 157
    externalizing disorder, 157, 159
    internalizing disorder, 157
    personality disorder, 154
    prevalence, 157
    psychosis, 154
    R/O, 155
    risk factor, 153, 158
    serious mental illness, 154
    severity, 155
    sex, 157
    significant impact, 155
    substance abuse disorder, 157
    unspecified, 156
    urgent health concern, 153
Metacognitive deficits hypothesis, 92
Mood disorder
    behavioral and social implications, 167–168
    bipolar disorder (*see* Bipolar disorder)
    cause delinquency, 176
    chronic irritability, 177
    cognitive and academic implications, 167
    competency, 180
    depression, 176
    depressive disorders, 163–165
    disruptive behavior disorder, 163–165
    dysregulation (*see* Mood dysregulation disorder)
    emotional instability, 177
    etiology and treatment, 165–166
    factors, 177
    internalizing disorders, 163
    risk assessment
        dangerousness, 179
        disruptive behavior, 178
        sophistication and maturity, 179
        substance use disorders, 178
        treatment amenability, 179
    variability, 176
Mood dysregulation disorder
    diagnosis and treatment, 173–174
    DSM-5, 168–171
    family relationships, 170
    implications, 170–171
    prevalence, 169
Multiple disability, 79
Multisystemic therapy (MST), 222

N
National Advisory Committee for Juvenile Justice and Delinquency Prevention, 62
National Comorbidity Survey, 223
Neoclassical theory, 42
Neuropsychological impairments, 49
Nondiscriminatory assessment, 76

O
Obsessive-compulsive disorder, 188
Offense type, 176
Olmstead v. L.C., 74
Oppositional defiant disorder (ODD)
    adolescents, 218
    characteristics, 216
    symptoms, 216
Orthopedic impairment, 79
Other Health Impairment (OHI), 79

P
Parens patriae, 58, 60, 69
Parental participation, 77
Parent management training, 221, 222
Parent training programs, 215
Persistent depressive disorder, 164
Personality disorders, 154
Personality trait theory, 44
Post-traumatic stress disorder (PTSD), 15, 189
    academic difficulty, 193, 194
    cognitive restructuring, 195
    diagnostic criteria, 193
    exposure therapy, 195
    functional implications, 194
    risk factors, 194
    stress inoculation training, 195

trauma-focused CBT, 195
treatment, 195
Practical skills, adaptive functioning, 88
Procedural due process, 77
Psychoanalytic and psychodynamic theories, 43
Psychological evaluation, 242–244
Psychological theory
    labeling theory, 44
    personality trait theory, 44
    psychoanalytic and psychodynamic theories, 43
    social learning theory, 44
    youth disability, 45

R

Rational choice theory, 42, 43
Reactive attachment disorder (RAD), 15
    diagnostic criteria, 197
    DSED, 198
    feature, 197
    functional and structural differences, 198
    functional implications, 199
    prevalence, 198
    risk factors, 198
    severe neglect cases, 198
    social difficulties, 199
    social skills development, 198
    subtypes, 197
    treatment, 199
Reading disability
    diagnosis and treatment, 123–126
    dyslexia, 123
    etiology, 124
    fMRIs, 124
    language, 124
    neurodevelopmental disorder, 124
    phonological awareness, 123
Recidivism, 142, 178
Rehabilitation Act (Section 504), 81–82
Remediation programs, 70, 203
Risk assessment
    actuarial assessment, 68
    ASD, 104
    communication disorder, 114
    dangerousness, 69, 93, 105, 179, 226
    disruptive behavior, 178
    intellectual disability, 93
    learning and emotional disabilities, 142–143
    sophistication and maturity, 69, 179, 227
    structured professional judgment, 68
    substance use disorders, 178
    treatment amenability, 179, 227
Rule out (R/O), 155

S

Schizophrenia, 154
School dropout, 137
School failure theory, 33, 92
School-to-prison pipeline, 34
Section 504 of the Rehabilitation Act, 81–82
Self-control theory, 47
Sequential Matching Memory Test, 19
Serious mental illness, 154
Shifting institutionalization, 75
Social and mental health difficulties, 137
Social control theory, 14, 47
Social-information processing model, 219
Social learning theory, 44
Social skills, 137, 138, 143
    adaptive functioning, 88
    training, 215
Society for the Reformation of Juvenile Delinquents, 57
Socioeconomic status (SES), 14
Sociological theory
    anomie theory, 46
    disorganization theory, 45–46
    strain theory, 46–47
Sophistication and maturity, 202
Special education, 121, 122, 127, 134, 135, 137, 139, 140
Specific learning disability (SLD), 79, 121, 122
    impact of, 132–133
    math disabilities, 126–128
    reading disabilities, 123–126
    writing disabilities, 128–132
Speech disorder, 108–109
Speech or language impairment (SLI), 79
Speech sound disorder, 108
Speech therapy, 110
Status offense, 12, 55, 59
Strain theory, 14, 46–47
Structured professional judgment, 68
Stuttering, 108
Substance use disorders, 159–160
Susceptibility theory, 33, 92
Suspension, 132

T

Tennard v. Dretke, 75
Theory of mind, 97
Trauma and stressor-related mental health disorders
    adjustment disorder (*see* Adjustment disorder)
    case study, 191–192

Trauma and stressor-related mental health disorders (*cont.*)
  juvenile justice system
    competency, 203
    depression and substance abuse, 200
    number of offenses, 201
    risk assessment, 202
    violence, 200
  PTSD
    cognitive restructuring, 195
    diagnostic criteria, 193
    exposure therapy, 195
    functional implications, 194–195
    risk factors, 194
    stress inoculation training, 195
    trauma-focused CBT, 195
    treatment, 195
  RAD (*see* Reactive attachment disorder (RAD))
Traumatic brain injury (TBI), 79
Treatment amenability, 143, 179, 202, 227
Treatment for Adolescents with Depression Study (TADS), 166
Treatment outcome assessment (TOA), 222

U
Unspecified anxiety disorder, 156

V
Violence, 168
Visual impairment, 80

W
Weak central coherence theory, 101
Wisconsin Card Sorting Test (WCST), 19
Writing disability
  ADHD, 130
  diagnosis and treatment, 130–132
  differential treatment hypothesis, 140
  dysgraphia, 129
  etiology, 130
  executive functioning, 130
  language, 128
  mental health, 131
  neuropsychological impairment, 130
  school failure hypothesis, 132, 140
  spelling skills, 129, 131
  susceptibility theory, 140
  written expression, 130, 131

Y
Yick Wo v. Hopkins, 74
Youth disability
  case study, 5–6
  characteristics, 3
  cognitive impairments, 7, 32, 34
  common disabilities, 4
  coordinating services, 245–246
  definition, 32
  delinquency, 36
  depression, 32
  differential treatment theory, 33
  disruptive behaviors, 36
  diversion, 241–242
  DSM-5 classification, 32
  educational disability, 35
  emotional disability, 34
  judicial impacts, 5
  juvenile justice system, 67–70, 240
  law enforcement, 240–241
  mental health disability, 35
  negative involvement, 34
  neuropsychological impairments, 33
  police contact, 240–241
  prevalence, 33
  psychological theories, 45
  punishment-oriented system, 31
  research literature, 4, 239
  school failure theory, 33
  susceptibility theory, 33
  thinking impairments, 32, 34
  zero tolerance policy, 34

Z
Zero reject, 76
Zero tolerance policy, 34